Assessment of Central Auditory Dysfunction

FOUNDATIONS AND CLINICAL CORRELATES

Assessment of Central Auditory Dysfunction
FOUNDATIONS AND CLINICAL CORRELATES

Edited by

Marilyn L. Pinheiro, Ph.D.

Professor of Neurosciences, Retired
Medical College of Ohio
Toledo, Ohio
Visiting Scientist
Dartmouth Medical School
Hanover, New Hamsphire

Frank E. Musiek, Ph.D.

Associate Professor of Otolaryngology, Audiology, and Neurology
Director of Audiology
Dartmouth-Hitchcock Medical Center
Hanover, New Hampshire

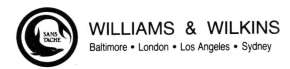

WILLIAMS & WILKINS
Baltimore • London • Los Angeles • Sydney

Senior Editor: John Butler
Associate Editor: Carol Eckhart
Copy Editor: Andrea Clemente
Design: JoAnne Janowiak
Illustration Planning: Reginald Stanley
Production: Raymond E. Reter

RC
394
.W63
A87
1985

Copyright ©, 1985
Williams & Wilkins
428 East Preston Street
Baltimore, MD 21202, U.S.A.

Printed in the United States of America

Library of Congress Cataloging in Publication Data

Main entry under title:
Assessment of central auditory dysfunction.

Includes bibliographies and index.
1. Word deafness. 2. Auditory evoked response. I. Pinheiro, Marilyn L. II. Musiek, Frank E. [DNLM: 1. Auditory Perception—physiology. 2. Evoked Potentials, Auditory. 3. Hearing Tests—methods. 4. Perceptual Disorders—diagnosis. WV 272 A846]
RC394.W63A87 1985   617.8   84-26955
ISBN 0-683-06887-3

Composed and printed at the
Waverly Press, Inc.

85 86 87 88 89
10 9 8 7 6 5 4 3 2 1

This book is dedicated to: *Clyde L. Nash, Jr., M.D., who gave me back my life.*

M.L.P.

And to: *Nellie (Glod) Musiek, for her love, inspiration, and care.*

F.E.M.

Foreword

During the past century, the concept of central auditory dysfunction has surfaced and resurfaced under a variety of labels: central deafness, word deafness, auditory memory deficit, auditory sequencing problem, auditory perceptual dysfunction, etc. By and large, early workers concentrated on the study of individual patients, detailing their exact deficits and residual capacities. The emphasis, especially during the close of the last century and the early years of the present century, was on localization of brain function. Patients with central auditory problems were studied primarily from this viewpoint. Viewed from today's relatively more sophisticated perspective, however, these early data suffered some limitations. Since possible peripheral auditory sensitivity deficits were seldom evaluated, it is not always clear, in retrospect, whether the patient's failure to make an appropriate behavioral response to auditory input was due to his inability to execute the appropriate central processes or to his inability to hear all or part of the auditory signal. A second factor complicating the interpretation of these early case studies was a common failure to control for the influence of extraauditory factors on the patient's behavior. It was not always clear, for example, whether the patient's failure to respond appropriately to a complex verbal command was due to his inability to process the auditory message, his inability to remember the entire message, or his inability to comprehend all the elements of the required task.

These two persistent problems, namely, the problems of concomitant peripheral hearing sensitivity loss and concomitant extraauditory dysfunction, were anticipated by the great English neurologist, Sir Henry Head, in his study of the phenomenon of "word deafness." In 1924, he wrote:

"Word deafness" . . . is shown particularly by inability to understand spoken words. Like a person in a foreign country, the patient hears the sounds, distinguishes one from another, but they convey to him no meaning . . . . But all attempts to demonstrate the existence of primary, uncomplicated "word deafness" . . . have failed completely. For in every instance where the clinical records are sufficiently detailed, either there was some want of perceptual capacity beyond that for words, or the patient was a straightforward example of "sensory" aphasia unable to execute both oral and written commands of a certain difficulty. (*Aphasia & Kindred Disorders of Speech*. New York, Hafner Publishing Co, 1926, vol 1, pp 118–119.)

In this passage, Head succinctly articulated the nature of the problems that continue, to this day, to complicate the measurement of central auditory dysfunction.

The modern era in central auditory assessment began in 1955 with the pioneering studies of Ettore Bocca and his colleagues in Italy, on patients with temporal lobe tumors. Bocca's group showed, for the first time, how speech audiometry could be sensitized to reveal abnormality in these patients whose auditory complaints were not otherwise striking. In the three decades since the Italians' initial report, we have seen two important developments: first, mushrooming estimates of the prevalence of central auditory dysfunction, especially in children and the elderly; second, the development of a wide variety of new techniques for the assessment of central auditory dysfunction.

Today, we find ourselves in the midst of great interest in the measurement of central auditory dysfunction, especially among speech and language pathologists, educators, neuropsychologists, and parents. At the same time, we are surrounded by an ever burgeoning technical armamentarium of test procedures and techniques. The time is certainly ripe for the present book. Drs. Pinheiro and Musiek have succeeded in leading us, carefully and step by step, through the complexities of the central auditory system, the variety of approaches to the assessment of central auditory dysfunction, and, finally, to an integration of theory and practice in actual patient evaluation. The present volume will be a valuable ally in the continuing effort to understand central auditory dysfunction and its implications for the amelioration of communicative disorders.

James Jerger, Ph.D.

Acknowledgments

I wish to acknowledge with deep gratitude the many years Dr. Joseph M. Foley, Professor of Neurology, Case Western Reserve Medical School, fostered my interest and supervised my training in the nervous system and encouraged my research in central auditory function and dysfunction. I would also like to express my appreciation to the Department of Neurosciences at the Medical College of Ohio at Toledo for the opportunities I had during my career there for furthering my work in central auditory research.

Much thanks is due my co-editor, Frank E. Musiek, Ph.D., for his enthusiasm, co-operation, and effort, without which this book would never have been completed.

The warm friendship and encouragement of Dr. Lurley J. Archambeau and his family and the understanding, caring, and support given me by Dr. John M. Croci were invaluable in providing me with the motivation and strength to carry on with this work during a long illness.

Most of all, the love and faith which my mother has always had in me were responsible for my doing the very best I could.

Marilyn L. Pinheiro

The editing of a book, as realized by those who have done this, is a most challenging endeavor. This task requires the work and support of many people. At the risk of omitting someone, I would like to acknowledge the contributions of the following individuals.

First, I would like to thank the co-editor of this book, Marilyn L. Pinheiro, not only for her invaluable help and contributions, but also for her encouragement to do work in the central auditory system.

Next, I would like to express my gratitude to Nathan A. Geurkink, M.D., Chief of Otolaryngology, who provided the necessary freedom and encouragement to combine clinical and academic work. Also, thanks are due to the other members of our otolaryngology staff, Samuel Doyle, M.D., Dudley Weider, M.D., Glenn Johnson, M.D., and Ruth West, R.N., for their interest and support and to the audiologists Karen Gollegy, M.A., and Karen Kibbe, M.A., for their clinical research work which has contributed to Chapters 12 and 13.

I would also like to acknowledge Robert Crichlow, M.D., Chairman of Surgery, for his many helpful comments and continuing interest in my career and Alex Reeves, M.D., Chief of Neurology, for his guidance and assistance in collecting research subjects. The friendship, valuable comments, and encouragement of Bill Rintelmann, Ph.D., throughout the development of the book were very much appreciated.

I would also like to acknowledge Sarah McCanna, Lynn Currier, and Cathy Coffin for their help in the manuscript preparation and organization.

Lastly, but most importantly, thanks are due to my wife Sheila and two sons, Erik and Justin, for their love, patience, and support.

Frank E. Musiek

Contributors

Robert Efron, M.D.
Professor of Neurology
Veterans Administration Hospital
Martinez, California

James W. Hall, III, Ph.D.
Associate Professor and Chief
Division of Audiology
Department of Otolaryngology
University of Texas Medical School
Houston, Texas

Paul Kileny, Ph.D.
Associate Clinical Professor
University of Alberta
Director, Department of Audiology
Glenrose Hospital
Edmonton, Alberta

Aage R. Møller, Ph.D.
Research Professor of Neurological Surgery
   and Physiology
Department of Neurological Surgery
University of Pittsburgh School of Medicine
Pittsburgh, Pennsylvania

Margareta B. Møller, M.D., Ph.D.
Associate Professor of Neurological Surgery
   and Otolaryngology
Department of Neurological Surgery
University of Pittsburgh School of Medicine
Pittsburgh, Pennsylvania

Frank E. Musiek, Ph.D.
Associate Professor of Otolaryngology, Au-
   diology, and Neurology
Director of Audiology
Dartmouth-Hitchcock Medical Center
Hanover, New Hampshire

Charles R. Noback, Ph.D.
Professor of Anatomy
Department of Anatomy and Cell Biology

Columbia University
College of Physicians and Surgeons
New York, New York

James O. Pickles, Ph.D.
Lecturer in Physiology
Department of Physiology
Medical School
University of Birmingham
Birmingham, England

Marilyn L. Pinheiro, Ph.D.
Professor of Neurosciences, Retired
Medical College of Ohio
Toledo, Ohio
Visiting Scientist
Dartmouth-Hitchcock Medical Center
Hanover, New Hampshire

Alexander G. Reeves, M.D.
Professor of Medicine (Neurology)
Professor of Anatomy
Chairman, Neurology Section
Dartmouth-Hitchcock Medical Center
Hanover, New Hampshire

William F. Rintelmann, Ph.D.
Professor and Chairman
Department of Audiology
Wayne State University School of Medicine
Detroit, Michigan

Henry Tobin, Ph.D.
Veterans Administration Medical Center
Fort Howard, Maryland

Jack A. Willeford, Ph.D.
Division of Audiology
Associate Professor and Director
Department of Communication Disorders
Colorado State University
Fort Collins, Colorado

Contents

CHAPTER 1

Introduction

FRANK E. MUSIEK, Ph.D.
MARILYN L. PINHEIRO, Ph.D.

There are about 30,000 auditory fibers in the eighth nerve. Proceeding in a rostral direction along the auditory afferent pathways, the number of nerve fibers increases until it reaches 250,000 in the auditory radiations between the nucleus of the medial geniculate and the primary auditory cortex. Together with this increase in the auditory neural substrate from the cochlea to the more central structures, there is an increase in the complexity of auditory processing. In spite of this evidence of complex auditory activity in the central nervous system, this area has not been studied anatomically, physiologically, or clinically as much as the peripheral end organ of hearing. Therefore, there are still many questions, but few answers, about the function of the central auditory nervous system.

It is logical to assume that auditory centers beyond the eighth nerve contribute to many facets of the hearing experience, but at present it is difficult to understand just what these contributions are. The pathogenesis of many hearing losses, once considered to be entirely peripheral, may have a central component (Morest, 1982). Also, auditory deprivation, especially when it occurs early in life, may interfere with appropriate neuronal development of the central auditory nervous system (Webster and Webster, 1977). In the later years of life many central nervous system neurons are lost, due to the aging process and the accumulative effects of damage related to noise, diseases, drugs, and metabolic and circulatory changes. These findings stress the immediate need for learning more about the assessment of central auditory function.

In addition, there is the challenge of studying specific problems that seem to involve central auditory processing skills. One example of such a problem is the large number of so-called learning-disabled children in the school systems. Also, there is a host of degenerative neurological disorders for which potential correlates to higher auditory function have never been investigated. The quest for more knowledge in such areas is creating demands for basic and clinical research on central auditory function. As recent anatomical studies have demonstrated, the brain has many areas of neural substrate sensitive to auditory stimulation (Galaburda and Sanides, 1980). Therefore, one may expect to discover central auditory dysfunction associated with many lesions and disorders outside the primary central auditory brainstem pathways and primary auditory cortex and its association areas. Thus, there are many compelling reasons to study the central auditory nervous system and its clinical assessment.

The best way to approach the study of the central auditory nervous system and its audiological evaluation is to develop a good foundation in neuroanatomy, neurophysiology, and disorders of the central nervous system. Because lesions and diseases of the central nervous system distant in origin from the primary auditory pathways and cortex may affect central auditory function, this foundation should not be limited to study of the central auditory system alone. The above fields of knowledge are crucial for understanding pathological correlates of audiological findings and for general central auditory test interpretation. An in-depth background in these basic subjects also serves to enhance intra- and interprofessional communications as well as comprehension of the patient's difficulties.

Next, cautious test selection should be used to compose a sensitive and reliable central auditory test battery. Electrophysiological and psychophysical test procedures should be included in the battery. One should be aware of the strengths and weaknesses of each central auditory task. This knowledge is best derived by establishing accurate normative data and by having the experience of running trials first on patients with known and well-defined lesions. One should learn exactly which facet of auditory function each central auditory task examines. One must also keep in mind the natural effects of aging and peripheral hearing losses on the results of both electrophysiological and psychophysical methods.

The first half of this book, Chapters 2 through 8, is organized to present the scientific bases and electrophysiologic procedures for central auditory nervous system assessment. The remaining chapters primarily deal with behavioral tests used in the assessment of central auditory dysfunction.

Although much of our knowledge of the structure of the central auditory system is based on animal research, Charles Noback emphasizes the human model of brain anatomy as much as possible in *Chapter 2*. His overview of the central auditory system begins in the cochlea where the eighth nerve fibers originate, and he traces the auditory pathway through its numerous central nuclei to auditory cortex. He concludes with a description of the limited amount that is known at present about the efferent auditory system. This chapter includes numerous clear and informative illustrations and gives the reader a basic introduction to this area of knowledge.

Another basic area for study is covered in *Chapter 3* by Aage Møller. This well-known researcher discusses in detail the physiological correlates of auditory brainstem function from the transformation of sound into electrical activity in the cochlea and eighth nerve through the nuclei of the ascending brainstem pathways. He describes the neural correlates of the auditory brainstem response (ABR), and recordings from various points of interest in the central auditory system are illustrated. This chapter provides a background for *Chapter 4* by Margareta and Aage Møller on the clinical applications of the ABR in many different lesions of the

eighth nerve and brainstem. Although the eighth nerve generally is not considered to be part of the central auditory system, its most common disorder, the acoustic schwannoma, often compresses, displaces, or in some manner affects the brainstem, thus affecting ABR results (Musiek and Gollegly, 1985). Chapter 4 is highlighted with many clinical case studies and discusses the advantages of digital filtering of the ABR. Both Chapters 3 and 4 cover a wide range of reference materials.

To complete the basic overview of the central auditory nervous system James Pickles describes the physiology of the cerebral auditory areas in *Chapter 5*. He covers tonotopic organization, binaural dominance, callosal connections, and neuronal responses in sound localization and other complex feature extraction activities attributed to auditory cortex. Behavioral studies accomplished on animals are reported, and the chapter concludes with a concise summary of the auditory processing activities which may involve the human auditory cortex.

While much of the work covered in Chapters 2, 3, and 5 was done on animals, this is often the only way these areas can be studied. However, the reader must keep in mind that the human brain, while sharing some of the basic attributes in structure and function with the animal model, is considerably different and much more complex.

In *Chapter 6* Paul Kileny presents the auditory electrophysiological techniques used for clinically assessing auditory cortical function in humans. He discusses both the middle latency and late vertex auditory potentials and illustrates the clinical correlates with a series of case studies.

Although the acoustic reflex is not often thought of as a central auditory test, the reflex is mediated at the level of the brainstem. Jay Hall's *Chapter 7* reveals that the acoustic reflex can be of great value in assessing central nervous system disorders. His coverage of this subject is thorough, with an excellent organization of much research and reference materials as well as relevant case studies.

Alexander Reeves writes an excellent summary of disorders of the central nervous system from the point of view of the neurologist. He provides some fundamental knowledge of the more common neurological disease processes to acquaint the reader with this area of study. He discusses the responses of the central nervous system in general to pathological processes, including the phenomena of momentum or progress of disease and remission or recuperation from disease. These two latter aspects of central nervous system disorders are important to the clinician who assesses central auditory function because the central auditory test battery is, in many cases, an excellent way to evaluate and follow this progress or recovery from disease. It is a noninvasive technique, usually easy for the patient to perform because it is not unpleasant nor painful. The central auditory test battery often may reveal subtle changes not detectable by other neurological examinations. Doctor Reeves correlates his description of diseases of the central nervous system at the levels of the cortex, basal ganglia, brainstem, cranial nerve nuclei, and cerebellum with their functional effects. This chapter should alert the reader to the many possible pathologies of the central nervous system and make him aware of the importance of this field of study for anyone involved in central auditory assessment. It is the correlation of disease processes, their anatomical sites (Chapter 2) and physiologic effects (Chapters 3 and 5), with the results of central auditory nervous system evaluations that makes the latter a worthwhile professional goal.

The remainder of this book focuses on the psychophysical (behavioral) tasks involved in assessing central auditory function. Binaural interaction, monaural and dichotic speech tests, and temporal ordering are discussed. A special chapter on the assessment of central auditory dysfunction in children is included, although this is an area in which relatively little has been accomplished due to the difficulties inherent in such investigations. This section of the book begins (Chapter 9) and ends (Chapter 15) with thought-provoking discussions relevant to problems in assessment of the central auditory nervous system.

In *Chapter 9* Robert Efron brings up some important areas for serious consideration. He reports on contralateral auditory deficits associated with unilateral cerebral lesions and points out the possibility that such effects may be related to the anterior temporal lobe and the auditory efferent system, a system about which little is known as to its specific role in central auditory processing. Doctor Efron encourages a reexamination of some long-standing theories, such as the right ear advantage in dichotic listening, the pooling of dichotic test data, and the interpretation of hemispheric specialization. He also alerts the reader to possible pitfalls when symmetrical hearing is taken for granted because the bilateral audiometric thresholds are the same and to problems with the assumptions related to earphone reversal. The possible effects of the subcortical auditory system on the results of dichotic tasks are brought to the reader's attention.

Henry Tobin gives an insightful review of binaural interaction, including fusion, integration, and lateralization in *Chapter 10*. He discusses the two well-known tasks of rapidly alternating speech and masking level differences. The interaural intensity difference for lateralization is examined as well. Although this task is not widely used, it appears to offer a clinically feasible and sensitive procedure to contribute to the central auditory test battery. Clinical examples and much reference material are included.

Monaural low redundancy speech tests probably have the longest history of any speech tasks used for the detection of central auditory lesions. In *Chapter 11* William Rintelmann covers this topic thoroughly and clearly with a detailed review of previous work accomplished on adults and children in this area of research. He illustrates with case studies and examples. This chapter includes discussion of the "rollover" phenomenon and speech tests, wherein speech signals are frequency-filtered or time-altered to degrade the stimulus. Competing message tasks are described also, and the effects of peripheral hearing loss and aging on central auditory tasks are carefully considered.

The next two chapters written by the editors cover two types of central auditory nervous system test procedures which may be the most sensitive psychophysical indices for detecting cerebral auditory dysfunction.

Frank Musiek presents a careful and complete analysis of dichotic speech tasks in *Chapter 12*. The acoustic factors affecting these tasks are explained, followed by a wealth of descriptions of clinical research data on the central nervous system findings in tasks of binaural interaction and binaural separation. In these categories the Staggered Spondee Words, Northwestern University test number 20, dichotic digits, Synthetic Sentence Identification with Contralateral Competing Message task, and Competing Sentences are examined and illustrated with results on clinical populations with central nervous system disorders. This area of dichotic listening probably has been explored in recent years more than any other area of central auditory processing. These tasks also have been employed more often clinically and appear to have great value in the central auditory test battery, provided the precautions noted in Chapters 9, 12, and 15 are heeded.

In *Chapter 13* Marilyn Pinheiro gives a well-rounded account of temporal ordering or sequencing tasks with a thorough review of the literature on normal and brain-damaged subjects. The author explains the many psychophysical variables involved in this type of task, including the kind of stimulus employed and the manner of temporal order judgments. Theories of probable subject encoding techniques, the anatomical/physiological bases for temporal ordering, and the problem of hemispheric dominance are scrutinized. Clinically useful sequencing tasks are described, and clinical data are given. This area is presently one of great interest because a temporal ordering or sequencing task generally is nonverbal, whereas other psychophysical central auditory tasks widely available involve the use of speech signals and, commonly, some kind of response entailing overt or covert speech.

In the opinion and experience of the editors dichotic speech tests and temporal ordering tasks discussed in Chapters 12 and 13, respectively, should not be omitted in the composition of a central auditory test battery. Both historically and futuristically these two types of tests appear to be very worthwhile for both basic research and clinical diagnosis of central auditory dysfunction.

Due to the paucity of research on central auditory function in children and its almost insurmountable difficulties, this book includes only one chapter entirely devoted to this area, although central auditory tests on children also are discussed briefly in some other chapters. Jack Willeford is the one investigator who has done much of the work on children using a test battery, and he brings his clinical experience to bear on this subject in *Chapter 14*. Children with learning disabilities are generally the target population for assessment of central auditory function in this age group. Dr. Willeford describes the manifestations of learning disorders in auditory-communicative behavior, academic performance, and social conduct. He discusses the relationship between central auditory dysfunction and language skills and the etiological implications of learning disorders, pointing out the clinical challenge in evaluating these children. The many central auditory tests applicable to children are noted and include filtered speech, pitch pattern sequences, Synthetic Sentence Identification with Ipsilateral or Contralateral Competing Messages, Performance Intensity Function, speech-in-noise, binaural fusion, Rapidly Alternating Speech, Masking Level Differences, and dichotic tasks such as digits, Staggered Spondee Words, Competing Sentences, Ipsi- and Contralateral Competing Sentences, and Environmental Sounds test. He also mentions the electrophysiological tests described in Chapters 4 and 6. The author then discusses the interpretation, implications, and limitations of such tests on children.

In the final chapter, *Chapter 15*, the editors comment on some important areas in the assessment of central auditory nervous system function, highlighting some salient features presented in earlier chapters. Such problems as instrumentation, stimulus material, normative data, and standardization of central auditory tests are brought to the attention of the reader. The relationship of age, whether young or old, hearing losses, and psychiatric disorders to central auditory evaluation are considered. Difficulties in statistical analysis of central auditory test results, location of lesions, and the clinician's frequently limited training in and knowledge of the basic areas of neuroanatomy, neurophysiology, and neurological disorders are brought up. The relationship between language and the tasks of the central auditory test battery is discussed. The central auditory test battery is seen as making a contribution to neurodiagnosis in skilled hands. Finally, there is an exploration of future needs and directions.

This book doubtlessly omits many worthy topics in the area of central auditory assessment. Remediation for central auditory problems is not covered because it does not fall into the category of assessment and, generally, is accomplished by a separate group of professionals. Also, it would require an entire book to discuss this one controversial subject.

However, it is hoped by the editors and chapter authors that this book provides some scientific background for central auditory assessment and that it offers the clinician enough material on various clinical procedures so that he may select and compose an appropriate test battery. We have attempted to present enough knowledge, old and new, in a well-organized and interesting manner to inspire the reader to pursue further the subject of assessment of the central auditory nervous system dysfunctions so that he may learn to become an expert and contribute his own clinical research to this fascinating and worthwhile area of study.

References

Galaburda A, Sanides F: Cytoarchitectonic organization of the human auditory cortex. *J Comp Neurol* 190:597–610, 1980.

Morest K: Degeneration in the brain following exposure to noise. In Hamernik R, Henderson D, Salvi R (eds): *New Perspectives on Noise Induced Hearing Loss.* New York, Raven Press, 1982.

Musiek F, Gollegly K: ABR in eighth nerve and low brainstem lesions. In Jacobsen J (ed): *The Auditory Brainstem Response.* San Diego, College Hill Press, 1985.

Webster D, Webster M: Neonatal sound deprivation affects brainstem auditory nuclei. *Arch Otolaryngol* 103:392–396, 1977.

CHAPTER 2

Neuroanatomical Correlates of Central Auditory Function

CHARLES R. NOBACK, Ph.D.

One of the most important facets of central auditory assessment is an in-depth background in auditory neuroanatomy. Dr. Charles Noback's chapter provides a clear and relevant account of the central nervous system's morphology related to audition.

INTRODUCTION

The objective of this chapter is to outline some salient features of the neuroanatomy of the auditory system with the primary focus on that in the human. Some of the morphological and conceptual aspects presented are based on evidence obtained from several primates and the cat, species in which experimental observations are available. Valuable reviews on the structural and functional aspects of the auditory system include Rasmussen and Windle (1960), Fields and Alford (1964), Whitfield (1967), Keidel and Neff (1975), Brugge and Geisler (1978), Strominger (1978), Naunton and Fernandez (1978), and Osen (1981).

The auditory system is morphologically organized into ascending and descending auditory pathways (Harrison and Howe, 1974a and b). Within these pathways a succession of levels (nuclei) are encompassed where neural processing occurs. From the **cochlea** to the **cerebral cortex**, these include, in order, the **organ of Corti, cochlear nuclei,** superior olivary nuclear complex, nuclei of **lateral lemniscus, inferior colliculus, medial geniculate body (nucleus),** and **auditory cortex (neocortex)** (Figs. 2.1 and 2.2). These levels are characterized by having tonotopic (cochleotopic) representations, which are expressed as "frequency maps." The neural

information from each cochlea is transmitted via a cochlear nerve to the cochlear nuclei. From the cochlear nuclei in the lower brainstem the neural signals are conveyed via both the contralateral (crossed) and ipsilateral (uncrossed) ascending pathways, with each pathway having a greater contralateral representation. At nearly all levels, the neural centers are interconnected by decussating axons or by **commissural fibers.** Many of the projections from the cochlear nuclei and nuclei of the superior olivary complex are via decussating fibers. These fibers decussate in the ventral tegmentum of the pons as the trapezoid body and in the dorsal tegmentum as the dorsal acoustic stria (Fig. 2.1). Between these two striae is an intermediate acoustic stria (Strominger, 1978). Commissural connections across the midline include the commissure of the nuclei of the lateral lemniscus, commissure of the inferior colliculus, and the fibers of corpus callosum between the auditory cortices.

The tracts of the auditory pathways include (1) the lateral lemniscus, located in the lateral **tegmentum** of the pons, which interconnects the cochlear nuclei and nuclei of the superior olivary complex with the inferior colliculus, (2) the **brachium of the inferior colliculus,** located in the lateral tegmentum of the midbrain, which interconnects the inferior colliculus with the medial geniculate body, and (3) the auditory radiation, which consists of fibers interconnecting the medial geniculate body with the auditory cortex in the temporal lobe.

The higher levels of the auditory pathways—comprising the inferior colliculus, medial geniculate body, and auditory cor-

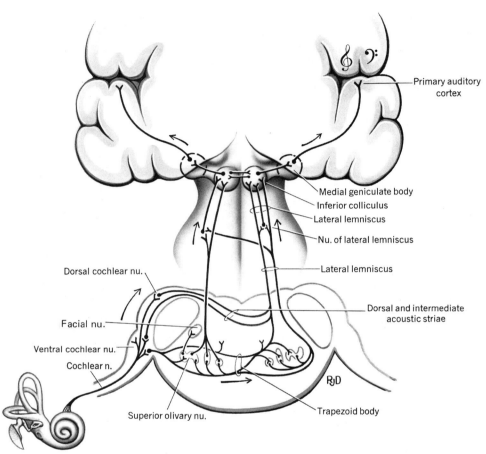

Figure 2.1. The ascending auditory pathways. The cross section is through the junctional zone between the pons and medulla. The nuclei comprising the superior olivary nuclear complex include from lateral to medial: lateral superior olivary nucleus (labeled), medial superior olivary nucleus, and nucleus of the trapezoid body. The periolivary nucleus surrounds the superior olivary nuclei. The ventral acoustic stria consists of fibers in the ventral tegmentum. (From Noback CR, Demarest RJ: *The Human Nervous System*, ed 3. New York, McGraw-Hill Book Co, 1981.)

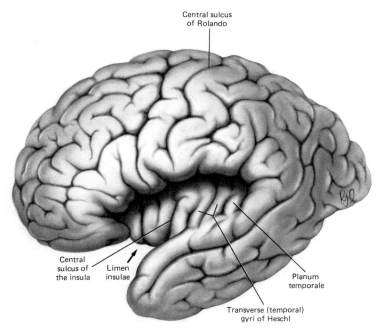

Central sulcus
of Rolando

Central
sulcus of   Limen
the insula   insulae

Planum
temporale

Transverse (temporal)
gyri of Heschl

Figure 2.2. Lateral view of the cerebrum with opercula bordering the lateral sulcus separated to expose the insula, transverse temporal gyri of Heschl, and planum temporale. (From Noback CR, Demarest RJ: *The Human Nervous System*, ed 3. New York, McGraw-Hill Book Co, 1981.)

tex—are considered to be organized into a core portion (projection) surrounded by a belt portion (projection). This division of the ascending auditory pathway is apparently characteristic of all mammals (Casseday et al, 1976). These two portions are not completely separate. The core portion terminates primarily but not exclusively in the primary auditory cortex, whereas the belt portion terminates primarily but not exclusively in the auditory cortex bordering the primary auditory cortex.

Within the confines of the ascending pathways are neurons comprising the descending auditory pathways (Fig. 2.3) (Rasmussen, 1944; Harrison and Howe, 1974b). The latter parallel the former sequentially from the higher to the lower levels, commencing with the auditory cortex and terminating in the organ of Corti in the cochlea. The precise roles of the descending auditory system have not been established with certainty. Through its excitatory and inhibitory influences, it is presumed to exert modulatory effects and to have significant roles in the neural processing within the ascending auditory system.

THE HAIR CELLS OF THE COCHLEA

Two types of neuroepithelial sensory cells, namely, the inner **hair cells** and outer hair cells of the organ of Corti, are the peripheral receptors of the auditory system (Fig 2.4). In man, the 3500 bottle-shaped inner hair cells are arranged in a single row and the 15,000 outer hair cells are arranged in three rows along the entire length of the cochlear coil. The nerve fibers of the cochlear nerve have synaptic connections at the basal ends of the hair cells.

A spatial representation of tonal frequencies is present sequentially along the length of the cochlear coil in the so-called tonotopic (cochleotopic) representation. The highest tones (high pitch, high frequencies) are "heard" at the base of the cochlea and the lowest tones (low pitch, low frequencies) near the apex of the coil.

The hairs of the hair cells are specialized microvilli, also called stereocilia (not true cilia). They are cylindrical organelles with a core component of tightly packed filaments (Hudspeth, 1983). Each outer hair cell has

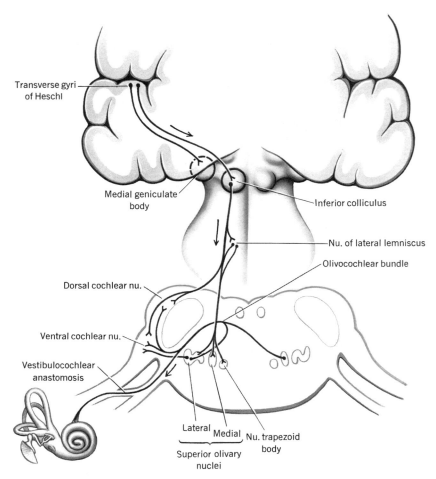

Figure 2.3.   The descending auditory pathways. The fibers of the olivocochlear bundle emerge from the medulla through the vestibular nerve and then pass via the vestibulocochlear anastomosis of the cochlear nerve. (From Noback CR, Demarest RJ: *The Human Nervous System*, ed 3. New York, McGraw-Hill Book Co., 1981.)

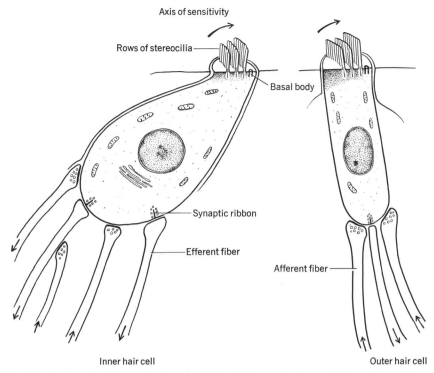

Figure 2.4. The hair cells of the spiral organ of Corti. The axis of sensitivity of a cochlear hair cell is in the direction of the basal body (after Wersall and Flock). (From Noback CR, Demarest RJ: *The Human Nervous System*, ed 3. New York, McGraw-Hill Book Co, 1981.)

from 80 to 100 microvilli, while each inner hair cell has from 40 to 60 microvilli. In the lateral side of microvilli is a **basal body** (Fig. 2.4), which is all that is left of a modified true cilium or **kinocilium** (a kinocilium is present in each cochlear hair cell during development, but it disappears, except for its basal body by the late fetal or circumnatal life). This arrangement of the hairs and the basal body imparts upon each hair cell a polarity and a bilateral symmetry.

The displacement (bending) of the hair toward or from the basal body defines the **axis of sensitivity** of each hair cell (Fig. 2.4). When the hairs are displaced along the axis of sensitivity toward the basal body ionic channels are opened in the plasma membrane, resulting in the membrane becoming selectively permeable so that the potential difference across the membrane decreases (depolarization). This is followed by the generation and spread of electric signal (receptor potential) toward the base of the cell. When the hairs are displaced away from the basal body the potential difference across the membrane decreases (hyperpolarization). The hair cell does not respond when the hairs are displaced along an axis perpendicular to that of the symmetry (axis of sensitivity). After the depolarization spreads to the base of the cell, channels that selectively admit Ca^{2+} ions open. The Ca^{2+} ions trigger the events, resulting in the fusion of neurotransmitter vesicles with the plasma membrane followed by the release of an as yet unknown neurotransmitter, which excites the axon terminals of the cochlear nerve fiber to generate generator potentials. Hair cells are called paraneurons because they have many of the properties of neurons but lack dendrites and axons.

The hair cells are the mechanoreceptors in which transduction of the mechanical energy of the sound waves into the generator (local) potentials of the hair cells occurs. These generator potentials excite the cochlear nerve endings to elaborate generator potentials. The hairs act both as transducers and as biologic amplifiers (Khanna and Tonndorf, 1978). Whereas the displacement amplitude of the tympanic membrane (eardrum) can range to atomic dimensions, the displacement of the **basilar membrane** of the organ of Corti is even smaller, and, in turn, the deflection of the hair along the axis of sensitivity is even less.

THE COCHLEAR NERVE

The cochlear nerve consists of two functional types of neurons, namely, (1) afferent neurons with their cell bodies located in the spiral (cochlear) **ganglion** and (2) efferent neurons (cochlear efferent neurons) with their cell bodies located in the superior olivary nuclear complex. In man, each of the 32,000 myelinated fibers in the cochlear nerve (Rasmussen, 1940) is characterized by having a myelin sheath which also encapsulates each cell body. The peripheral processes of the afferent neurons commence at their synaptic endings with the hair cells, while all their central processes terminate within the dorsal and ventral cochlear nuclei (Fig. 2.5) (Rose et al., 1960). In the squirrel monkey, there is a regional difference within the cochlear nerve, with the fibers innervating the basal region of cochlear coil being larger than those innervating the apical region (Romand et al, 1981). From their origin in the superior olivary complex, the efferent fibers course successively through the vestibular nerve, **vestibulocochlear** anastomosis within the internal acoustic meatus, and the cochlear nerve (Fig. 2.3). These efferent fibers comprise the so-called **olivocochlear bundle** (see later on Descending Auditory Pathway).

Two types of spiral ganglion neurons have been described: (1) Type I neurons are large myelinated bipolar neurons with a round nucleus, prominent nucleolus, and many ribosomes and (2) type II neurons are small usually unmyelinated neurons with a lobated nucleus, small nucleolus, and filamentous cytoplasm (Spoendlin, 1978). The vast majority of afferent neurons in man is the type I neuron (Nomura, 1976). In the cat 95% of the neurons are type I, and 5% are type II neurons (Spoendlin, 1978). As indicated by anatomical studies (Spoendlin, 1978) and from physiological evidence (Kiang et al, 1982), there is virtually a complete segregation of these two types with respect to their peripheral innervation. The peripheral fibers of the type I neurons have synaptic connections with the inner hair

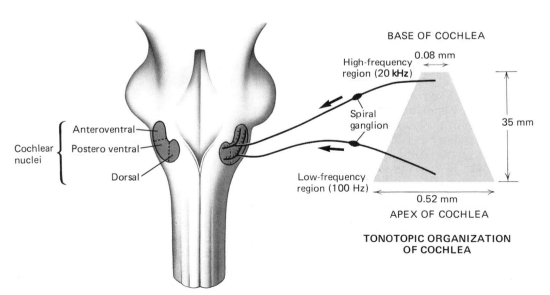

Figure 2.5. Diagram illustrating the tonotopic projections of the fibers of the cochlear nerve from the basilar membrane of the cochlea to the cochlear nuclei. The dimensions of the uncoiled basilar membrane are indicated. (From Noback CR, Demarest RJ: *The Human Nervous System,* ed 3. New York, McGraw Hill, 1981.)

cells and those of the type II neurons with the outer hair cells. In essence, the less numerous type II neurons innervate the large population of outer hair cells. In contrast, the more numerous type I neurons innervate the smaller population of inner hair cells. Each inner hair cell is innervated by about 20 unbranched type I individual afferent fibers. Each outer hair cell is innervated by branches of several type II neurons, each of which participates in innervating about 10 outer hair cells (Spoendlin, 1978). Thus, the innervation of the inner hair cells is characterized by great divergence (1:20) and for the outer hair cells by great convergence (10:1).

COCHLEAR NUCLEI

The afferent nerve fibers of the cochlear nerve terminate in the cochlear nuclear complex (cochlear nuclei) located on the outer aspect of the inferior cerebellar peduncle (Fig. 2.5). This complex consists of two main divisions—a dorsal cochlear nucleus and a ventral cochlear nucleus (Bacsek and Strominger, 1973). The latter is divided into a rostral segment, called the anteroventral cochlear nucleus (subnucleus), and the caudal segment is called the posteroventral cochlear nucleus (subnucleus). The cochlear nerve enters this complex at the junction of the anteroventral and posteroventral nuclei. Each nerve fiber divides within the complex into an ascending branch terminating in the anteroventral nucleus and a descending branch terminating in the posteroventral or in the dorsal cochlear nuclei (Fig. 2.5) (Osen, 1970; Moskowitz and Liu, 1972; Kane, 1978; Moore and Osen, 1979). The cochlear fibers are arranged tonotopically with the low-frequency fibers from the apex of the coil located on the superficial aspect of the nuclei and with the high-frequency fibers from the base of the coil located on the deep aspect of the nuclei. Thus each of the fibers of the cochlear nerve innervates all three cochlear nuclei in a tonotopic organization (Fig. 2.5).

Studies of Nissl preparations have revealed nine distinct neuronal cell body types in the cochlear complex of the cat (Osen, 1969)—namely, small spherical cell, large spherical cell, globular cell, multipolar cell, small cell, octopus cell, pyramidal cell, giant cell, and granule cell. On the basis of evidence obtained from Golgi preparations (Brawer et al, 1974) and from electrophysiological studies (Godfrey et al, 1975a and b), these cells have been characterized by their electrophysiological properties and their afferent and efferent connections. They are differentially and not homogeneously distributed within the nuclei . The morphological and functional features of the cell types have not been analyzed to the same extent in the primate and man. Apparently variations exist in different species. For example, no dichotomy is observed between small and large spherical cells in the macaque and man (Strominger and Strominger, 1971). Giant cells are not present in the squirrel monkey (Moskowitz, 1969).

The main targets for the projections from the cochlear complex in the cat, according to Osen (1981), may be summarized in the following way. The axons of the pyramidal cells and multipolar cells project as far rostral as the contralateral inferior colliculus. The spherical cells have axons coursing directly to both the ipsilateral and the contralateral medial superior olivary nuclei and to the ipsilateral lateral superior olivary nucleus. The globular cells have axons projecting to the contralateral nucleus of the **trapezoid body**, whose neurons project to the lateral superior olivary nucleus. The octopus cells have axons terminating in the periolivary nuclei. The combination of ipsilateral and contralateral projections from each cochlear nuclear complex is involved with the binaural input to the superior olivary complex (see later on) and nuclei of the lateral lemniscus.

The cochlear centers in the lower brainstem include the cochlear nuclei, superior olivary nuclear complex, and nuclei of lateral lemniscus. They are strategically located between the organ of Corti and the higher centers with their core-belt organization (including the inferior colliculus, medial geniculate body, and auditory cortex). The neurons of the cochlear nuclei project to centers on both the same and opposite sides. The neurons which first receive and process biaural input from both organs of Corti are those in the superior olivary complex. Efferent projections from the superior olivary to the cochlear nuclei and to the organ of Corti are routes involved in the central control of primary afferent input.

Superior Olivary Nuclear Complex

This complex comprises the lateral superior olivary nucleus, medial superior olivary nucleus, nucleus of the trapezoid body, and the periolivary nuclear group—all located in ventral tegmentum of the lower pons (Fig. 2.1). The periolivary group is composed of diffusely and poorly differentiated groupings of cells in the vicinity of the superior olivary nuclei; they have been subdivided into subnuclei (see Strominger, 1978).

Nerve fibers associated with the auditory system pass through the tegmentum of the lower pons. The origin and course of these fibers as demonstrated in the monkey, chimpanzee, man (Strominger, 1973, 1978), and other mammals (Osen, 1981; and others) are outlined in the following short review. The axons from the dorsal cochlear nucleus course in the dorsal acoustic stria (bypass the superior olivary complex), ascend in the contralateral lateral lemniscus, and terminate in the central nucleus of the inferior colliculus. The axons from the anteroventral cochlear nucleus pass through the trapezoid body and terminate in the ipsilateral lateral superior olivary nucleus, contralateral nucleus of the trapezoid body, bilaterally in the periolivary nuclear complex, and bilaterally in the medial superior olivary nuclei. The axons from the posteroventral cochlear nucleus course in the intermediate acoustic stria and terminate bilaterally in the periolivary nuclear complex, in the ipsilateral lateral superior olive, and in the contralateral nucleus of the trapezoid body. Evidence indicates that some fibers from the cochlear nuclei ascend in the contralateral auditory pathway (lateral lemniscus and brachium of the inferior colliculus) and terminate in the medial geniculate body of the rhesus monkey and chimpanzee (Strominger et al, 1977). The neurons of the nucleus of the trapezoid body project to the lateral superior olivary nucleus. These nuclei in primates and man are described by Moskowitz (1969), Moore and Moore (1971), and Strominger and Hurwitz (1976).

The tonotopically organized medial and lateral superior olivary nuclei are involved with the processing of localization of sound in space. The medial nucleus responds mainly to low-frequency sounds, while the lateral nucleus responds to all auditory frequencies (Tsuchitani and Boudreau, 1966). Each of these nuclei is composed of bipolar neurons, with each pole having a dendritic process. As previously noted, these bipolar cells receive inputs from the spherical and globular cells of the cochlear nuclei. These connections are precisely organized, with one pole of each neuron receiving neural input from the ipsilateral cochlear nuclei and the other pole from the contralateral cochlear nuclei. Thus, when a sound from one side of the body reaches the one ear a fraction of a second prior to the other ear farther away, this temporal difference is thus conveyed to the bipolar neurons of the superior olivary nuclei so that one pole of a neuron receives the information at a different time than the other pole. These interaural time and intensity differences are important clues for the localization of sound in space (Whitfield, 1967). The resulting activity within the central nervous system can then "interpret" the localization of the source of the sound in space (Boudreau and Tsuchitani, 1973; Tsuchitani, 1978). The neurons of the lateral superior olivary nuclei project bilaterally, and the medial superior olivary nuclei project ipsilaterally via fibers in the lateral lemniscus to the central nucleus of the inferior colliculus. The periolivary nuclei are primarily associated with the descending auditory pathway and with the cochlear efferent bundle to the organ of Corti.

Nuclei of the Lateral Lemniscus

These nuclei are aggregations of cells located within the lateral lemniscus. Two nuclei—dorsal and ventral—are designated in the primates and man. An additional nucleus, called the intermediate nucleus, is present in the cat (Bruno-Bechtold et al, 1981; Glendenning et al, 1981). The dorsal nucleus receives fibers from the superior olivary complex, from the contralateral dorsal nucleus of the lateral lemniscus via the commissure, and only a few from the cochlear nuclei. In contrast, the ventral nucleus receives many fibers from the contralateral ventral cochlear nucleus and only a few fibers from the superior olivary complex.

The intermediate nucleus receives some fibers from both the cochlear nuclei and superior olivary complex. These nuclei of the lateral lemniscus project their output to the central nucleus of the inferior colliculus.

Lateral Lemniscus

The lateral lemniscus is composed of ascending and descending fibers. The ascending fibers include crossed fibers from the cochlear nuclei, both crossed and uncrossed fibers from the lateral superior olivary nucleus, and uncrossed fibers from the medial superior olivary nucleus. These ascending fibers along with those from the nuclei of the trapezoid body terminate in the central nucleus of the inferior colliculus (Goldberg and Moore, 1967). The descending fibers in the lateral lemniscus originate in the central nucleus of the inferior colliculus and terminate mainly in the superior olivary complex of the same side and bilaterally in the cochlear nuclei.

Ear Reflexes

The audiomotor reflexes (middle ear reflexes) are associated with changes in the tone of the stapedius muscle, which is innervated by the facial (seventh) cranial nerve, and the tensor tympani muscle, which is innervated by the trigeminal (fifth) cranial nerve (Borg, 1973). The role of these reflexes is to protect the organ of Corti from excessive stimulation by dampening the amplitude of the vibrations by exerting tension on the ear ossicles. Loud sounds result in reflex contraction of the stapedius muscle (inserts on stapes) in man (Djupesland, 1980). The tensor tympani muscle (inserts on malleus) contracts only when the loud sound is of such high intensity that it produces a startle defense reaction; the latter is accompanied by the contraction of the muscles of facial expression (Djupesland, 1980). (For detailed discussion see Chapter 7.)

INFERIOR COLLICULUS

As a consequence of its location and neural connections astride the auditory pathways, the inferior colliculus has been called the obligatory relay nuclear complex. The subdivision of the upper auditory pathway into a core portion and a belt portion is expressed in the division of the inferior colliculus into central nucleus (core) and peripheral gray matter (belt). The latter has been variously subdivided by different authors (Harrison and Howe, 1974a and b). This colliculus of the rhesus monkey, chimpanzee, and human has been divided into three parts: (1) a large central nucleus (core), (2) an external nucleus bordering the central nucleus laterally and rostrally (belt), and (3) a pericentral nucleus bordering the central nucleus caudally and dorsally (belt) (Strominger, 1978). The central nucleus in the monkey (FitzPatrick, 1975) and in the human (Geniec and Morest, 1971), as revealed by Golgi studies, is characterized by a laminar arrangement of its disk-shaped neurons oriented in parallel with its afferent fibers. The bilateral inferior colliculi are interconnected by the commissure of the inferior colliculus. The central nucleus is a tonotopically organized laminated structure (Harrison, 1978).

The following summarizes the general connections of the inferior colliculus (Harrison, 1978; Strominger, 1978; Adams, 1979; Osen, 1981). The ascending input from the lower auditory centers is conveyed via the lateral lemniscus to the central nucleus. Some descending input is derived directly from the auditory cortices of both sides. The central nucleus projects its output to the tonotopically organized ventral subdivision and medial division of the medial geniculate body (Moore and Goldberg, 1966). In addition, it also projects to the peripheral gray matter (belt) of the colliculus, to the periaqueductal gray matter, to the periolivary nuclei, to the trapezoid body, and bilaterally to the cochlear nuclei (Osen, 1981).

The belt nuclei receive other inputs from the spinothalamic **tract** ("pain fibers") and the medial lemniscus ("touch fibers"). The main projection of the belt nucleus is rostrally to the nonlaminated medial and lateral subnuclei of the medial geniculate body.

In the monkey, a small fascicle passes through the commissure of the inferior colliculus and contralateral brachium of the inferior colliculus to terminate in some regions of the medial geniculate body as does the ipsilateral projection (Moore and Goldberg, 1966); some fibers in this fascicle terminate in all nuclei of the contralateral inferior colliculus.

The **superior colliculus** receives some stimuli from the auditory system: This input is integrated into the reflexes influencing the position of the head and eyes (Gordon, 1972).

MEDIAL GENICULATE BODY

Several schemas exist parcelling the medial geniculate body. A most useful terminology especially for functional correlations is that of Morest (1964) based primarily on Golgi studies in the cat—namely, dorsal, ventral and medial divisions. According to Burton and Jones (1976), the medial geniculate body in the primates (based on Nissl studies in the squirrel monkey and rhesus monkey) consists of a medial (magnocellular) division and a lateral (principal or parvocellular) division. The latter is further parcelled into posterolateral, anterolateral, and ventral subdivisions. Of importance, is that the ventral subdivision gives a hint, on the basis of cytoarchitectural criteria, of having a laminar organization. The lateral division, especially ventral subdivision, which is tonotopically organized, is considered to be included in the core portion; it receives input from the central nucleus of the inferior colliculus. The medial division and ventral subdivision of the medial geniculate body are functionally characterized as receiving input from the central nucleus of the inferior colliculus, and, in addition, projections from the spinothalamic pathway ("pain") and medial lemniscus ("touch"), fastigial nucleus of the cerebellum (related to audiovisual area of cerebellum), and superior colliculus. All nonlaminated portions of the medial geniculate body (auditory belt portion) receive input from the belt regions of the inferior colliculus.

The core portion of the medial geniculate body projects fibers in the auditory radiations to the primary auditory cortex (areas 41 and 42). The nonlaminated nuclei are considered to project to the cortical belt area. There are no commissural fibers interconnecting the medial geniculate bodies of the two sides.

The **pulvinar** of the thalamus has reciprocal connections with the temporal cortex (Trojanoski and Jacobson, 1975). Their functional significance is not known.

THE AUDITORY CORTEX

The human auditory cortex is located on the superior surface of the temporal lobe facing the lateral fissure; it includes portions of the planum temporale (Fig. 2.2). Click-evoked potentials were obtained in the human in these cortical regions and portions of the frontal and parietal opercula (Celesia, 1976). The auditory cortex may be divisible into (1) a primary auditory cortex or core portion and (2) several surrounding cortical fields or belt portion, all of which receive projections from the medial geniculate body. The primary auditory cortex occupies the transverse temporal gyri of Heschl (area 41, Figs. 2.2 and 2.6), which are separated by the supratemporal **sulcus**. Only one **gyrus** of Heschl is present when this sulcus is absent. The surrounding belt cortical fields include areas 42 and 22 (Fig. 2.6).

Recent studies of the cerebral cortex have redefined the organization of the sensory cortices, especially with the discovery of many more topographically organized representations of the skin, retina of the eye, and cochlea of the ear in the classical association cortex (for these advances, refer to Merzenich and Kaas, 1980; Schmitt et al, 1981; Jones, 1981; and Merzenich, 1982). Observations based on experimental analyses of the auditory cortex of two primates—rhesus monkey and owl monkey—have uncovered significant data of relevance to the human auditory cortex (Woolsey and Walzl, 1944; Walzl, 1947; Merzenich and Brugge, 1973; Imig et al, 1977; Merzenich and Kaas, 1980; Woolsey, 1982). For the auditory system, at least five or seven (or more) separate delineated representations are present in the cortex of primates (Merzenich, 1982). These are more than just expressions of cochleotopic (tonotopic) representations as such but apparently are expressions of other perceptual dimensions as, for example, sound localization and distance of the vocalizing object from the listener (Suga, 1978; Merzenich, 1982).

The primary auditory cortex, konio-cortex, is tonotopically organized in the human, with the highest frequencies located caudomedially and the lowest frequencies located

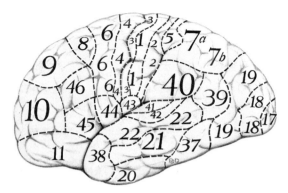

Figure 2.6.   Cytoarchitectural map of the lateral surface of the human cerebral cortex. (Numbers represent the areas of Brodmann). (From Noback CR, Demarest RJ: *The Human Nervous System*, ed 3. New York, McGraw-Hill Book Co, 1981.)

rostrolaterally. The belt portions including area 22 have several fields. Physiological responses indicate that some of these fields have tonotopic representations, which are less accurately delineated than in the primary auditory cortex. Experimental evidence in the cat indicates that the cortex has functional columnar organization similar to that described for the visual cortex. These columns may be expressed in the primary auditory cortex as frequency columns (Merzenich et al, 1975) or as binaural interaction columns with input from both ears (Imig and Adrian, 1977). (For further discussion see Chapter 5.)

The auditory cortex has intrahemispheric and interhemispheric connections through association and commissural fibers. Data on these connections have been determined in the rhesus monkey by Pandya et al (1969), Jones and Powell (1970), and Karol and Pandya (1971). A sequential series of reciprocal connections commencing with the primary auditory have been described by Jones and Powell (1970). The *first sequence* comprises projections from the primary auditory cortex to the cortical belt areas and to area 8 of the frontal lobe (Fig. 2.6). Area 8 is the frontal eye field which is the cortical area for voluntary scanning movement of the eye. The *second sequence* comprises fibers from the belt area to area 22 of the superior temporal gyrus and from area 8a to area 9 of the frontal lobe (Fig. 2.6). The *third sequence* comprises fibers projecting from the supratemporal gyrus to the area of the supratemporal sulcus and from area 9 to areas 10 and

12 of the frontal lobe. In the monkey the area bordering the supratemporal sulcus is a multisensory region where auditory input is integrated with inputs from the visual and somesthetic cortices. This multisensory cortex is presumably the progenitor of **Wernicke's area** of the human cortex, which consists of the angular gyrus (area 39), supramarginal gyrus (area 40), and portions of area 22. Intrahemispheric fibers arise in lamina III of the cortex and terminate in all laminae (Szentagothai, 1978).

The auditory cortices of the two cerebral hemispheres are interconnected by commissural fibers passing through the anterior commissure and corpus callosum (Pandya et al, 1969). The lateral portions of the primary auditory cortex are largely devoid of connections. The source of the anterior commissural fibers is the rostral half of the superior temporal gyrus and the adjacent cortex of the supratemporal plane. The commissural fibers from the caudal part of the superior temporal gyrus and adjacent auditory cortex of the supratemporal plane pass through the caudal part of the body of the corpus callosum (rostral to the splenium). The commissural fibers arise from laminae II through VI of the cortex and terminate in all laminae of the opposite cortex (Szentagothai, 1978).

CLAUSTRUM

The "enigmatic" **claustrum** is a band of gray matter located between the cortex of the insula and the lenticular nucleus. Recently it has been established that the claustrum has reciprocal connections with the visual cortex, somesthetic cortex, and auditory cortex of the cat but not with the thalamic relay nuclei, such as the geniculate bodies (Olson and Graybiel, 1980; LeVay and Sherk, 1981). A portion of the claustrum receives projections from the auditory cortex and contains neurons which are responsive to auditory stimulation (Olson and Graybiel, 1980). The functional role of the claustrum is, as yet, unknown.

DESCENDING AUDITORY PATHWAY

Parallel to the ascending auditory pathway is the descending (centrifugal) pathway (Fig. 2.3). These centrifugal projections comprise in order from cortex to organ of Corti: (1) corticogeniculate fibers from the auditory cortex to the medial geniculate body; (2) corticocollicular fibers from the auditory cortex to the inferior colliculus, and some other brainstem structures; (3) collicular efferent fibers from the inferior colliculus to the nuclei of the lateral lemniscus and the superior olivary nuclei and to the dorsal and ventral cochlear nuclei; (4) superior olivary-cochleonuclear fibers from the periolivary nucleus to the dorsal and ventral cochlear nuclei; and (5) the cochlear efferent bundle of fibers from the superior olivary complex to the cochlear nerves beneath the hair cells of the organ of Corti. Note there is no geniculocollicular projection.

The precise role of the descending pathway is, as yet, poorly understood (Osen, 1981). Its fibers are presumably integrated into feedback loops of various degrees of complexity and are involved with processing and sharpening the influences conveyed by the ascending pathway through excitatory and inhibitory activities. The result is to channel essential neural information (enhance the signals) and inhibit unwanted neural information (suppress noise). (See Chapter 9.)

The three descending projections from the auditory cortex comprise those to the medial geniculate body, inferior colliculus, and pontine nuclei (corticopontine fibers). In general, the geniculate projections in primates originate in lamina VI of the cortex, with each cortical subdivision reciprocating its ascending projection from the medial geniculate body by a descending projection to the medial geniculate body (Diamond, 1978; Kelly and Wong, 1981). Thus, each auditory cortical area projects back to the source of its afferent fibers in the medial geniculate body. These interconnections are incorporated into short feedback loops (Forbes and Moskowitz, 1974; Oliver and Hall, 1978). A small projection from the auditory cortex to the pulvinar of the **thalamus** is present in the owl monkey (FitzPatrick and Imig, 1978). The corticocollicular projection arises from lamina V of the primary auditory cortex and bypasses the medial geniculate body (Diamond, 1978). These fibers terminate bilaterally in the pericentral nucleus and not in the central nucleus of the inferior colliculus (Jones et al, 1976). The corticopontine fibers are presumed to be integrated into circuits involving the audiovisual areas of the cerebellum (Osen, 1981). In the cat, cells in lamina V and VI project to the medial geniculate body and cells in lamina V to the inferior colliculus; each cell projects to one of these two structures, but none projects to both structures (Kelly and Wong, 1981; Wong and Kelly, 1981).

The centrifugal fibers from the inferior colliculus descend in the lateral lemniscus and terminate in the superior olivary complex (colliculoolivary fibers) and in the cochlear nuclei (colliculocochleonuclear fibers) (Casseday et al, 1976). The colliculoolivary projection terminates primarily in the periolivary nucleus of the same side in the region from which crossed fibers of the olivocochlear bundle orginate (see later on). The region from which uncrossed olivocochlear fibers originate has not been demonstrated (Osen, 1981). The colliculocochlear nuclear projections terminate bilaterally in the dorsal and ventral nuclei of both sides. The olivocochleonuclear fibers terminate in the cochlear nuclei.

The olivocochlear bundle of fibers to the organ of Corti consists of two tracts [details determined in the cat (Iurato et al, 1978; Warr, 1978)]. The first tract originates from small cells located in the margin of the lateral superior olivary nucleus. These fibers are primarily uncrossed unmyelinated axons which terminate on the peripheral process of the spiral ganglion afferent cells beneath the inner hair cells of the organ of Corti (Fig. 2.3). The second tract originates from large medially located cells in the periolivary nuclei. These fibers are primarily crossed myelinated axons which terminate on the peripheral processes of spiral ganglion cells beneath the outer hair cells (Fig. 2.4). The olivocochlear bundle affects the afferent cochlear fibers. Electric stimulation of these fibers in the medulla reduces the auditory nerve activities to sound stimulation (Galambos, 1956; Keidel and Neff, 1975).

References

Adams JC: Ascending projections to the inferior colliculus. *J Comp Neurol* 183:519–538, 1979.

Bacsek RD, Strominger NL: The cytoarchitecture of the human anteroventral cochlear nucleus. *J Comp Neurol* 147:281–290, 1973.

Borg E: On the neuronal organization of the acoustic middle ear reflex. A physiological anatomical study. *Brain Res* 49:101–123, 1973.

Boudreau JC, Tsuchitani C: *Sensory Neurophysiology with Special Reference to the Cat.* New York, van Nostrand, 1973.

Brawer JR, Morest DK, Kane EC: The neuronal architecture of the cochlear nucleus of the cat. *J Comp Neurol* 155:251–300, 1974.

Brugge JF, Geisler CD: Auditory mechanisms in lower brainstem. *Annu Rev Neurosci* 1:363–394, 1978.

Bruno-Bechtold JK, Thompson GC, Masterton RB: HRP study of the organization of auditory afferents ascending to central nucleus of inferior colliculus. *J Comp Neurol* 197:705–722, 1981.

Burton H, Jones EG: The posterior thalamic region and its cortical projections in New World and Old World monkey. *J Comp Neurol* 168:249–302, 1976.

Casseday JH, Diamond IT, Harting JK: Auditory pathways to the cortex in Tupaia glis. *J Comp Neurol* 166:303–380, 1976.

Celesia GG: Organization of auditory cortical areas in man. *Brain* 99:403–414, 1976.

Diamond IT: The auditory cortex. In Naunton RF, Fernandez C (eds): *Evoked Electrical Activity in the Auditory Nervous System.* New York, Academic Press, 1978, pp 463–485.

Djupesland G: The acoustic reflex. In Jerger JF, Northern JL (eds): *Handbook of Clinical Impedance Audiometry.* New York, American Electromedics Corp, 1980.

Fields WS, Alford BR (eds): *Anatomic Relationships of the Ascending and Descending Auditory Systems,* Springfield, IL, Charles C Thomas, 1964.

FitzPatrick KA: Cellular architecture and topographic organization of the inferior colliculus of the squirrel monkey. *J Comp Neurol* 164:185–207, 1975.

FitzPatrick KA, Imig TJ: Projections of the auditory cortex upon the thalamus and midbrain in the owl monkey. *J Comp Neurol* 177:537–556, 1978.

Forbes B, Moskowitz N: Projections of auditory responsive cortex in squirrel monkey. *Brain Res* 67:239–254, 1974.

Galambos R: Suppression of auditory nerve activity by stimulation of efferent fibers to cochlea. *J Neurophysiol* 19:424–437, 1956.

Geniec P, Morest DK: The neuronal architecture of the human posterior colliculus—a study with the Golgi method. *Acta Otolaryngol [Suppl] (Stockh)* 295:1–33, 1971.

Glendenning KK, Bruno-Bechtold JK, Thompson GC, Masterton RB: Ascending auditory afferents to the nuclei of the lateral lemniscus. *J Comp Neurol* 197:673–703, 1981.

Godfrey DA, Kiang NYS, Norris BF: Single unit activity in the posteroventral cochlear nucleus of the cat. *J Comp Neurol* 162:247–268, 1975a.

Godfrey DA, Kiang NYS, Norris BE: Single unit activity in the dorsal cochlear nucleus of the cat. *J Comp Neurol* 162:269–284, 1975b.

Goldberg JM, Moore RY: Ascending projections of the lateral lemniscus in the cat and monkey. *J Comp Neurol* 129:143–156, 1967.

Gordon B: The superior colliculus of the brain. *Sci Am* 227:72–82, 1972.

Harrison JM: The auditory system of the brain stem. In Naunton RF, Fernandez C (eds): *Evoked Electrical Activity in Auditory Nervous System.* New York, Academic Press, 1978, pp 353–371.

Harrison JM, Howe MF: Anatomy of the afferent auditory nervous system in mammals. In Keidel WD, Neff WD (eds): *Handbook of Sensory Physiology.* Berlin, Springer-Verlag, 1974a, vol 7, pp 283–336.

Harrison JM, Howe MF: Anatomy of the descending auditory system (mammalian). In Keidel WD, Neff WD (eds): *Handbook of Sensory Physiology.* Berlin, Springer-Verlag, 1974b, vol 7, pp 336–388.

Hudspeth AJ: The hair cells of the inner ear. *Sci Am* 248:54–64, 1983.

Imig TJ, Adrian HO: Binaural columns in the primary field (A1) of cat. *Brain Res* 13:338–359, 1977.

Imig TJ, Ruggero MH, Kitzes LM, Javel E, Brugge JF: Organization of auditory cortex in the owl monkey. *J Comp Neurol* 192:293–332, 1977.

Iurato S, Smith C, Eldredge D, et al: Distribution of crossed olivocochlear bundle in chinchilla's cochlea. *J Comp Neurol* 182:57–76, 1978.

Jones DR, Cassaday JH, Diamond IT: Further study of parallel auditory pathways in the tree shrew *Tupaia glis. Anat Rec* 184:438–439, 1976.

Jones EG: Anatomy of the cerebral cortex. In Schmitt FO, Worden FG, Adelman G, Dennis SG (eds): *The Organization of the Cortex.* Cambridge, MA, MIT Press, 1981, pp 199–236.

Jones EG, Powell TPS: An anatomical study of conveying sensory pathways within the cerebral cortex of the monkey. *Brain* 93:793–820, 1970.

Kane ES: Primary afferents and the cochlear nucleus. In Naunton RF, Fernandez C (eds): *Evoked Electrical Activity in the Auditory Nervous System.* New York, Academic Press, 1978, pp 337–351.

Karol EA, Pandya DN: The distribution of the corpus callosum in the rhesus monkey. *Brain* 94:471–486, 1971.

Keidel WD, Neff WD (eds): Auditory systems. In *Handbook of Sensory Physiology.* Berlin, Springer Verlag, 1975, Vol 5.

Kelly JP, Wong D: Laminar connections of the cat's auditory cortex. *Brain Res* 212:1–15, 1981.

Khanna SM, Tonndorf J: Physical and physiological principles controlling auditory sensitivity in primates. In Noback CR (ed): *Sensory Systems of Primates.* New York, Plenum, 1978, pp 23–53.

Kiang NYS, Rho JM, Northrup CC, Liberman, MC, Ryugo DK: Hair cell innervation by spiral ganglion cells in adult cats. *Science* 217:175–177, 1982.

LeVay S, Sherk H: The visual claustrum of the cat. *J Neurosci* 1:956–1002, 1981.

Merzenich MM: Organization of primate sensory forebrain structures: a new perspective. In Thompson RA, Green SR (eds): *New Perspectives in Cerebral Localization.* New York, Raven Press, 1982, pp 47–62.

Merzenich MM, Brugge JF: Representation of the cochlear partition of the superior temporal plane of the macaque monkey. *Brain Res* 50:275–296, 1973.

Merzenich MM, Kaas JH: Principles of organization of sensory-perceptual systems in mammals. *Prog Psychobiol Physiol Psychol* 9:1–42, 1980.

Merzenich MM, Knight PL, Roth GL: Representation of cochlea within primary auditory cortex in the cat. *J Neurophysiol* 38:231–249, 1975.

Moore JK, Moore RY: A comparative study of the superior olivary complex in the primate brain. *Folia Primatol* 16:35–51, 1971.

Moore JK, Osen KK: The cochlear nuclei in man. *Am J Anat* 154:393–418, 1979.

Moore RY, Goldberg JM: Projections of the inferior colliculus in the monkey. *Exp Neurol* 14:429–438, 1966.

Morest DK: The neuronal architecture of the medial geniculate body of the cat. *J Anat (Lond.)* 98:611–630, 1964.

Moskowitz N: Comparative aspects of some features of the central auditory system of primates. Comparative and evolutionary aspects of the vertebrate central nervous system. *Ann NY Acad Sci* 167:357–369, 1969.

Moskowitz N, Liu J: Central projections of the spiral ganglion in the squirrel monkey. *J Comp Neurol* 144:335–344, 1972.

Naunton RF, Fernandez C (eds): *Evoked Electrical Activity in the Auditory Nervous System.* New York, Academic Press, 1978.

Nomura Y: Nerve fibers in the human organ of Corti. *Acta Otolaryngol* 82:317–324, 1976.

Oliver DL, Hall WC: The medial geniculate body of the tree shrew, *Tupaia glis.* II. Connections with the neocortex. *J Comp Neurol* 182:459–494, 1978.

Olson CR, Graybiel AM: Sensory maps in the claustrum of the cat. *Nature* 288:479–481, 1980.

Osen KK: Cytoarchitecture of the cochlear nuclei in the cat. *J Comp Neurol* 136:453–484, 1969.

Osen KK: Course and termination of the primary afferents in the cochlear nuclei of the cat. An experimental anatomical study. *Arch Ital Biol* 108:21–51, 1970.

Osen KK: The auditory system. In Brodal A (ed): *Neurological Anatomy in Relation to Clinical Medicine,* ed 3. New York, Oxford University Press, 1981, pp 602–639.

Pandya DN, Hallett M, Mukherjee SK: Intra- and extrahemispheric connections of the neocortical auditory system in the rhesus monkey. *Brain Res* 14:49–65, 1969.

Rasmussen AT: Studies of the VIII cranial nerve. *Laryngoscope* 50:67–83, 1940.

Rasmussen GL: Anatomic relationships of the ascending and descending auditory systems. In Fields WS, Alford BR (eds): *Neurological Aspects of Auditory and Vestibular Disorders.* Springfield, IL, Charles C Thomas, 1944, pp 5–23.

Rasmussen GL, Windle W (eds): *Neural Mechanisms of the Auditory and Vestibular Systems.* Springfield, IL, Charles C Thomas, 1960.

Romand R, Romand MR, Marty R: Regional difference in fiber size in the cochlear nerve. *J Comp Neurol* 198:1–5, 1981.

Rose JE, Galambos R, Hughes JB: Organization of frequency sensitive neurons in the cochlear complex of the cat. In Rasmussen G, Windle W (eds): *Mechanisms of the Auditory and Vestibular Systems.* Springfield, IL, Charles C Thomas, 1960, pp 116–136.

Schmitt FO, Worden FG, Adelman G, Dennis SG (eds): *The Organization of the Cerebral Cortex.* Cambridge, MA, MIT Press, 1981, 592 pp.

Spoendlin H: The afferent innervation of the cochlea. In Naunton RF, Fernandez C (eds): *Evoked Electrical Activity in the Auditory Nervous System.* New York, Academic Press, 1978, pp 21–41.

Strominger NL: The origins, course and distribution of the dorsal and intermediate striae in the rhesus monkey. *J Comp Neurol* 147:209–274, 1973.

Strominger NL: The anatomical organization of the primate auditory pathways. In Noback CR (ed): *Sensory Systems of Primates.* New York, Plenum Press, 1978, pp 53–91.

Strominger NL, Hurwitz JL: Anatomical aspects of the superior olivary complex. *J Comp Neurol* 170:485–498, 1976.

Strominger NL, Nelson LR, Dougherty WJ: Second order auditory pathways in the chimpanzee. *J Comp Neurol* 172:349–366, 1977.

Strominger NL, Strominger AI: Ascending brain stem projections of the anteroventral cochlear nucleus of the rhesus monkey. *J Comp Neurol* 143:217–242, 1971.

Suga N: Specialization of the auditory system for reception and processing of species-specific sounds. *Fed Proc* 37:2342–2354, 1978.

Szentagothai J: The neuron network of the cerebral cortex: a functional interpretation. *Proc R Soc Lond [Biol]* 201:219–248, 1978.

Trojanoski JJ, Jacobson S: A combined horseradish perioxidase autoradiographic investigation of reciprocal connections between superior temporal gyrus and pulvinar in the squirrel monkey. *Brain Res* 85:347–353, 1975.

Tsuchitani C: Lower-auditory brain stem structures of the cat. In Naunton RF, Fernandez C (eds): *Evoked Electrical Activity in the Auditory Nervous System.* New York, Academic Press, 1978, pp 373–401.

Tsuchitani C, Boudreau JC: Single unit analysis of cat superior olive S segment with tonal stimuli. *J Neurophysiol* 29:684–697, 1966.

Walzl EM: Representation of the cochlea in the cerebral cortex. *Laryngoscope* 57:778–787, 1947.

Warr WB: The olivocochlear bundle: its origin and

terminations in the cat. In Naunton RF, Fernandez C (eds): *Evoked Electrical Activity in the Auditory Nervous System.* New York, Academic Press, 1978, pp. 43–65.

Whitfield IC: *The Auditory Pathways.* Baltimore, Williams Wilkins, 1967.

Wong D, Kelly JP: Differentially projecting cells in individual layers of the auditory cortex: a double-labeling study. *Brain Res* 230:362–366, 1981.

Woolsey CN (ed): *Multiple Auditory Areas. Cortical Sensory Organization.* Clifton, NJ, Humana Press, 1982, vol 3.

Woolsey CN, Walzl EM: Topical projection of the cochlea to the cerebral cortex of the monkey. *Am J Med Sci* 207:685–686, 1944.

Physiology of the Ascending Auditory Pathway with Special Reference to the Auditory Brainstem Response (ABR)

AAGE R. MØLLER, Ph.D.

Dr. Møller presents the background for **auditory brainstem response (ABR).** *Necessarily, this includes a review of tonotopic organization and* **frequency tuning curves** *in the cochlea and brainstem, respectively. An overview of electrical potentials in the ear provides the basis for discussion of single nerve fiber activity, the recording of farfield and nearfield potentials, and the neural generators of the ABR.*

The use of auditory brainstem responses (ABR) in clinical diagnosis is based upon knowledge of the anatomy and physiology of the auditory system. Most of the knowledge of physiology of the auditory brainstem has been gained from the results of animal experiments in which recordings of neuro-electric potentials have provided important information about coding of sounds in the nervous system and the transformation of information in the sound waves that reach the ear. This knowledge has been acquired basically by recording the discharge patterns of single nerve fibers and cell bodies. The recording of compound action potentials, which reflect the electrical activity of many nerve elements, has contributed to knowledge about the gross organization of the auditory system.

TRANSFORMATION OF SOUNDS IN THE COCHLEA

Sounds within the audible range which reach the ear set the fluid in the cochlea into motion and, subsequently, a traveling wave motion is set up on the basilar membrane. This traveling wave starts at the base of the cochlea and increases in amplitude as it progresses towards the apex. At a certain point it rapidly decreases in amplitude. The distance it travels before it reaches its peak is a direct function of the frequency (or spectrum) of the sound; low frequencies travel greater distances toward the apex than high frequencies.

The hair cells which are located along the basilar membrane and which translate motion of the basilar membrane into a neural code in the auditory nerve fibers respond in accordance with the frequency content of the stimulating sound. Pure tone stimuli of different frequencies activate different groups of nerve fibers; sounds of higher intensity activate more nerve fibers than do those of lower intensity.

When it recently became possible to measure the vibration velocity of the basilar membrane at low sound intensities in cochleas which had been minimally damaged as the result of the recording itself, the tuning shown was nearly as sharp as the **frequency tuning curves (FTC)** of single auditory nerve fibers (Sellick et al, 1982; Khanna and Leonard, 1982).

Frequency threshold curves [also known as frequency tuning curves (FTC)] of single auditory nerve fibers obtained in an experiment in a cat are shown in Figure 3.1. The frequency of lowest threshold is known as the **characteristic frequency (CF)** of the particular fiber (Katsuki et al, 1958; Kiang et al, 1965). The curves in Figure 3.1 were selected to represent CF throughout the entire audible frequency range of the cat. Russell and Sellick (1978) recorded electrical potentials intracellularly from inner hair cells and found a frequency selectivity at threshold that was similar to that of FTC of single auditory nerve fibers.

Frequency threshold curves, such as those shown in Figure 3.1, show within which ranges (areas) of frequency and intensity the different nerve fibers respond with an increase in discharge rate. If a tone within that area is presented and at the same time another tone is presented, this second tone can decrease the discharge rate of the response evoked by the first tone (Nomoto et al, 1964; Sachs and Kiang, 1968). Figure 3.2 shows the frequency-intensity areas where a second tone can suppress the neural activity evoked by a tone at CF just above threshold. It has been shown that two-tone inhibition is pres-

ent in intracellular recordings from inner hair cells (Sellick and Russell, 1979). This indicates that the underlying mechanism is related to the vibration of the basilar membrane itself.

Associating frequency with a specific place on the basilar membrane is one way of coding frequency and is known as the "place principle" of frequency discrimination (Bekesy, 1941, 1960; Zwislocki, 1980). Another, and perhaps more important, way of coding frequency in the auditory nerve is through phase-locking of nerve impulses to the wave form of the sound (Tasaki, 1954; Wever, 1949; Brugge et al, 1969; Arthur et al, 1971; Anderson et al, 1971). This is illustrated in Figure 3.3, which shows nerve impulses recorded from a single auditory nerve fiber in response to a pure tone. It is seen that nerve impulses occur in the same phase of the sine wave, but not all waves give rise to a nerve impulse.

It is not only pure tones that give rise to phase-locking. More complex sounds also evoke nerve impulses in accordance with the wave form of the sound, and the frequency selectivity of single auditory nerve fibers can be determined using broadband stimuli (de Boer, 1967, 1968; Møller, 1978a, b, 1983a). The frequency selectivity determined at stimulus levels *above* threshold decreases

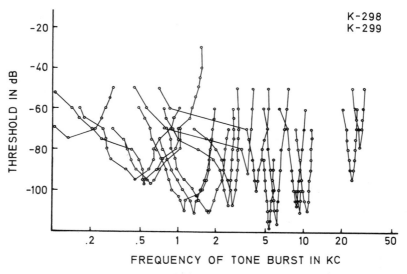

Figure 3.1. Frequency threshold curves (FTC) obtained by recording from single auditory nerve fibers in a cat. The individual curves represent different fibers. (From Kiang NYS, Watanabe T, Thomas EC, Clark LF: Discharge patterns of single fibers in the cat's auditory nerve. In: *Research Monograph 35.* Cambridge, MA, MIT Press, 1965.)

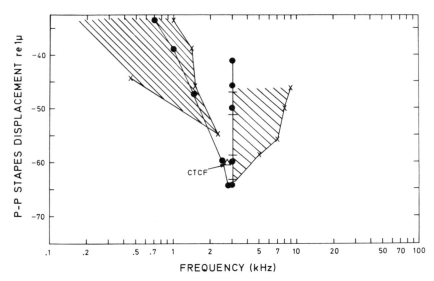

Figure 3.2. Frequency threshold curve (*solid circles*) and suppression areas of a typical auditory nerve fiber (*hatched area*). The suppression areas were determined as those areas where a decrease in the discharge rate of the response was noted in response to a tone with frequency and intensity marked *CTCF*. (From Sachs MB, Kiang NYS: Two-tone inhibition in auditory nerve fibers. *J Acoust Soc Am* 43:1120–1128, 1968.)

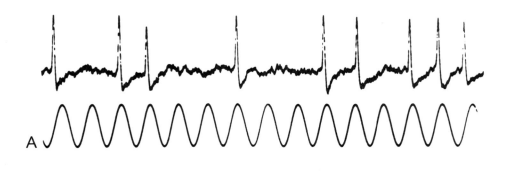

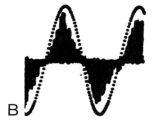

Figure 3.3. Responses of a cochlear nerve fiber to stimulation with a low-frequency tone (300 Hz). (*A*) Discharges and tone shown together. (*B*) Period histogram of the discharges locked to a certain phase of the stimulus tone combined with an inverted histogram locked to the tone shifted 180°. (From Arthur RM, Pfeiffer RR, Suga N: Properties of two tone inhibition in primary auditory neurons. *J Physiol (Lond)* 212:593–609, 1971.)

with increasing stimulus intensity (Møller, 1977, 1978a,b, 1983a), and the center frequency shifts downward (Fig. 3.4). These changes are less pronounced in fibers with CF below 1,500 Hz, and fibers with CF below 1000 Hz show practically no change in their tuning properties with change in stimulus intensity.

The significance of temporal coding of frequency becomes obvious when the discharge patterns of single auditory nerve fibers in response to sounds such as vowels are studied. It has been assumed that the coding of the spectrum of complex sounds in the discharge patterns of auditory nerve fibers, in general, describes the distribution of vibration amplitudes along the basilar membrane, that is, that the coding of sounds is related to the distribution of energy over the frequency of the sound (spectrum). However, it seems from studies (Sachs and Young, 1979; Young and Sachs, 1979) that it is the temporal structure of complex sounds such as vowels that conveys the in-

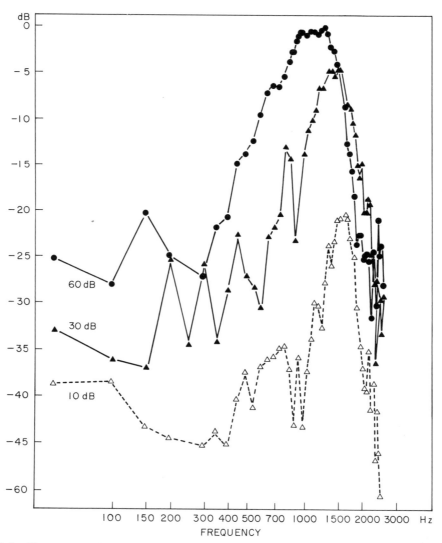

Figure 3.4. Frequency selectivity curves of single rat cochlear nerve fibers obtained using broadband noise of three different intensities as the stimuli (From Møller AR: Frequency selectivity of phase-locking of complex sounds in the auditory nerve. *Hear Res* 11:267–284, 1983a.)

INVOICE NUMBER	G48804		
INVOICE DATE	7/07/86		
CUSTOMER ORDER NO.			
ORDER RECEIVED DATE	7/07/86		
PAGE NUMBER	1	SHIPMENT NUMBER	MP7S788

QUANTITY ORDERED	ORDER STATUS	QUANTITY SHIPPED	LIST PRICE
1 BKS		1	

ARGEABLE WGT/LBS	TRANSPORTATION CHARGES	B.L. NO.	DATE SHIPPED		
			MO.	DAY	YR.
2	.94		7	9	

SS CO.   FULFILLMENT

formation about the spectrum envelope (formant frequencies), as well as the fundamental voice frequency (pitch), to higher nervous centers to a greater extent than does the spatial distribution of vibration amplitude along the basilar membrane.

The fact that the wave on the basilar membrane travels relatively slowly from base to apex of the cochlea implies that different nerve fibers are excited in a specific temporal order. A loud broadband transient sound, such as a **click sound,** therefore, will first activate those nerve fibers that are tuned to high frequencies and then will successively activate those that are tuned to lower frequencies. The importance of this in coding of complex sounds is not known, but it has recently been suggested that it may have a significance in how temporal information in the firing patterns of auditory nerve fibers is used to extract information about the frequency of sounds (Loeb et al, 1983). While the functional importance of this sequential excitation of auditory nerve fibers has yet to be proven experimentally, it is clearly of practical value in interpreting the results of experiments in which broadband transient sounds, such as click sounds, are used to test the auditory system by measuring its electrical responses (such as ABR). The travel time on the basilar membrane will contribute to the total **latency** of the response. The value of this latency depends upon the location on the basilar membrane from which the response is mainly evoked, and that may vary due to the spectrum of the sound; for instance, when broadband clicks are used as the stimulus, the latency will be affected by the presence of a high-frequency hearing loss.

ASCENDING AUDITORY PATHWAY

Responses from Single Nerve Cells

Most FTC (obtained using pure tone stimuli) of nerve cells in the two most peripheral nuclei of the ascending auditory pathway (cochlear nucleus and superior olive) are similar in shape to those of single auditory nerve fibers (Rose et al, 1959; Møller, 1969, 1983b; Guinan et al, 1972), but they are slightly wider (Møller, 1972a). Some nerve cells, however, show FTC with two peaks (Rose et al, 1959; Møller, 1983b). In more central nuclei (inferior colliculus and medial geniculate), FTC are of a variety of shapes, many of which are wide and some of which are narrow. The functional significance of FTC of neurons of nuclei at higher levels has not yet been clearly established.

At all levels of the ascending auditory pathway the neural activity evoked by sound stimulation can be inhibited by other sounds. In the auditory nerve, activity evoked by tones at center frequency can be inhibited (or, more correctly, suppressed) by tones within a range of frequencies slightly higher than center frequency and also by tones below center frequency (Nomoto et al, 1964; Sachs and Kiang, 1968; Sachs, 1969) (see Fig. 3.2). A similar pattern of inhibition is present in the cochlear nucleus, but, in addition, spontaneous activity can usually be inhibited (Rose et al, 1959). Some cells in the cochlear nucleus show a more complex pattern of inhibition (Greenwood and Maruyama, 1965; Møller, 1971, 1976a). It is difficult to study inhibition in higher order auditory nuclei because of the influence of anesthesia on the results, but studies in unanesthetized animals have shown a complex pattern of excitation and inhibition, which in many neurons varies with such factors as attention.

While the patterns of response of all auditory fibers are similar except for their frequency tuning, it is a general rule that neurons in the nuclei of the ascending auditory pathway can be classified into different groups based on their patterns of responding to certain stimuli (see, e.g., Kiang et al, 1973). One of the first such classifications of neurons in the cochlear nucleus was based on their responses to **tonebursts** (Pfeiffer, 1966). Four classes of neurons were identified on the basis of the shapes of the poststimulus time (PST) histograms. (See also Chapter 2)

When sounds more complex than pure tones are used as stimuli, it becomes apparent that the most characteristic feature of single nerve cells throughout the ascending auditory pathway is frequency tuning. Information carried in the discharge patterns of single auditory nerve fibers is transformed in various ways by the nuclei of the ascending auditory pathway. This is most apparent when complex sounds of broad spectrum and varying intensity or frequency are used as stimuli. Thus, the response of neurons in the nuclei of the ascending auditory pathway to sounds that vary rapidly is much more complex than is their response to stimulation with pure tones of steady frequency. This has been studied particularly in neurons in the cochlear nucleus (Møller, 1972a,b, 1974c) and to some extent in those of the inferior colliculus (Rees and Møller, 1983) and medial geniculate (Kallert, 1974; see also Møller, 1983b). Neurons in the cochlear nucleus respond better to changes in amplitude or frequency than they do to steady-state tones. Neurons in the cochlear nucleus reproduce the modulation frequency in their discharge pattern when stimulated by amplitude-modulated tones over a wide range of stimulus intensities (Møller, 1974a,b; 1976a,b). There is for each neuron a particular modulation frequency that is reproduced best, and in many neurons 1 to 2 dB modulation can result in

a 100% modulation of the discharge rate. The modulation frequencies at which neurons in the cochlear nucleus respond best vary from neuron to neuron between about 100 and 500 Hz (Fig. 3.5). In some neurons the modulation is reproduced for low modulation frequencies up to a certain **modulation frequency** above which the modulation of the discharge rate decreases with further increase in modulation frequencies. In other neurons modulation is reproduced in the discharge pattern only within a relatively narrow range of modulation frequencies. This can also be expressed in the way that neurons in the cochlear nucleus are tuned to different modulation frequencies. The interplay between inhibition and excitation has been studied in the cochlear nucleus neurons using **amplitude-modulated tones or noise** (Møller, 1975a,b, 1976a,b) (see also Møller, 1983b).

Studies of the responses of cells in the

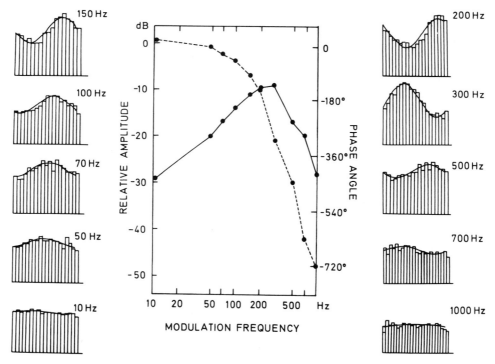

Figure 3.5. Period histogram of the response of a neuron in the cochlear nucleus to amplitude-modulated tones of different frequencies (given by legend numbers) and the modulation transfer function showing the relative amplitude of the modulation of this histogram as a function of the modulation frequency (*solid line*). The phase angle between the modulation of the stimulus tone and the modulation of the histogram is also shown (*dashed line*). (From Møller AR: Coding of sounds in lower levels of the auditory system. *Q Rev Biophys* 5:59–155, 1972a.)

cochlear nucleus to tones, the frequencies of which are varied slowly over a wide range that includes the response area of the unit, show that nerve impulses are elicited when the tone is within the response area of the unit. This is illustrated in Figure 3.6 which shows a histogram of the nerve impulses as a function of the frequency. The shapes of these histograms change in such a way that they become narrower and higher as the rate of change is increased up to a certain rate, above which they become broader and decrease in height (Møller, 1971, 1972b, 1974c). This means that at a certain rate of change in frequency, more nerve impulses are evoked within a narrower range of frequencies as the rate of change is increased up to a certain rate; above this rate of change nerve impulses are again evoked over a wider frequency range. The range of rate of change in frequency that produces the highest histogram varies from unit to unit. Fibers of the auditory nerve do not show such an enhancement of the response to tones with rapidly varying frequency (Sinex and Geisler, 1981).

Only a few neurons in the inferior colliculus respond to sustained tones and noise, but most units respond to click sounds and the onset of tonebursts. Units respond preferentially to contralateral stimulation, but there is a complex interaction between ipsilateral and contralateral stimulation in many units. Units in the inferior colliculus show a similar dependence on rate of change (as seen in the response patterns of single neurons in the cochlear nucleus) when stimulated with tones for which the frequency or amplitude varies rapidly, but the change is more varied from unit to unit and more complex in nature (Rees and Møller, 1983). Neurons in the inferior colliculus also respond to amplitude modulation, but these neurons respond best to modulation frequencies that are two to four times lower than the best modulation frequencies of neurons of the cochlear nucleus (Rees and Møller, 1983). Most of the nerve cells in the ventral and medial divisions of the geniculate body respond to tonebursts and clicks presented to the contralateral ear (Aitkin and Webster, 1972; Aitkin, 1973), and many are excited binaurally or are binaurally or ipsilaterally suppressed. Their response pattern is complex, and only a few units will respond to continuous tones or noise. The response to more complex sounds such as an animal's own vocalization has also been studied (Symmes et al, 1980).

Tonotopic Organization

Nerve cells in the nuclei of the ascending auditory pathway are arranged anatomically according to the frequency to which they are tuned. This tonotopic or cochleotopical organization is a result of an orderly branching of auditory nerve fibers. An example of this is shown in Figure 3.7, where the cochlear nucleus of a cat is represented. In each of the three subdivisions of this nucleus (anteroventral, posteroventral, and dorsal) neurons are arranged according to center frequency from high to low frequencies in the dorsoventral, posteroanterior, and mediolateral directions. A microelectrode passed through the anteroventral and dorsal divisions of the nucleus from posterior to anterior encounters cells that are tuned to frequencies from high to low. This tonotopic organization implies that individual auditory nerve fibers innervate limited areas of the auditory nuclei. This type of organization is found in all auditory brainstem nuclei (Merzenich and Kaas, 1980).

ELECTRICAL POTENTIALS OF THE EAR AND THE AUDITORY NERVOUS SYSTEM

Potentials Recorded Directly from the Ear and the Auditory Nerve

While recordings from single nerve fibers and nerve cells in the various nuclei have contributed greatly to our understanding of the transformation of sounds in the auditory nervous system, only gross potentials can be recorded in man. We shall here describe the gross potentials from the ear and the auditory nervous system and relate these potentials to various functional aspects of the auditory system.

There are three different sound-evoked potentials that can be recorded from the cochlea: **cochlear microphonic (CM)**, the **summating potential (SP)**, and the **compound action potential (CAP)**. The CM potential is generated by the hair cells and is essentially a replica of the acoustic wave form. The SP is also generated by the hair

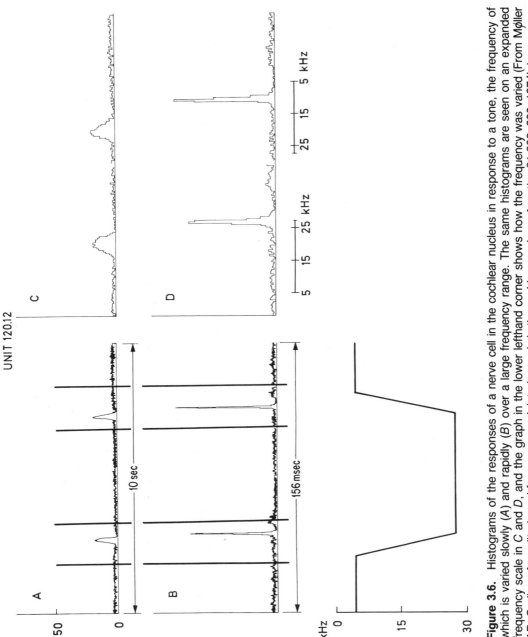

Figure 3.6. Histograms of the responses of a nerve cell in the cochlear nucleus in response to a tone, the frequency of which is varied slowly (A) and rapidly (B) over a large frequency range. The same histograms are seen on an expanded frequency scale in C and D, and the graph in the lower lefthand corner shows how the frequency was varied (From Møller AR: Coding of amplitude and frequency modulated sounds in the cochlear nucleus. *Acustica* 31:292–299, 1974b.)

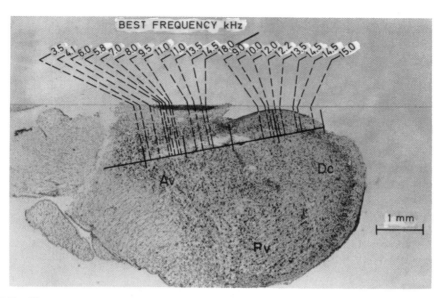

Figure 3.7. Tonotopical organization of the cochlear nucleus in a cat. The different CF of units encountered by a microelectrode passing through the cochlear nucleus in a caudal-rostral direction is illustrated. *Av*, anterior ventral cochlear nucleus; *Dc*, dorsal cochlear nucleus; *Pv*, posterior ventral cochlear nucleus. (From Rose JE, Galambos R, Hughes JR: Microelectrode studies of the cochlear nuclei in the cat. *Bull Johns Hopkins Hosp* 104:211–251, 1959.)

cells, and it is a slow potential that follows the envelope of the stimulus (see Dallos, 1973). The CAP is generated by the auditory nerve. Each of these potentials can be recorded by placing electrodes on the round window membrane, inside the cochlea, or on the cochlear capsule. The CM is best seen when a continuous pure tone is used as the stimulus, while the SP is best illustrated when a burst of a high-frequency tone is used after the CM has been removed by filtering.

In the small animals usually used in auditory experiments the CAP contains two negative peaks (N_1 and N_2), while in man it essentially contains only one peak (N_1). Figure 3.8 shows the N_1N_2 potential recorded from the round window of a rat in response to click sounds. The N_2 is generated by the cochlear nucleus (see Fisch and Ruben, 1962; Møller, 1983c). Because the N_1 of the CAP is assumed to represent a summation of the discharges of many nerve fibers (Kiang et al, 1976; Antoli-Candela and Kiang, 1978), these potentials are best seen when many nerve fibers are activated simultaneously in such a way that the discharges of individual fibers occur at precisely the same time.

The latency of the CAP recorded from the round window or the auditory nerve depends upon the travel time on the basilar membrane, the synaptic delay in the hair cell receptors (about 0.7 msec), and the neural conduction time from the distal end of the nerve to the site of recording. Although these latencies are only slightly influenced by stimulus intensity, it is a well-known finding that the latency of the CAP of the auditory nerve evoked by clicks or tonebursts decreases as a function of sound intensity. Therefore, there must be additional sources of latency.

In fact, we know of at least two such intensity-dependent sources of latency. Although the stimulus sound, e.g., in the form of a click or toneburst, may have a very rapid rise time, the motion of the basilar membrane rises relatively slowly due to its frequency selectivity. Since the amplitude of the basilar membrane vibration has to rise to a certain level before the threshold of the hair cells is reached, the latency of the response will depend upon the sound intensity. Also, the neural excitation process involves a generator potential that has to reach a certain level before a nerve impulse is elicited. The rate of rise of this generator

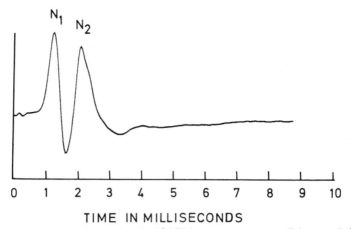

TIME IN MILLISECONDS

Figure 3.8. The compound action potential (CAP) in response to a click sound. The results were obtained by recording from the round window in a rat.

potential is a function of the intensity of the stimulus. The result is that it takes a longer time for the firing threshold of the neuron to be reached in response to a sound of low intensity than it does when the stimulus is of high intensity. The fact that the discharges of auditory nerve fibers innervating the hair cells located in the basal end of the basilar membrane have a higher degree of synchronization also contributes to the decrease in latency with increasing sound intensity. This results in the CAP in response to low-frequency sounds gradually being dominated by the activity of nerve fibers activated by more basal hair cells as the sound intensity is increased. Near threshold the excitation is limited to the area of highest response—for low-frequency sounds, in the apical portion of the basilar membrane—and the CAP near threshold is consequently generated by nerve fibers originating in the apical portion of the basilar membrane. Thus, the larger change in latency of the response to low-frequency sounds as a function of sound intensity is due to the shift of the peak of the envelope of the traveling wave toward the base of the cochlea. This becomes evident when **band-pass-filtered clicks** are used to assess the latencies of the CAP. The latencies of the rat CAP in response to bandpass-filtered clicks with different center frequencies are shown in Figure 3.9 as a function of sound intensity. It is evident that the latencies of the low-frequency clicks are longer than those

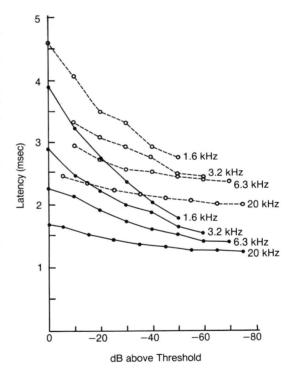

Figure 3.9. Latency of the CAP (N_1, *solid lines*; N_2, *dashed lines*) peaks in response to ⅓-octave bandpass-filtered clicks. The center frequencies of the filters are given by legend numbers. The duration of the clicks that were fed into the bandpass filters was 5 μsec. The results were obtained by recording from the round window in a rat. (From Møller AR: *Auditory Physiology.* New York, Academic Press, 1983b.)

of the high-frequency clicks in accordance with the longer travel time on the basilar membrane of low-frequency sound. It may also be seen that there is a larger change in latencies with change in sound intensity for low-frequency clicks than for high-frequency clicks. A contributing factor for this can be found in the fact that the basilar membrane is nonlinear, which results in the point of maximal excitation on the basilar membrane being shifted toward the base when the ear is stimulated with a low-frequency sound (Møller, 1977, 1978a,b, 1983a). This has been shown by using continuous amplitude-modulated sounds. Such sounds can be used to study the conduction time from the basilar membrane to, e.g., the auditory nerve or cochlear nucleus (Møller, 1981) when cross-correlation techniques are employed to analyze the recorded potentials. The obtained results resemble the response to transient sounds with some important differences. The reason is that amplitude-modulated sounds continuously exceed the threshold level of firing of the auditory neurons, so that the amplitude modulation varies only the probability of when the threshold is exceeded. The latency values obtained using this technique are independent of the rate of the rise of the generator potential (see Møller, 1973, 1975b, 1981). Thus, the change in latency values using this technique mainly reflects the shift in the location of the maximal vibration along the basilar membrane. This method, however, has not yet been applied clinically.

When stimuli of broad spectrum (such as unfiltered clicks) are used, interpretation of the response becomes more complex, and many times the curves showing latency as a function of sound intensity (such as those in Fig. 3.9) have two different slopes, so that the part representing low intensities is less steep than that representing high intensities. The response also depends upon the polarity of the sound (**rarefaction** vs **condensation clicks**) (Peake and Kiang, 1962).

Direct recording of the CAP from the auditory nerve in patients undergoing neurosurgical operations has recently been shown to be valuable in monitoring auditory function during operations in the posterior fossa (Møller and Jannetta, 1983a, 1984a).

Potentials Recorded from the Auditory Nervous System

Compound action potentials can also be recorded from other nerve tracts and nuclei of the ascending auditory pathway in response to transient stimuli. When recorded from other parts of the auditory nervous system, such CAP are usually referred to as evoked potentials or event-related potentials. When recording from the surface of nuclei, slow potentials are seen in addition to the sharp peaked response (CAP). These slow potentials are assumed to be generated by dendrites. The electrical activity that can be recorded from the surface of the cortex is of two kinds, namely a spontaneous activity and a stimulus-evoked activity (or evoked potentials). Usually the spontaneous activity is of a larger amplitude than the evoked potentials, but the latter can be retrieved by presenting many stimuli together with the use of signal-averaging technique. The evoked potentials are mainly postsynaptic potentials rather than synchronized firings. These are slower than those that are generated by neurons in more peripheral structures of the ascending auditory pathway. In the cortex excitatory postsynaptic potentials have rise times of several milliseconds and fall times of 10 to 30 msec. Inhibitory postsynaptic potentials are still slower and may last 70 to 150 msec. The latency of the evoked response from different fiber tracts and nuclei of the ascending auditory nervous system in animal experiments has played an important role in studies of the organization of the auditory nervous system (Kemp et al, 1937; Jungert, 1958). Recently, such recordings have also been performed during neurosurgical operations on human beings in order to identify the neural generators of the ABR (Møller and Jannetta, 1981, 1982a,b,c; Møller et al, 1981; Hashimoto et al, 1981; Spire et al, 1982).

Farfield Potentials Recorded from the Scalp (ABR)

The principal clinical usefulness of the auditory potentials depends upon the possibility of recording them from electrodes placed on the scalp. Such electrodes will record the **farfield** of the **potentials** generated by the various structures of the ascending auditory pathway.

Farfield potentials are in many ways different from the potentials recorded from electrodes placed directly on the structure that generates the potentials (which is usually referred to as the nearfield). Farfield potentials have a much smaller amplitude than **nearfield potentials**, and the wave form depends relatively little upon the distance to the source. Farfield potentials often contain contributions from many sources (nuclei and nerve tracts). It is convenient to think of the sources of such farfield potentials as **dipoles** (Goff et al, 1978). In addition to the magnitude of the potentials of these sources, the dimension and orientation of these dipoles also determine the amplitude of the farfield potentials. There is no simple relationship between the amplitude of the potentials recorded near the source (nearfield potentials) and those recorded at a distance from the source (farfield potentials). The amplitude of farfield potentials depends upon a number of factors in addition to the distance to the source, such as the extension and orientation of the equivalent dipole of the source in relation to the recording electrodes. By using bipolar recording technique and comparing the results obtained from many locations on the scalp it has been possible to identify cortical sources of evoked potentials. Auditory evoked potentials recorded from the scalp have been classified according to their latencies into short latency (0 to 10 msec), middle latency (20 to 80 msec), and long latency (100 to 500 msec).

Recording of the auditory brainstem response (ABR) for clinical diagnostic purposes was introduced by Sohmer and Feinmesser (1967) and Jewett and Williston (1971). The way that the ABR is usually recorded, namely, differentially between one electrode placed on the mastoid and one placed on the vertex or forehead, adds to the difficulty in interpreting the recorded potentials because both electrodes record sound-evoked potentials. This means that the results of this **differential recording** reflect the difference between the potentials recorded by the two electrodes. Since the latencies of the potentials picked up by the two electrodes often differ slightly, the resulting recording shows peaks that do not necessarily

have the same latencies as the nearfield potentials (Terkildsen et al, 1974; Møller and Jannetta, 1983c). In contrast, when recording nearfield potentials usually only one of the recording electrodes is active while the other, the reference electrode, is placed on a location where the stimulus-evoked potentials are negligible.

It is the latency of the various components of the ABR that has been found to be the most important parameter in the clinical use of these potentials, since this seems to increase as a result of many disease processes that affect the system tested (Stockard and Rossiter, 1977; Stockard et al, 1977, 1978a, 1980; Starr and Achor, 1975; Starr and Hamilton, 1976). (See Chapter 4.) However, this latency also depends upon several non-pathological factors, such as the stimulus parameters (Stockard et al, 1978b), body temperature (Stockard et al, 1978a), and various other factors, such as anesthetics used during the recording.

NEURAL GENERATORS OF ABR

The auditory brainstem-evoked potentials recorded from scalp electrodes during the first 10 msec in response to transient sounds are assumed to originate in the ear and neural structures of the ascending auditory pathway. The individual peaks of the ABR are assumed to reflect the sequential activation of the auditory nerve and nerve tracts and nuclei of the ascending auditory pathway.

The exact origin of each of the peaks in the ABR has been the subject of numerous studies. Simultaneous recordings from the scalp and nerve tracts and nuclei of the ascending auditory pathway in animals were made (Buchwald and Huang, 1975; Achor and Starr, 1980a; Britt and Rossi, 1980), and the effects of known lesions on the ABR recorded from scalp electrodes were studied (Achor and Starr, 1980b; Rossi and Britt, 1980) in order to correlate the ABR with its origin in the auditory nervous system. Recordings have also been made in human subjects with lesions of assumed known type and location (Starr and Achor, 1975; Starr and Hamilton, 1976; Stockard et al, 1977, 1980).

There is general agreement that peak I in the ABR originates in the auditory nerve.

This is supported by studies in which the potentials recorded from the scalp electrode were compared to those recorded from the inner ear (**promontorium**) (Portmann et al, 1980; Gersdorff, 1982). These studies showed that peak I had the same latency as the sharp negative peak recorded from the ear. The most simplistic hypothesis regarding the origin of the subsequent peaks assigns the second peak to the cochlear nucleus, the third to the superior olivary complex, the fourth to the lateral lemniscus, and the fifth peak to the inferior colliculus (Thornton, 1978). Others have arrived at more complex interpretations, indicating more than one source for each of the peaks in the ABR and more than one peak receiving contributions from a particular source (Starr and Achor, 1975; Starr and Hamilton, 1976; Achor and Starr, 1980a; Stockard and Rossiter, 1977).

Recently, the results of recording simultaneously from scalp electrodes and various parts of the ascending auditory pathway in patients undergoing neurosurgical operations have shed new light on the origin of the different components of the ABR (Møller et al, 1981; Møller and Jannetta, 1981, 1982a,b,c, 1983a,b; Hashimoto et al, 1981; Spire et al, 1982). These experiments showed that the compound action potentials recorded from the intracranial portion of the auditory nerve have a latency that is about 1 msec longer than that of peak I (Møller et al, 1981; Møller and Jannetta, 1981). Figure 3.10 shows examples of potentials recorded from the intracranial portion of the auditory nerve near the porus acusticus at different sound intensities. It is seen that the potentials recorded from the nerve are triphasic potentials, with an initial positive peak followed by a large negative peak which is followed by a smaller positive peak. This is in agreement with what can be expected from recording from the surface of a long nerve (i.e., the second derivative of the action potential).

Figure 3.11 shows results of recording intracranially from the human eighth nerve near the **porus acusticus** (*A*), near its entrance into the brainstem (*B*), and from a location on the brainstem presumably overlying the superior olivary complex (*C*). The ABR recorded simultaneously from the vertex-mastoid electrodes are shown in *D*. The potentials recorded close to the brainstem

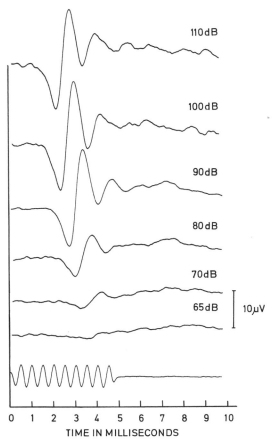

Figure 3.10. Recordings from the eighth nerve in a patient undergoing neurosurgery for hemifacial spasm showing the response at different stimulus intensities (from 60 to 100 dB). The stimulus was a 5-msec-long, 2000-Hz toneburst. (From Møller AR, Jannetta PJ: Compound action potentials recorded intracranially from the auditory nerve in man. *J Exp Neurol* 74:862–874, 1981.)

are smaller in amplitude than those recorded from the distal part of the nerve and have an initial positivity followed by a negative peak that appears with about a 0.5 msec longer latency than those recorded near the porus acusticus, in agreement with the assumption that the potentials represent propagated activity in a nerve. The difference in latency represents conduction time in the nerve between the porus acusticus and its entry into the brainstem. Comparison of the potentials recorded intracranially with the ABR recorded simultaneously shows that the main negative peak of the potentials that

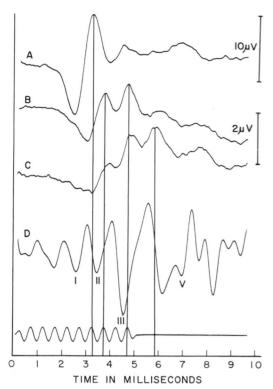

Figure 3.11. Recordings from different locations on the human eighth nerve and brainstem compared to the ABR recorded simultaneously. *A*, Recording from the eighth nerve near the porus acusticus. *B*, Recording from the brainstem near the entrance of the eighth nerve. *C*, Recording from a location on the brainstem about 4 mm medial and caudal to the entrance of the eighth nerve into the brainstem. *D*, ABR recorded differentially between a location immediately above the ipsilateral pinna and the vertex. The stimuli were 2000-Hz tonebursts of 5-msec duration at 90 dB SPL presented at intervals of 130 msec. The upper amplitude calibration relates to curve *A* and the other to curves *B* and *C*. (From Møller AR, Jannetta PJ: Neural generators of the brainstem auditory evoked potentials (BAEP). In: *Proceedings of the Second International Evoked Potentials Symposium.* Cleveland, OH, 1985.)

are recorded from the nerve appears with nearly the same latency as that of peak II in the ABR. These results were taken to show that in man the auditory nerve is the generator of both peaks I and II of the ABR. These results have been confirmed by others (Spire et al, 1982). However, results obtained in animal studies show that only the first

peak in the auditory response recorded from the scalp is generated by the auditory nerve and that the second peak is generated by the cochlear nucleus (Buchwald and Huang, 1975). The reason for this discrepancy between animals and man is that the experimental animals, usually used in auditory research, have a much shorter auditory nerve (due to their small head size) than does man: 0.5 cm or less compared to 2.5 cm in man. Thus, the long delay between the response of the distal portion of the eighth nerve and that of the intracranial portion of the eighth nerve in man is because the eighth nerve in man is about 2.5 cm long (Lang, 1981), and its fibers are relatively slow conducting (Engstrom and Rexed, 1940; Lazorthes et al, 1961).

The potentials from the eighth nerve in man recorded close to the brainstem (Fig. 3.11*B*) show a second negativity, which presumably represents activity of second-order neurons in the cochlear nucleus, and a slow potential on which these peaks are superimposed. This slow potential is assumed to represent the dendritic potentials that originate in the cochlear nucleus. The second negative peak appears with about the same latency as peak III in the ABR recorded simultaneously from scalp electrodes (*D*). These results were confirmed in other studies in which ABR recorded from scalp electrodes and intracranial recordings of auditory evoked potentials made in patients undergoing neurosurgical operations were compared (Møller and Jannetta, 1982b, 1983b, 1984a).

Recordings from the brainstem at a location overlying the superior olivary complex (Fig. 3.11*C*) also show a slow potential on which three negative peaks are riding. The two earliest of these peaks have approximately the same latencies as the two negative peaks seen in the recording from the eighth nerve near its entrance into the brainstem. The third peak, appearing about 1 msec after the second, is presumed to represent activity of third-order neurons, presumably located in the superior olivary complex. This third peak has a latency that approximately matches that of peak IV in the ABR recorded from scalp electrodes.

Recordings from the inferior colliculus and its vicinity in patients undergoing neurosurgical operations revealed a complex origin for peak V (Møller and Jannetta, 1982c). The response obtained from the contralateral inferior colliculus showed an initial surface-positive peak that most likely was generated by the lateral lemniscus. The latency of this peak was very close to that of the ABR's peak V. This positive potential was followed by a slow negativity on which several peaks could be seen. The rising phase of this negativity had about the same latency as the slope following wave V seen in the ABR (Fig. 3.12A). The slow potential following peak V in the ABR, known as Davis SN_{10} (Davis and Hirsch, 1976), had about

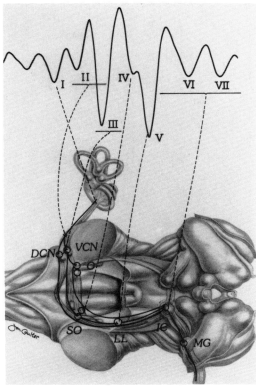

Figure 3.13. Schematic outline of the main neural generators of the ABR in man.

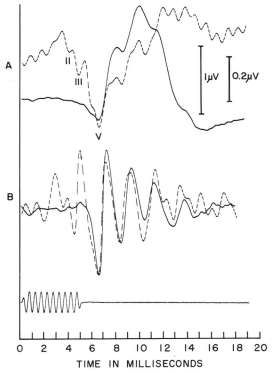

Figure 3.12. Recordings from the vicinity of the inferior colliculus (*solid lines*) and differentially from scalp electrodes placed on the vertex and over the clavicula (*dashed lines*). *A*, Digital low-pass filtering with a triangular weighting function 0.8 msec wide. Lefthand calibration relates to the recording made intracranially, and the righthand calibration relates to the recording made on the vertex. *B*, Same data as in *A* but after attenuating low-frequency components through digital filtering. (From Møller AR, Jannetta PJ: Auditory evoked potentials recorded from the cochlear nucleus and its vicinity in man. *J Neurosurg* 59:1013–1018, 1983b.)

the same appearance in time as the slow negative potential recorded from the inferior colliculus. The peaks that were seen superimposed on this slow potential coincided in time with peaks VI and VII of the ABR recorded simultaneously (Fig. 3.12B).

The results of studies on the neural generators of the ABR are summarized in Figure 3.13, which shows typical ABR together with a simplified picture of the ascending auditory pathway. The principal neural generators of the different peaks are indicated. It must be emphasized that the different peaks, except peaks I and II, receive contributions from more than one anatomical structure. In particular, the sources of peak V seem to be very complex. The fact that there is both a crossed and an uncrossed central auditory pathway complicates matters further. The schematic diagram shown in Figure 3.14 must be taken, therefore, as a simplified illustration of the neural generation of the ABR in man.

In comparing the responses from the au-

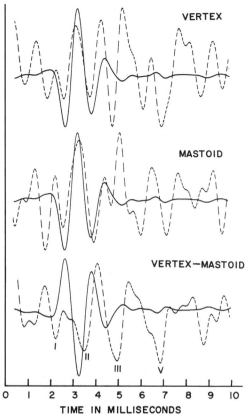

VERTEX

MASTOID

VERTEX—MASTOID

I
II
III   V

TIME IN MILLISECONDS

Figure 3.14. Auditory nerve (proximal). Comparison between recordings made intracranially from the eighth nerve (*solid lines*) and those made simultaneously from the vertex and from a position immediately above the pinna ("mastoid") using a noncephalic reference (*dashed lines*). In the upper and middle tracings negativity is shown as an upward deflection for the intracranial response as well as for the scalp response. The bottom tracing also shows the difference between the scalp (vertex-mastoid) recording (shown with vertex-negativity upward) and the intracranial recording, but the intracranial recording is shown inverted (negativity is a downward deflection). The recording from the nerve was done at a location medial to the porus acusticus. All curves were subjected to digital filtering to attenuate the slow components. The stimuli were 1-msec long tonebursts at 100 dB presented at intervals of 120 msec. The amplitude scale was the same in the recording from the scalp where noncephalic reference electrodes were used (two upper tracings).

between the vertex (or forehead) and the mastoid, may not be the ideal way of recording when it comes to correlating the responses of specific structures of the auditory nervous system with the potentials that can be recorded using scalp electrodes. The reason is that in this method both the mastoid and the vertex electrodes are active (Terkildsen et al, 1974; Møller and Jannetta, 1984b). Although the mastoid electrode records mainly the earlier peaks (I to III), it also records peak V, but with a lower amplitude than the vertex electrode. The vertex electrode mainly records later peaks (V to VII), but usually earlier peaks are also clearly visible in a recording made from a vertex electrode. It is important that the peaks in the potentials recorded from the two electrodes often have slightly different latencies. This can be seen when recordings are made from the vertex and the mastoid using a reference electrode placed on the body below the neck (noncephalic reference). Examples of recordings using such a noncephalic reference made during an operation (in which recordings also were obtained from the auditory nerve) are shown in Figure 3.14. It is seen that the potentials recorded intracranially do not occur with precisely the same latencies as do the peaks in the ABR recorded differentially between the vertex and the mastoid. A much better temporal match is obtained when the potentials recorded intracranially were compared to the potentials recorded from the scalp independent of the mastoid and vertex using noncephalic references. Similar results were obtained when comparing recordings from the inferior colliculus with potentials recorded from the scalp (Møller and Jannetta, 1984b).

The results of animal experiments indicate that the amplitude of evoked potentials recorded from the ascending auditory pathway is likely to depend upon such properties of the neural pathway as the degree of synchrony of the discharges of many nerve fibers or cell bodies to transient sound. This means that nerve tracts, in which the discharges of many fibers occur in perfect synchrony and in which **synaptic transmission** has a high safety factor, are the biggest contributors to the recorded evoked potentials. Thus, it may be that the evoked potentials reflect the activities of certain special parts of the ascending auditory pathway, namely, that part containing fast conducting fiber

ditory nerve and from other structures of the ascending auditory pathway, it becomes apparent that the way the ABR is usually recorded clinically, namely, differentially tracts and synapses with a high safety factor. Such pathways may constitute only a small portion of the entire auditory pathway. We do not know the relative importance of such fast conducting pathways compared to more slowly conducting pathways in which the discharges to transient stimuli may take place with a lesser degree of synchrony among different nerve fibers or cell bodies and in which synaptic transmissions have a smaller safety factor. These factors add to the difficulty in evaluating the relative significance of changes in the evoked potentials in relation to changes in the normal function of the auditory brainstem.

References

Achor LJ, Starr A: Auditory brain stem responses in the cat. I. Intracranial and extracranial recordings. *Electroencephalogr Clin Neurophysiol* 48:154–173, 1980a.

Achor LJ, Starr A: Auditory brain stem responses in the cat. II. Effects of lesions. *Electroencephalogr Clin Neurophysiol* 48:174–190, 1980b.

Aitkin LM: Medial geniculate body of the cat: responses to tonal stimuli of neurons in medial division. *J Neurophysiol* 36:275–283, 1973.

Aitkin LM, Webster WR: Medial geniculate body of the cat: organization and responses to tonal stimuli of neurons in ventral division. *J Neurophysiol* 35:365–380, 1972.

Anderson DJ, Rose JE, Hind JE, Brugge JF: Temporal position of discharges in single auditory nerve fibers within the cycle of a sine-wave stimulus: frequency and intensity effects. *J Acoust Soc Am* 49:1131–1139, 1971.

Antoli-Candela F Jr, Kiang NYS: Unit activity underlying the N_1 potential. In Naunton RF, Fernandez C (eds): *Evoked Electrical Activity in the Auditory Nervous System.* New York, Academic Press, 1978, pp 165–189.

Arthur RM, Pfeiffer RR, Suga N: Properties of two tone inhibition in primary auditory neurons. *J Physiol (Lond)* 212:593–609, 1971.

Békésy G von: Uber die tresrung Schwingungsamplitude der Gehorknochelchen mittels eine Kapacitieren Soude. *Akust Z.* 6:1–16, 1941.

Békésy G von: *Experiment in Hearing.* New York, McGraw-Hill, 1960.

Britt RH, Rossi GT: Neural generators of brain stem auditory evoked responses. Part I. Lesion studies. *Neurosci Abstr* 6:594, 1980.

Brugge JF, Anderson DJ, Hind JE, Rose JE: Time structure of discharges in single auditory nerve fibers of the squirrel monkey in response to complex periodic sounds. *J Neurophysiol* 32:386–401, 1969.

Buchwald JS, Huang ChM: Far-field acoustic responses: origins in the cat. *Science* 189:382–384, 1975.

Dallos P: *The Auditory Periphery.* New York, Academic Press, 1973.

Davis H, Hirsh S: The audiometric utility of brain stem responses to low-frequency sounds. *Audiology* 15:181–195, 1976.

de Boer E: Correlation studies applied to the frequency resolution of the cochlea. *J Aud Res* 7:209–217, 1967.

de Boer E: Reverse correlation. I. A heuristic introduction to the technique of triggered correlation with application to the analysis of compound systems. *Proc K Ned Akad Wet Ser C Biol Med Sci* 71:472–486, 1968.

Engstrom H, Rexed B: Uber die Kaliber Verhaltnisse der Nerven Fasern im N. Stato-acusticus des Menchen. *Z Mikrosk Anat Forsch* 47:448–455, 1940.

Fisch UP, Ruben RJ: Electrical acoustical response to click stimulation after section of the eighth nerve. *Acta Otolaryngol (Stockh)* 54:532–542, 1962.

Gersdorff MCH: Simultaneous recordings of human auditory potentials: transtympanic electrocochleography (ECoG) and brainstem-evoked responses (BER). *Arch Otorhinolaryngol* 234:15–20, 1982.

Goff WR, Allison T, Vaughan HG Jr: The functional neuroanatomy of event related potentials. In Callaway E, Tueting P, Koslow SH (eds): *Event Related Brain Potentials in Man.* New York, Academic Press, 1978, pp 1–18.

Greenwood DD, Maruyama N: Excitatory and inhibitory response areas of auditory neurons in the cochlear nucleus. *J Neurophysiol* 28:863–892, 1965.

Guinan JJ, Guinan SS, Norris BE: Single auditory units in the superior olive complex. I. Responses to sounds and classifications based on physiological properties. *Int J Neurosci* 4:101–120, 1972.

Hashimoto I, Ishiyama Y, Yoshimoto T, Nemoto S: Brainstem auditory evoked potentials recorded directly from human brain-stem and thalamus. *Brain Res* 104:841–859, 1981.

Jewett DL, Williston JS: Auditory evoked far fields averaged from the scalp of human. *Brain* 94:681–696, 1971.

Jungert S: Auditory pathways in the brain stem: a neurophysiological study. *Acta Otolaryngol [Suppl] (Stockh)* 138:1–67, 1958.

Kallert S: Telemetrische Mikroelectrodenuntersuchungen am Corpus geniculatum mediale der Wachen Katze. Dissertation. Nürnberg, West Germany, 1974.

Katsuki Y, Sumi T, Uchiyama H, Watanabe T: Electric responses of auditory neurons in cat to sound stimulation. *J Neurophysiol* 21:569–588, 1958.

Kemp EH, Coppee GE, Robinson EH: Electric responses of the brainstem to unilateral auditory stimulation. *Am J Physiol* 120:304–315, 1937.

Khanna SM, Leonard DGB: Basilar membrane tuning in the cat cochlea. *Science* 215:305–306, 1982.

Kiang NYS, Morest DK, Godfrey DA, Guinan JJ, Kane EC: Stimulus coding at caudal levels of the cat's auditory nervous system. I. Response characteristics of single units. In Møller AR (ed): *Basic Mechanisms in Hearing.* New York, Academic Press, 1973, pp 455–478.

Kiang NYS, Moxon EC, Kahn AR: The relationship of gross potentials recorded from the cochlea to single unit activity in the auditory nerve. In Ruben RJ, Elberling C, Salomon G (eds): *Electrocochleography.* Baltimore, University Park Press, 1976, pp 95–115.

Kiang NYS, Watanabe T, Thomas EC, Clark LF: Discharge patterns of single fibers in the cat's auditory nerve. In: *Research Monograph 35.* Cambridge, MA, MIT Press, 1965.

Lang J: Facial and vestibulocochlear nerve, topographic anatomy and variations, In Samii M, Jannetta PJ (eds): *The Cranial Nerves.* New York, Springer-Verlag, 1981, pp 363–377.

Lazorthes G, Lacomme Y, Ganbert J, Planel H: La constitution du nerf auditif. *Presse Med* 69:1067–1068, 1961.

Loeb GE, White MW, Merzenich MM: Spatial cross-correlation: a proposed mechanism for acoustic pitch perception. *Biol Cybern* 47:149–163, 1983.

Merzenich MM, Kaas JH: Principles of organization of sensory-perceptual systems in mammals. In Sprague JM, Epstein AM (eds): *Progress in Psychobiology and Physiological Psychology*. New York, Academic Press, 1980, vol 9, pp 1–42.

Møller AR: Unit responses in cochlear nucleus of the rat to pure tones. *Acta Physiol Scand* 75:530–541, 1969.

Møller AR: Unit responses in the rat cochlear nucleus to tones of rapidly varying frequency and amplitude. *Acta Physiol Scand* 81:540–556, 1971.

Møller AR: Coding of sounds in lower levels of the auditory system. *Q Rev Biophys* 5:59–155, 1972a.

Møller AR: Coding of amplitude and frequency modulated sounds in the cochlear nucleus of the rat. *Acta Physiol Scand* 86:223–238, 1972b.

Møller AR: Statistical evaluation of the dynamic properties of cochlear nucleus units using stimuli modulated with pseudorandom noise. *Brain Res* 57:442–456, 1973.

Møller AR: Responses of units in the cochlear nucleus to sinusoidally amplitude modulated tones. *Exp Neurol* 45:104–117, 1974a.

Møller AR: Coding of amplitude and frequency modulated sounds in the cochlear nucleus. *Acustica* 31:292–299, 1974b.

Møller AR: Coding of sounds with rapidly varying spectrum in the cochlear nucleus. *J Acoust Soc Am* 55:631–640, 1974c.

Møller AR: Dynamic properties of excitation and inhibition in the cochlear nucleus. *Acta Physiol Scand* 93:442–454, 1975a.

Møller AR: Latency of unit responses in the cochlear nucleus determined in two different ways. *J Neurophysiol* 38:812–821, 1975b.

Møller AR: Inhibition and excitation in the cochlear nucleus using amplitude modulated tones. *Exp Brain Res* 25:307–321, 1976a.

Møller AR: Dynamic properties of the responses of single neurons in the cochlear nucleus. *J Physiol (Lond)* 259:63–82, 1976b.

Møller AR: Frequency selectivity of single auditory-nerve fibers in response to broadband noise stimuli. *J Acoust Soc Am* 62:135–142, 1977.

Møller AR: Frequency selectivity of the peripheral auditory analyzer studied using broadband noise. *Acta Physiol Scand* 104:24–32, 1978a.

Møller AR: Responses of auditory nerve fibers to noise stimuli show cochlear nonlinearities. *Acta Otolaryngol (Stockh)* 86:1–8, 1978b.

Møller AR: Neural delay in the ascending auditory pathway. *Exp Brain Res* 43:93–100, 1981.

Møller AR: Frequency selectivity of phase-locking of complex sounds in the auditory nerve. *Hear Res* 11:267–284, 1983a.

Møller AR: *Auditory Physiology*. New York, Academic Press, 1983b.

Møller AR: On the origin of the compound action potentials (N_1,N_2) of the cochlea of the rat. *J Exp Neurol* 80:633–644, 1983c.

Møller AR, Jannetta PJ: Compound action potentials recorded intracranially from the auditory nerve in man. *J Exp Neurol* 74:862–874, 1981.

Møller AR, Jannetta PJ: Comparison between intracranially recorded potentials from the human auditory nerve and scalp recorded auditory brainstem responses. *Scand Audiol* 11:33–40, 1982a.

Møller AR, Jannetta PJ: Auditory evoked potentials recorded intracranially from the brainstem in man. *J Exp Neurol* 78:144–157, 1982b.

Møller AR, Jannetta PJ: Evoked potentials from the inferior colliculus in man. *Electroencephalogr Clin Neurophysiol* 53:612–620, 1982c.

Møller AR, Jannetta PJ: Monitoring auditory functions during cranial nerve microvascular decompression operations by direct recording from the eighth nerve. *J Neurosurg* 59:493–499, 1983a.

Møller AR, Jannetta PJ: Interpretation of brainstem auditory evoked potentials: results from intracranial recordings in humans. *Scand Audiol* 12:125–133, 1983b.

Møller AR, Jannetta PJ: Auditory evoked potentials recorded from the cochlear nucleus and its vicinity in man. *J Neurosurg* 59:1013–1018, 1983c.

Møller AR, Jannetta PJ: Monitoring auditory nerve potentials in operations in the cerebellopontine angle. *Otolaryngol, Head Neck Surg* 92(4): 434–439, 1984.

Møller AR, Jannetta PJ: Neural generators of the brainstem auditory evoked potentials (BAEP). In: *Proceedings of the Second International Evoked Potentials Symposium*. Cleveland, OH, in press, 1985.

Møller AR, Jannetta PJ, Bennett M, Møller MB: Intracranially recorded responses from human auditory nerve: new insights into the origin of brainstem evoked potentials. *Electroencephalogr Clin Neurophysiol* 52:18–27, 1981.

Nomoto M, Suga N, Katsuki Y: Discharge pattern and inhibition of primary auditory nerve fibers in the monkey. *J Neurophysiol* 27:768–787, 1964.

Peake WT, Kiang NYS: Cochlear responses to condensation and rarefaction clicks. *Biophys J* 2:23–34, 1962.

Pfeiffer RR: Classification of response patterns of spike discharges for units in the cochlear nucleus: tone-burst stimulation. *Exp Brain Res* 1:220–235, 1966.

Portmann M, Cazals Y, Negrevergme M, Aran J: Transtympanic and surface recordings in the diagnosis of retrocochlear disorders. *Acta Otolaryngol (Stockh)* 89:362–369, 1980.

Rees A, Møller AR: Responses of neurones in the inferior colliculus of the rat to AM and FM tones. *Hear Res* 10:301–330, 1983.

Rose JE, Galambos R, Hughes JR: Microelectrode studies of the cochlear nuclei in the cat. *Bull Johns Hopkins Hosp* 104:211–251, 1959.

Rossi GT, Britt RH: Neural generators of brainstem evoked responses. Part II. Electrode recording studies. *Neurosci Abstr* 6:595, 1980.

Russell IJ, Sellick PM: Intracellular studies of hair cells in the mammalian cochlea. *J Physiol (Lond)* 284:261–290, 1978.

Sachs MB: Stimulus-response relations for auditory-nerve fibers: two-tone stimuli. *J Acoust Soc Am* 45:1025–1036, 1969.

Sachs MB, Kiang NYS: Two tone inhibition in auditory nerve fibers. *J Acoust Soc Am* 43:1120–1128, 1968.

Sachs MB, Young ED: Encoding of steady-state vowels

in the auditory nerve: representation in terms of discharge rate. *J Acoust Soc Am* 66:470–479, 1979.

Sellick PM, Russell IJ: Two tone suppression in cochlear hair cells. *Hear Res* 1:227–236, 1979.

Sellick PM, Patuzzi R, Johnstone BM: Measurement of basilar membrane motion in the guinea pig using the Mossbauer technique. *J Acoust Soc Am* 72:131–141, 1982.

Sinex DG, Geisler CD: Auditory fiber responses to frequency-modulated tones. *Hear Res* 4:127–148, 1981.

Sohmer H, Feinmesser M: Cochlear action potentials recorded from the external ear in man. *Ann Otol Rhinol Laryngol* 76:427–428, 1967.

Spire JP, Dohrmann GJ, Prieto PS: Correlation of brainstem evoked response with direct acoustic nerve potential, pp. 159–167. In Courjon J, Manguiere F, Reval M (eds): *Advances in Neurology: Clinical Applications of Evoked Potentials in Neurology.* New York, Raven Press, 1982, vol 32.

Starr A, Achor LJ: Auditory brain stem responses in neurological diseases. *Arch Neurol* 32:761–768, 1975.

Starr A, Hamilton A: Correlation between confirmed sites of neurological lesions and abnormalities of far field auditory brain stem responses. *Electroencephalogr Clin Neurophysiol* 41:595–608, 1976.

Stockard JJ, Rossiter VS: Clinical and pathological correlates of brain stem auditory response abnormalities. *J Neurol* 7:316–325, 1977.

Stockard JJ, Sharbrough FW, Tinker JA: Effect of hypothermia on the human brain stem auditory evoked responses. *Am J Neurol* 3:368–370, 1978a.

Stockard JJ, Stockard JE, Sharbrough FW: Detection and localization of occult lesions with brain stem auditory responses. *Mayo Clin Proc* 52:761–769, 1977.

Stockard JJ, Stockard JE, Sharbrough FW: Nonpathologic factors influencing brainstem auditory evoked potentials. *Am J EEG Technol* 18:177–209, 1978b.

Stockard JJ, Stockard JE, Sharbrough FW: Brain stem auditory evoked responses in clinical neurology—methodology, interpretations, clinical applications. In Aminoff MJ (ed): *Electrodiagnosis in Clinical Neurology.* New York, Churchill-Livingstone, 1980, pp 370–413.

Symmes D, Alexander GE, Newman JD: Neural processing of vocalizations and artifical stimuli in the medial geniculate body of the squirrel monkey. *Hear Res* 3:133–146, 1980.

Tasaki I: Nerve impulses in individual nerve fibers of the guinea pig. *J Neurophysiol* 17:97–122, 1954.

Terkildsen K, Osterhammel PO, Huis in't Veld F: Far field electrocochleography, electrode positions. *Scand Audiol (Stockh)* 3:123–129, 1974.

Thornton ARD: Interpretation of cochlear nerve and brain stem responses. In Naunton RF, Fernandez C (eds): *Evoked Electrical Activity in the Auditory Nervous System.* New York, Academic Press, 1978, pp 429–442.

Wever EG: *Theory of Hearing.* New York, Wiley, 1949.

Young ED, Sachs MB: Representation of steady-state vowels in the temporal aspects of the discharge patterns of populations of auditory nerve fibers. *J Acoust Soc Am* 66:1381–1403, 1979.

Zwislocki JJ: Five decades of research on cochlear mechanics. *J Acoust Soc Am* 67:1679–1685, 1980.

CHAPTER 4

Auditory Brainstem-Evoked Responses (ABR) in Diagnosis of Eighth Nerve and Brainstem Lesions

MARGARETA B. MØLLER, M.D., Ph.D.
AAGE R. MØLLER, Ph.D.

Drs. Margareta and Aage Møller describe auditory brainstem-evoked responses (ABR) including details on peak identification, filtering, and neural generators. They note the influence of peripheral hearing loss on the ABR and discuss diagnosis using interaural latency differences and interpeak latency. They summarize work on ABR in assessment of eighth nerve tumors, cerebellopontine angle tumors, syndromes of vascular compression at the brainstem, intra- and extraaxial brainstem lesions, as well as general neurological disorders.

INTRODUCTION

During the past decade auditory brainstem responses (ABR) have taken their place in the batteries of tests used to assist in the diagnosis of several disorders affecting the auditory nervous system (Clemis and McGee, 1979; Fisher et al, 1982; Josey et al, 1980; Kinney and Nodar, 1980; Møller and Møller, 1983; Rosenhall, 1981; Selters and Brackmann, 1979; Stockard and Rossiter, 1977; Stockard et al, 1980; Thomsen et al, 1978). Recently this technique has also proven to be of value in the diagnosis of disorders which do not affect the auditory system directly (Chiappa et al, 1980; Seales et al, 1979). While most places where this technique is used follow the same general principles in performing the ABR, differ-ences in the type of sound used, the way the averaged wave form is processed, interpretation of the recorded wave forms, and the features of the recorded wave forms used in the actual diagnosis vary considerably from place to place (Stockard et al, 1980). In the past, changes in the latency of peak V of the ABR have been most often used in diagnosis. However, the wave morphology and latencies of other peaks also provide important diagnostic information.

CONSIDERATION OF PERIPHERAL HEARING LOSS

Normative data on ABR are usually obtained from young people without ear or neurological disorders. There are a number of factors that affect the ABR that are not necessarily related to the disorders which the test is used to diagnose.

Conductive Hearing Loss

When the ABR is used in the diagnosis of disorders affecting the auditory nervous system, it is desirable that disorders affecting the middle ear and the inner ear have as little effect as possible on the ABR wave form and, specifically, that they affect the latencies of the different peaks as little as possible (Stockard et al, 1978). It is well known that in a normal ear the latencies of the different peaks depend upon the stimulus sound intensity. Since a conductive type of hearing loss has the same effect on the recording of ABR as reducing the sound intensity, it follows that a conductive hearing loss will influence the latency of the peaks in the ABR. Also, a conductive hearing loss usually affects different frequencies differently; therefore, its effect on the stimulus used in recording ABR becomes more complex when using a broadband stimulus, such as click sounds, than when using narrowband sounds such as tonebursts or bandpass-filtered clicks. When click sounds are used in persons with normal hearing, the entire frequency range of the click sounds may contribute to the response. When the same sound is used in an ear with a conductive loss affecting a certain frequency range more than other frequency ranges, different parts of the click spectrum will dominate in eliciting the response. This may give rise to a complex change in the response pattern, and its effect cannot easily be offset. When tonebursts are used as the stimulus to record ABR, a conductive hearing loss may be compensated for by increasing the sound intensity by an amount equal to the hearing loss at the frequency of the stimulus used in ABR testing.

Sensorineural Hearing Loss

The advantage in using narrowband stimuli, such as tonebursts, in measuring ABR becomes even more pronounced in patients with cochlear hearing loss. Such a hearing loss most commonly affects the higher frequencies. Since the high-frequency part of the click spectrum contributes heavily to the auditory brainstem response in the normal ear, a loss of the high-frequency part of the spectrum will have the effect of reducing the stimulus intensity. Therefore, it will be the lower frequency components of the click spectrum that dominate the response of the ear with a high-frequency impairment because that means that the responses of more apically located regions of the basilar membrane dominate the ABR. Depending upon the degree of high-frequency hearing loss, the latency will be prolonged due to the longer travel time on the basilar membrane. Such a latency shift is indistinguishable from an increased neural conduction time, if just the latency of peak V is used in interpreta-

tion. Hearing loss attributable to impairment of cochlear function often is associated with recruitment of loudness, further complicating efforts to compensate for it. For example, it is not possible to compensate for a sensorineural hearing loss simply by increasing the sound intensity level of a click stimulus as it is for a conductive hearing loss. However, if pure tone stimuli are used, even a severe sensorineural hearing loss does not cause much change in the ABR pattern because of the recruitment of loudness and the fact that the location on the basilar membrane from which the response is elicited is independent of the hearing loss.

A correction factor has been used to compensate for the latency shift due to hearing loss when click sounds are used as stimuli. This correction factor (used in interaural latency comparisons) has been applied in patients with a sensorineural hearing loss exceeding 50 dB at 4 kHz (Selters and Brackmann, 1977). For each additional 10 dB hearing loss, 0.1 msec is subtracted from the observed latency of wave V.

Some investigators have suggested that the problem presented by high-frequency hearing loss can be remedied by using the interpeak (I–V) latency measure instead of using the latency of peak V alone (Coats and Martin, 1977; Selters and Brackmann, 1977; Eggermont et al, 1980. Use of the latter procedure is based upon the assumption that the appearance of peak I corresponds to the time of greatest excitation of the auditory nerve, which in many cases may be difficult to verify, thus making the accuracy of this procedure uncertain.

Identification of Peak I of the ABR

Identification of peak I can be facilitated by several means. One of these is to use a special recording electrode arrangement, with electrodes placed so that the mastoid-mastoid potential is recorded. Another possibility is to place a special electrode in the ear canal near the tympanic membrane, although this requires use of an extra recording channel and thus adds to the complexity of the recording procedure (Coats, 1974).

Filtering of ABR

Optional filtering of the recorded potentials provides still another way of improving proper identification of peak I and all other peaks. Most commercial equipment for this purpose makes use of electronic filtering and averaging to provide sufficient reduction of the background activity for satisfactory identification of the various peaks. The degree of filtering that is useful is limited, however, because filtering also causes a shift of the peaks in time. The shift is dependent on the spectrum of the peaks and is not the same for all peaks (see Doyle and Hyde, 1981a; Dawson and Doddington, 1973). Also, the spectral content of the different peaks varies from person to person, which makes it impossible to compensate for this shift by introducing correction factors. This problem limits the use of electronic filtering in enhancing the peak pattern of the ABR.

There are other filters available that do not have the drawbacks of the simple electronic filters. One is a special electronic filter with linear phase shift, the Bessel filter (Doyle and Hyde, 1981a), and another is the digital filter (Doyle and Hyde, 1981b; Møller, 1983; Møller et al, 1981c). Because Bessel electronic filters are so difficult to create while digital filters can be designed fairly easily and with much greater flexibility, the latter have become an economic solution to the problem of filtering ABR. Digital filters are implemented on digital computers to filter the averaged wave form. An additional advantage is the ability to apply different types or degrees of filters to the same recording, whereas separate recordings must be made for each filter setting when electronic filters are used. Digital filters can be designed without any phase shift to operate in the frequency (spectral) domain or in the time domain. They can suppress background noise and enhance certain features of the wave pattern at the same time (Møller, 1983a).

Neural Generators of ABR

Recordings made intracranially from the auditory nerve in man (Møller et al, 1981a, b, 1982a,b; Møller and Jannetta, 1982a) have shown that the auditory nerve is the generator of both wave I and wave II and that wave III is principally generated by the ipsilateral cochlear nucleus (Møller and Jannetta, 1983). Wave IV mainly represents activity in the superior olivary complex, and wave V has a complex origin with the sharp

tip originating in the fiber tracts of the lateral lemniscus and the following slow vertex negativity in the inferior colliculus (Møller and Jannetta, 1982a; see also Møller, Chapter 3). These results have changed the previously accepted hypothesis which assumed that only wave I was generated by the auditory nerve and that wave II corresponded to neural activity in the cochlear nucleus (Thornton, 1978; see also Møller, 1985).

ABR IN DIAGNOSIS OF EIGHTH NERVE TUMORS

Auditory brainstem responses (ABR) have been shown to be the most sensitive means of revealing disorders involving the auditory nerve and the nuclei and fiber tracts of the ascending auditory pathways in the brainstem. In many if not most cases acoustic tumors (schwannomas) grow medially into the cerebellopontine angle (CPA) and affect the lower brainstem (pons) by displacement or compression. The effects of eighth nerve, CPA, and low pontine lesions on the ABR are often similar. The CPA tumor makes up the majority of extraaxial lesions affecting the brainstem. ABR is now in common use and is an important part of the test battery for the detection of tumors of the eighth nerve and CPA. The most frequently used diagnostic feature of ABR is the deviation from normal in the latencies of the different peaks. The use of ABR in a more systematic study to detect tumors of the eighth nerve was first described by Selters and Brackmann (1977) and later by Clemis and McGee (1979). In patients with confirmed tumors of the auditory nerve the most consistently reported finding was a prolonged latency of wave V recorded from the affected side. Also, only wave I may be present or waves III to V may have reduced amplitudes or be absent altogether in recordings ipsilateral to the tumor (Rosenhamer, 1977; Eggermont et al, 1980; Josey et al, 1980; Rosenhall, 1981; Hyde and Blair, 1981; Shanon et al, 1981). Recently, however, it has been shown that the most typical changes in ABR in patients with acoustic nerve tumors are prolonged latencies and/or reduced amplitudes of ABR waves II and III (Møller and Møller, 1983). These prolonged latencies of waves II and III are then reflected as a prolongation of wave V.

Interaural Latency Difference for Wave V

The interaural latency difference (ILD) is perhaps the most commonly studied parameter of ABR. The diagnosis of a retrocochlear lesion is made when the latency of wave V of the ABR is significantly prolonged relative to normal laboratory values, or when the ILD for wave V is greater than 0.3 msec (Selters and Brackmann, 1977; Møller and Møller, 1983). The absence of wave V on the affected side is also a strong indication of retrocochlear pathology. Selters and Brackmann (1977) found wave V absent in 45% of their patients with acoustic nerve tumors. Similar findings were reported by Eggermont et al (1980) and Rosenhall (1981), who could identify wave V only in 35 and 43%, respectively, of their patients. Clemis and McGee (1979), on the other hand, used tonebursts and failed to identify wave V in only 16% of their patients with acoustic nerve tumors.

Figure 4.1 shows the distribution of corrected ILD for wave V (from Selters and Brackmann's data, 1977) for 46 patients with acoustic nerve tumors and 54 patients with cochlear hearing losses. There is a clear separation between tumor and nontumor groups. Also, the most common finding in the tumor group is an absent wave V, while in those patients in which wave V is present, the ILD is uniformly between 0.5 and 4.0 msec.

In the study by Møller and Møller (1983) of 27 patients with CPA tumors the ILD was calculated for both wave III and wave V. In four of these patients no measurements could be made because one patient was deaf on the tumor side prior to surgery, one patient had bilateral tumors, and two patients had no identifiable wave V (8%). Results of measuring the interaural latency differences for waves III and V in the remaining 23 patients are shown in Figure 4.2. When the ILD was used to evaluate retrocochlear involvement, it was found that 21 of the patients had prolonged ILD (greater than 0.3 msec), and only two patients had ILD that were 0.3 msec or less. It is interesting that in 11 patients the increase in the ILD of wave III was the same as the increase in latency for wave V (less than a 0.3 msec difference), indicating that the prolonged la-

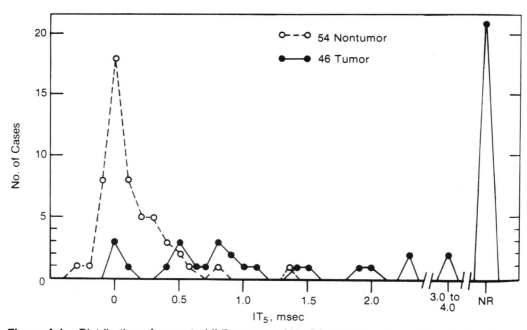

Figure 4.1. Distribution of corrected ILD for wave V in 54 patients with cochlear hearing loss and 46 patients with acoustic nerve tumors. There is a clear separation between the tumor and nontumor group. (From Selters WA, Brackmann DE: Acoustic tumor detection with brain stem electric response audiometry. *Arch Otolaryngol* 103:181–187, 1977. Copyright 1977, American Medical Association.)

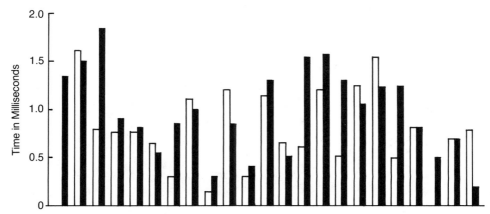

Figure 4.2. Interaural latency difference for wave III (*open bars*) and wave V (*solid bars*) in 23 patients with acoustic nerve tumors for whom ILD could be calculated. ILD less than 0.3 msec is considered normal. In 11 patients the increase in ILD of wave III was the same as the increase of wave V. In four patients ILD of wave V was larger than for wave III, while in four patients the opposite was found. (From Møller MB, Møller AR: Brainstem auditory evoked potentials in patients with cerebellopontine angle tumors. *Ann Otol Rhinol Laryngol* 92:645–650, 1983.)

tency found for wave III is merely transferred to wave V. The ILD for wave III ranged from 0.5 msec to as much as 1.6 msec. In four patients the ILD was prolonged for both waves III and V but was larger for wave V than it was for wave III. In four patients the opposite was the case—the ILD was largest for wave III. The only explanation for this may be that the tumor interfered with the efferent auditory system. In two patients the ILD for wave III was normal, and only wave V was abnormal.

Although the latency of wave V is commonly used in the detection of tumors because it is the largest, most robust, and the most easily detected of all waves in the brainstem potentials, this does not mean that the latency of wave V is the most suitable parameter to study in the diagnosis of auditory nerve lesions. Computer enhancement of ABR (Møller, 1980, 1985) has made it possible to accurately identify all the different waves without introducing any time shift, and it is thus possible to utilize the latency information as well as amplitude changes of earlier waves more precisely for diagnostic purposes.

Interpeak Latency

In order to minimize the effect of the hearing loss that almost always accompanies auditory nerve lesions, the interpeak latency

interval (IPL) from wave I to wave V has been used instead of absolute latencies or ILD. The IPL is regarded to be a more accurate measure of "central conduction time" (Coats and Martin, 1977) and is not influenced by stimulus intensity. However, IPL measurements require identification of wave I, and wave I could be identified in only 42% of patients with sensorineural hearing losses in results obtained by Hyde and Blair (1981).

In view of recent findings on neural generators of ABR a tumor affecting the auditory nerve would be expected to cause prolonged latencies mainly of wave II, while the IPL of waves III to V should remain normal, except in cases in which a large tumor compresses or displaces the brainstem. The results of ABR recording from 27 patients with surgically confirmed tumors of the cerebellopontine angle showed that such is indeed the case (Møller and Møller, 1983). In 24 (92%) of these patients, latency abnormalities were observed on the wave generated by the proximal portion of the auditory nerve, namely wave II. As may be seen in Figure 4.3, in 22 of the 26 patients who had hearing on the affected side, the IPL of waves I to III was abnormal, ranging from 2.3 to as much as 4.15 msec, while only in 4 patients was the IPL of waves I to III normal (less than 2.3 msec). Two of these four patients had prolonged IPL of waves III to V only

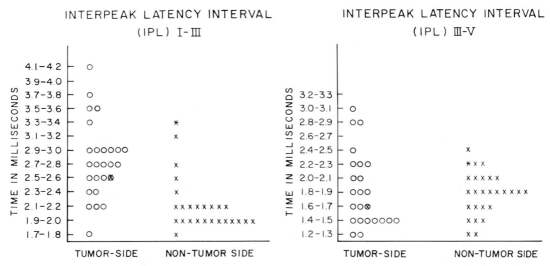

Figure 4.3. Distribution of IPL for waves I to III and III to V in 26 patients with surgically confirmed acoustic nerve tumors. (Patient indicated by *asterisk* had bilateral tumors due to von Recklinghausen's disease.) (From Møller MB, Møller AR: Brainstem auditory evoked potentials in patients with cerebellopontine angle tumors. *Ann Otol Rhinol Laryngol* 92:645–650, 1983.)

(greater than 2.1 msec), and two had abnormal interaural latency differences (greater than 0.3 msec) for both waves III and V. Thus, in 26 patients who had measurable hearing and confirmed tumors, the results of recording ABR indicated the presence of pathology in all cases.

Recordings of ABR from three patients with acoustic nerve tumors are shown in Figures 4.4 to 4.6. The upper tracing in each figure shows the results from the unaffected side and the lower tracing from the tumor side. The unfiltered responses for each ear are shown in Figure 4.5. In all three cases the prolongation in latencies between waves I and III are clearly evident, while the IPL for waves III to V are normal.

The observation that some patients with CPA tumors also had a broad and split wave III suggested that there is probably more than one generator of wave III. Five of the patients with prolonged IPL of waves I to III also had prolonged IPL of waves III to V on the affected side; this may reflect the fact that the tumors were large and possibly compressed or displaced the brainstem. A common finding in patients with auditory nerve tumors, in addition to a prolonged latency, was reduced amplitude of wave II. In most cases the wave morphology of waves III, IV, and V was normal.

Eggermont et al (1980) correlated measurements of the IPL for waves I to V and the ILD for wave V in 45 patients with CPA lesions. When both criteria were used, a tumor detection score of 95% was achieved. The ABR indicated pathology in 92 to 100% of patients with verified tumors of the cerebellopontine angle when abnormal latencies of wave V, absent wave V, or increased interpeak latency interval of wave I to wave V were the criteria for pathology (Clemis and McGee, 1979; Thomsen et al, 1978; Kinney and Nodar, 1980; Møller and Møller, 1983).

Selters and Brackmann (1977), Nodar and Kinney (1980), Rosenhamer (1977), Rosenhall (1981), Zappulla et al (1981), and Musiek et al (1983) have shown that large tumors in the posterior fossa also can cause abnormal ABR when the responses are recorded from the contralateral side. The changes observed included prolonged latencies, reduced amplitudes, or abnormal wave morphology. In our study (Møller and Møller, 1983) we found that five patients also had prolonged IPL of waves I to III, and four patients had prolonged IPL of waves III to V on the unaffected side. One of these patients had bilateral tumors which naturally influenced conduction time on both sides. Latencies of the early waves from the

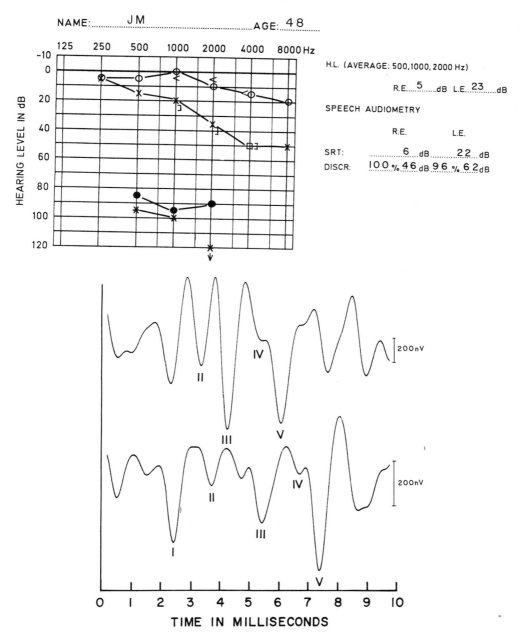

Figure 4.4. Results from audiometry and ABR in a patient with a medium sized acoustic nerve tumor on the left side. Upper tracing of ABR is from the nonaffected side and the lower tracing from the tumor side. The IPL for waves I to III are prolonged, while the IPL of waves III to V is normal. (Negative up, positive down on this and subsequent ABRs.) (From Møller MB, Møller AR: Brainstem auditory evoked potentials in patients with cerebellopontine angle tumors. *Ann Otol Rhinol Laryngol* 92:645–650, 1983.)

unaffected side may be abnormal due to the fact that large tumors in the posterior fossa cause displacement of the cerebellum. Because the flocculus is attached to the eighth cranial nerve, displacement of the cerebellum can also cause some stretching of the nerve on the nontumor side. Similar observations have been made regarding the ves-

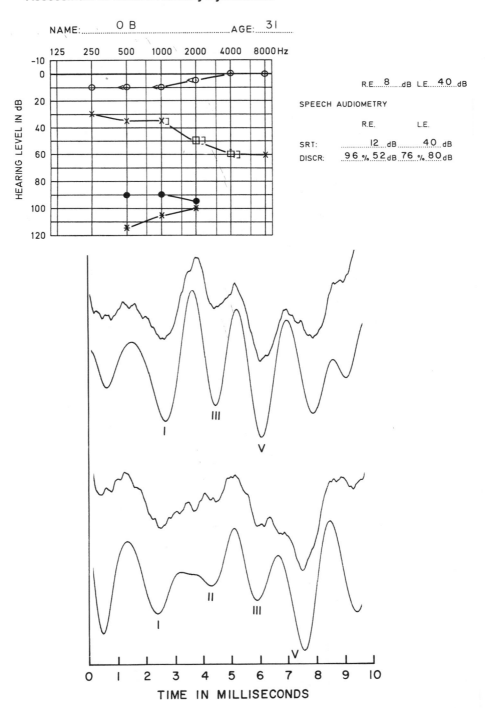

Figure 4.5. Results from audiometry and ABR in a patient with a left-sided acoustic nerve tumor. Upper tracings show unfiltered and digitally filtered recordings from the unaffected side, and the two lower tracings are unfiltered and filtered recordings from the tumor side. There is both prolonged latency and decreased amplitude of wave II, while the IPL for waves III to V is normal. (From Møller MB, Møller AR: Brainstem auditory evoked potentials in patients with cerebellopontine angle tumors. *Ann Otol Rhinol Laryngol* 92:645–650, 1983.)

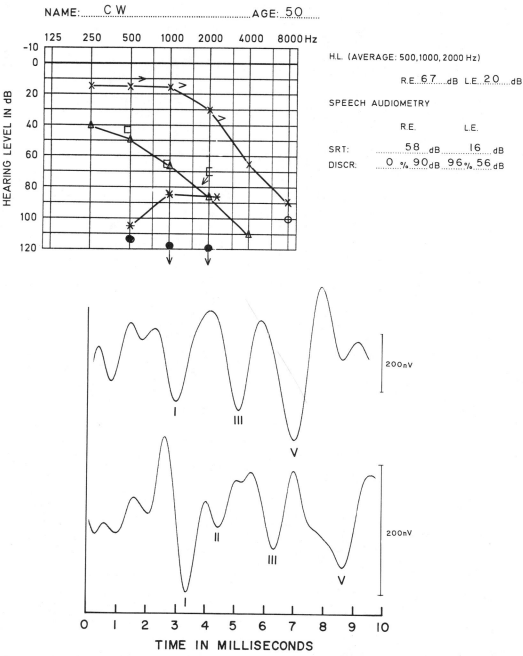

Figure 4.6. Results from audiometry and ABR in a patient with a right-sided acoustic nerve tumor. Upper tracing of ABR is from the unaffected side. Lower tracing is from the tumor side and shows increased IPL for waves I to III, while IPL for waves III to V is normal. (From Møller MB, Møller AR: Brainstem auditory evoked potentials in patients with cerebellopontine angle tumors. *Ann Otol Rhinol Laryngol* 92:645–650, 1983.)

tibular function on the unaffected side (Dr. Furman, personal communication, 1984).

In some studies of ABR changes in patients with cerebellopontine angle tumors a close correlation between the size of the tumor and abnormal latencies was found (Selters and Brackmann, 1977; Clemis and McGee, 1979; Eggermont et al, 1980; Hyde and Blair, 1981). Large tumors caused greater changes in ABR than small, intracanalicular tumors. Rosenhamer (1977) and Rosenhall (1981), on the other hand, found no such correlation, reporting total absence of ABR, even when the lesion was intracanalicular.

From the above discussion it is obvious that measuring ABR is an excellent way to diagnose lesions in the posterior fossa and, in particular, tumors affecting the eighth cranial nerve. It has been shown, however, that ABR frequently give false-positive results when measured in patients evaluated for a suspected eighth nerve lesion. Clemis and McGee (1979) found 34% of ABR to be false-positive, while in other studies (Selters and Brackmann, 1979; Glasscock et al, 1979) the percentage of false-positive tests varied between 8 and 16%. The determination that the ABR are false indications of pathology is always based on negative radiographic findings, particularly on computerized tomography. However, small tumors, especially those growing in the internal auditory canal, may not be detected even with the most advanced scanners, and it may be that patients with positive ABR findings but negative radiological findings may have small, not yet visible tumors. Only by more advanced radiological techniques (such as posterior fossa cisternography using air or metrizamide as contrast) is it possible to rule out the presence of such small tumors. Since this radiological test is invasive, it is not advisable or even suitable to perform it routinely on all patients with abnormal findings on ABR. Instead it is better to reevaluate the patients with such ABR changes after a period of 6 to 12 months, since acoustic tumors grow slowly. Other factors in the variance in false-positive rates may be related to differences in stimuli and recording parameters, as well as criteria for determining abnormality.

It is important to remember that other parameters, such as the threshold for the middle ear acoustic reflex and vestibular tests, can support the presence or absence of eighth nerve pathology. However, because false-negative findings on ABR in patients with acoustic neuromas have been reported to be only 0 (Kinney and Nodar, 1980) to 2.3% (Selters and Brackmann, 1979), ABR is currently the most sensitive test for detection of eighth nerve and CPA tumors.

ABR IN VASCULAR COMPRESSION AT THE BRAINSTEM

With increasing age, the brain sags caudally and the arteries become tortuous or ectatic due to arteriosclerosis or to deterioration of vascular collagen. Thus, the nerves of the cerebellopontine angle are subject to mechanical stresses, such as pulsatile compression from elongated arteries. This compression causes syndromes of hyperactive function leading to altered function or progressive loss of function of the nerves, depending upon the site of contact and the rate at which such neurovascular contact increases. Thus, a number of cranial nerve dysfunctions have been demonstrated to be due to vascular compression, including trigeminal neuralgia (N V), hemifacial spasm (N VII), and glossopharyngeal neuralgia (N IX + N X). Microvascular decompression of these nerves has been shown to relieve these symptoms (Jannetta, 1981a,b, 1982a,b). The audiovestibular nerve in the cerebellopontine angle is also subject to the same forces, and its compression can lead to tinnitus, disequilibrium, sensorineural hearing loss, and vertigo. In patients who present with such symptoms the case history is as important as the different tests (including middle ear acoustic reflex thresholds, decay tests, vestibular tests, and ABR) in arriving at a correct diagnosis.

Several studies have been published which deal with the anatomical relationship between loops of the anterior inferior cerebellar artery (AICA) in the cerebellopontine angle and the audiovestibular and facial nerve bundles (Sunderland, 1945; Salah et al, 1978; Mazzoni and Hansen, 1970). Ouaknine (1981) found that there is a loop of AICA or one of its branches in 80 to 100% of the cerebellopontine angles of specimens studied, and in 36% the loop was located between cranial nerves VII and VIII (Fig. 4.7). Normally these arterial loops do not cause any trouble, but if they become elongated as a result of arteriosclerotic processes, they may cause irritative disturbances of these nerves.

ABR changes in patients with vascular

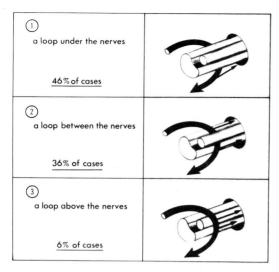

1. a loop under the nerves

46% of cases

2. a loop between the nerves

36% of cases

3. a loop above the nerves

6% of cases

Figure 4.7. Principal types of neurovascular contact between the loop of AICA (anteroinferior cerebellar artery) and NVII and NVIII in the cerebellopontine angle in cadavers. (From Ouaknine GE: Microsurgical anatomy of the arterial loops in the pontocerebellar angle and the internal acoustic meatus. In Samii M, Jannetta PJ (eds): *The Cranial Nerves.* New York, Springer-Verlag, 1981, pp 378–390.)

compression of the audiovestibular nerve are similar to those seen in patients with acoustic nerve tumors. The changes are, however, more discrete than those seen in patients with tumors. The most common findings are an increased latency and reduction of amplitude of wave II. In some cases, wave III also shows these changes (see Figs. 4.9 and 4.10).

Figure 4.8 shows an example of ABR in a patient with an eighth nerve lesion. The patient suffered a slowly progressive sensorineural hearing loss with intense tinnitus without any feeling of fullness or ear pressure. He also experienced constant and disabling vertigo and nausea. These symptoms had been present for 2½ yr at the time he was first seen, and he had had no relief of symptoms with conventional medical treatment. ABR showed an increased latency of wave II of 0.3 msec and an absent wave III on the affected side, while the latency of wave V was normal. In surgery it was found that the eighth nerve was compressed by an artery at the root entry zone. Microvascular decompression of the nerve resolved the ver-

tigo and tinnitus. Pure tone and speech audiometry revealed a significant improvement in hearing and a marked increase in the discrimination score from 16% preoperatively to 72% 2 months postoperatively.

Preoperative evaluation of 14 patients who underwent microvascular decompression for eighth nerve syndromes such as tinnitus, vertigo, or both (Jannetta et al, 1984) showed 6 patients with decreased amplitudes of wave II or waves I to III on the affected side. Three patients had prolonged IPL of waves I to III, and three patients had changes mainly in the latencies of wave V. Figures 4.9 and 4.10 illustrate typical changes in ABR seen in patients with disabling vertigo and tinnitus; these ABR changes are very similar to those seen in patients with acoustic nerve tumors.

In a few patients in this series the abnormal ABR patterns observed preoperatively, i.e., increase in amplitude of wave II and decrease in latency of waves II and III (Fig. 4.10), returned to normal postoperatively. This shows that decompression of the audiovestibular nerve can eliminate not only the symptoms but also restore objectively measurable function of the eighth nerve.

Hemifacial Spasm (HFS)

Cryptogenic hemifacial spasm is a hyperactive dysfunction of the facial nerve caused by cross-compression at the root entry zone (REZ) of the facial nerve (Gardner, 1962; Gardner and Sava, 1972; Jannetta, 1970, 1981a). The spasm is usually present only on one side of the face, occurs more commonly in women than in men, and is more frequently found on the left side. The close anatomical relationship between the seventh and eighth cranial nerves makes it likely that an arterial abnormality causing facial nerve damage may influence also the propagation properties of the eighth nerve with changes in both latency and morphology of the ABR pattern.

In order to evaluate auditory nerve function in patients with hemifacial spasm, ABR were recorded from both the affected side and the unaffected side of 39 patients seen consecutively who underwent microvascular decompression surgery (Møller et al, 1982b). ABR in these patients showed that the latencies of wave III and wave V were signifi-

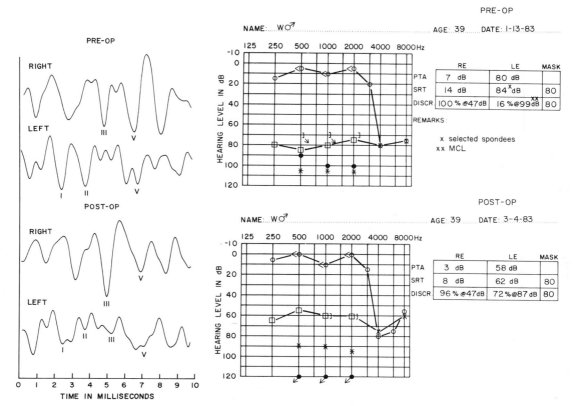

Figure 4.8. Results from audiometry and ABR pre- and postoperatively in a patient with disabling vertigo, tinnitus, and hearing loss in the left ear. The ABR from the left ear shows increased latency of wave II (0.3 msec) and absent wave III but with normal latency of wave V. Postoperatively ABR is improved regarding waves I and II, but shows abnormal latencies of waves III, IV, and V. SRT improved from 84 to 62 dB, and the discrimination score increased 56%. Also, the threshold for the acoustic middle ear reflex returned to normal when stimulating the left ear. (Postoperative tests were done 2 months after microvascular decompression (MVD) of the left audiovestibular nerve). (From Møller MB, Møller AR: Acoustic nerve microvascular decompression. In Jacobson JT (ed): *The Auditory Brainstem Response*. San Diego, College-Hill Press, 1985, pp 407–410.

cantly prolonged ($p < 0.05$) on the spasm side when compared to the latencies on the unaffected side. In some patients only IPL for waves I to III were affected (Fig. 4.11), while in other patients IPL of waves III to V were also prolonged. The morphology of the wave pattern was often found to be abnormal, with reduced amplitudes of wave II and wave III. Wave III was often broad and split, indicating desynchronized activity in the proximal portion of the auditory nerve and cochlear nucleus (see Fig. 4.12). The changes in latency and morphology of ABR in patients with hemifacial spasm resemble those seen in multiple sclerosis (Stockard et al,

1980; Chiappa et al, 1980) and acoustic nerve tumors.

Trigeminal Neuralgia

Elongation of arteries in the posterior fossa can also cause a hyperactive dysfunction of the trigeminal nerve (cranial nerve V), causing severe attacks of pain. Trigeminal neuralgia occurs more commonly on the right side and more frequently in women than in men. The offending blood vessel is most often a loop of the superior cerebellar artery (Jannetta, 1982a), which impinges upon the anterosuperior portion of the tri-

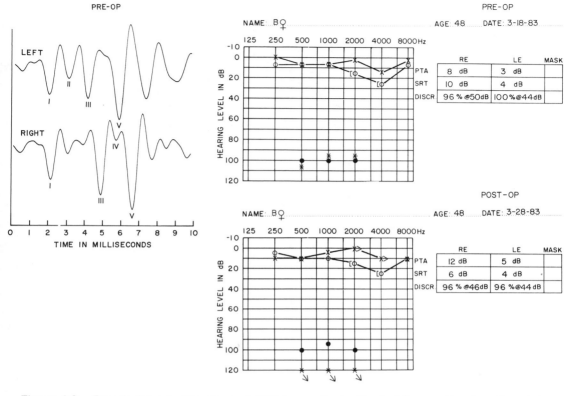

Figure 4.9. Results from audiometry and ABR in a patient with disabling positional vertigo, right side. ABR show that wave II is broad with reduced amplitude, and the latency of wave III is subsequently prolonged 0.7 msec. IPL of waves III to V is normal. The audiogram shows a mild sensorineural deficit in the right ear which is unchanged postoperatively. The patient had MVD of the right audiovestibular nerve, and a compressing artery was found at the caudal portion of the vestibular nerve.

geminal nerve. A common finding on ABR measurements in patients operated upon for microvascular decompression is either a prolonged latency of wave III on the affected side or prolonged IPL of waves III to V on the contralateral side. These results imply that pulsatile pressure from arteries at the brainstem causes changes in the ABR on the affected side when the blood vessel is impinging on the eighth nerve or contralateral changes when the vessel also is in contact with superficial structures at the brainstem.

ABR IN DIAGNOSIS OF GENERAL NEUROLOGICAL DISORDERS OF THE BRAINSTEM

ABR have been extensively used to evaluate patients with demyelinating disorders of the brainstem, such as multiple sclerosis, progressive multifocal leucoencephalopathy, and pontine myelinolysis.

Multiple Sclerosis

ABR has been shown to be helpful in patients with unclear historical and/or clinical findings who initially present themselves with a single nonbrainstem central nervous system focus. Abnormal ABR findings in these patients may provide evidence of a second clinically unsuspected site of involvement, thereby leading to a correct diagnosis of multiple sclerosis.

Starr and Achor (1975) first described the results of measuring ABR in four patients with clinically manifested multiple sclerosis. All four patients had abnormal test results.

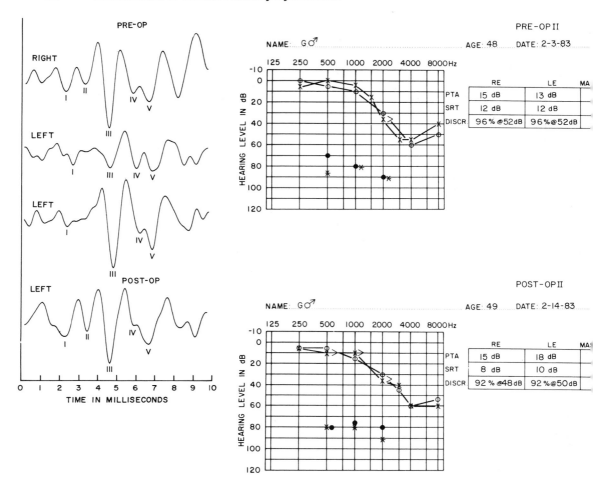

Figure 4.10.   Results from audiometry (pre- and postoperative) and ABR (pre- and postoperative) in a patient with left-sided tinnitus, vertigo, and atypical left face pain. ABR from the left ear shows absent wave II, reduced amplitude of wave III, and prolonged latencies of waves IV and V preoperatively. The patient underwent MVD of N VIII and was asymptomatic for 1 yr and then had recurrent vertigo and tinnitus in the left ear. Lower two tracings show second pre- and postoperative ABR from the left ear. Wave II is absent, while waves III to V are normal. Postoperatively ABR is normalized, and the patient is asymptomatic for vertigo and tinnitus.

The most common finding was a reduction in amplitudes of waves II to V in three patients, while in one patient wave V was absent in one ear.

A more systematic study of ABR changes in patients with multiple sclerosis was done by Stockard et al (1977). In patients with a confirmed diagnosis of multiple sclerosis with signs of brainstem dysfunction and involvement of visual pathways and myelopathy of the spinal cord, ABR were found to be abnormal (93%). The abnormalities of the ABR involved prolonged latencies of waves III to V, or reduced amplitudes of wave V, or both latency and amplitude changes (see Fig. 4.13). Musiek et al (1984) reported wave V amplitudes smaller than wave I in several patients with multiple sclerosis.

In a later study, Stockard et al (1980) evaluated 135 patients with clinical evidence of a single nonbrainstem lesion, such as unilateral optic neuritis or spinal cord myelopathy. Eighty patients were tested during

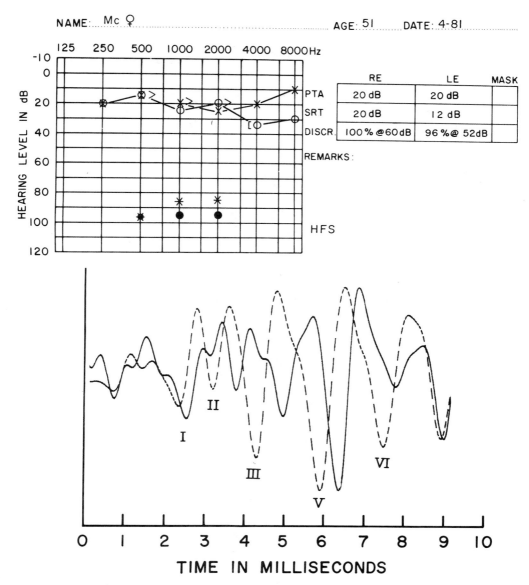

Figure 4.11. Results from audiometry and ABR from a patient with left-sided hemifacial spasm. *Solid line* is the recording from the spasm side, while *dotted line* is from nonaffected side. Waves I and II have abnormal configuration with 0.7 msec delay. Wave III is consequently delayed (ILD III = 0.7 msec) with reduced amplitude. (From Møller MB, Møller AR, Jannetta PJ: Brainstem auditory evoked potentials in patients with hemifacial spasm. *Laryngoscope* 92:848–852, 1982b.)

their first attack of symptoms, and, of those, nine were found to have abnormalities in the ABR. Within 3 yr all nine patients developed clinically definite multiple sclerosis. Of the total group of 135 patients, 31 had abnormal ABR, and within 1 to 3 yr almost half of these had clinically defined multiple sclerosis. In 104 patients with normal ABR, only 13 patients (12%) developed manifest disease. All patients with pontine myelinolysis who were tested had marked abnormalities in their ABR (Stockard and Sharbrough, 1978). On the other hand, patients with progressive supranuclear palsy (degen-

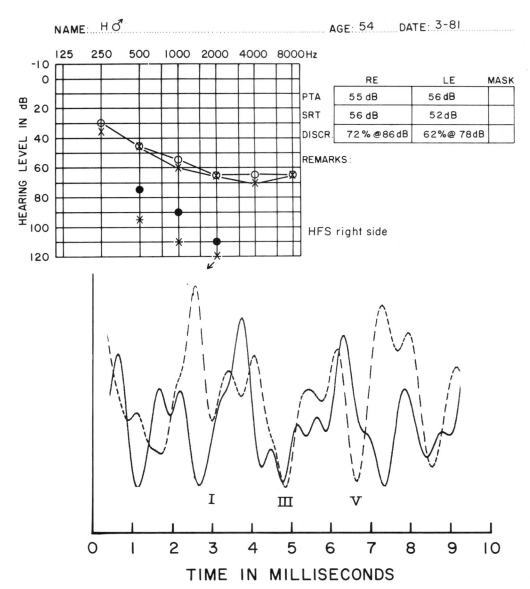

NAME: H ♂   AGE: 54   DATE: 3-81

	RE	LE	MASK
PTA	55 dB	56 dB	
SRT	56 dB	52 dB	
DISCR.	72% @86dB	62%@ 78dB	

REMARKS:

HFS right side

TIME IN MILLISECONDS

Figure 4.12. Results from audiometry and ABR in a patient with right-sided hemifacial spasm. *Solid line* is ABR from the spasm side, while *dotted line* is from the nonaffected side. Waves I and II are fused, and wave III has abnormal configuration, with a broad, split wave form and increased latency "transferred" to wave V. The threshold of the middle ear acoustic reflex is elevated when stimulating the left, consistent with facial nerve abnormality on the right side.

eration of pontine and midbrain tegmentum nuclei with sparing of the white matter) were found to have normal ABR. The same was true for patients with Wernicke's encephalopathy. (These patients have scattered lesions in the gray matter of the brainstem around the fourth ventricle but no involvement of white matter.)

Chiappa et al (1980) evaluated 202 multiple sclerosis patients with ABR. Contrary to the findings of Stockard et al (1980), Chiappa et al found abnormal ABR in only

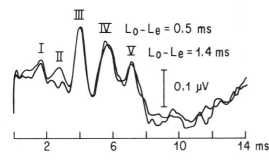

Figure 4.13. Typical ABR findings in a patient with multiple sclerosis. There are prolonged latencies of both wave III (0.5 msec) and wave V (1.4 msec). Stimulus used was 60-dB clicks. *Lo*, latency observed; *Le*, latency expected. (From Stockard JJ, Stockard JE, Sharbrough FW: Detection and localization of occult lesions with brain stem auditory responses. *Mayo Clin Proc* 52:761–769, 1977.)

32% of their patients. In those with signs of brainstem involvement ABR were abnormal in 57%, while in those without brainstem symptoms, despite definite diagnoses of multiple sclerosis, ABR were abnormal in only 19%. Figure 4.14 (from Chiappa et al, 1980) shows a spectrum of ABR abnormalities found in patients with multiple sclerosis. These abnormalities were unilateral in 45% of the cases.

Hausler and Levine (1980) correlated ABR with the ability to discriminate interaural time or intensity differences in 29 patients with definite multiple sclerosis. They found that 18 patients had abnormal ABR in this group, and 13 had abnormal (ranging from 50 to as much as 280 μsec) interaural time discrimination, despite normal hearing on the pure tone audiogram. They concluded that the abnormalities in ABR in patients with multiple sclerosis might indicate incorrect timing at the level of the brainstem. However, there was no correlation between changes in ABR and interaural intensity discrimination.

Thus, there are certain discrepancies in the reports of the incidences of ABR abnormalities in patients with multiple sclerosis. Nonetheless, it is clear that the ABR is of clinical value in identifying auditory brainstem involvement in neurological lesions of the brainstem. ABR can also be used to

follow the clinical remission of patients with multiple sclerosis during therapy (Stockard et al, 1977).

Intrinsic Brainstem Lesions

Neoplasms of the brainstem occur rather uncommonly. In the majority of cases these tumors are more accurately diagnosed by clinical examination and radiological evaluation than by ABR, but ABR can, in some instances, provide additional information regarding the site and extension of the tumor within the brainstem.

According to current knowledge regarding neural generators of the human ABR, we expect tumors involving principally the pontomedullary junction and the area around the fourth ventricle to cause prolonged latencies of wave III and, consequently, of all the later waves. Figures 4.15 and 4.16 show ABR in two patients with low brainstem tumors. Lesions of the midbrain may affect the latencies of waves IV and V, while rostral midbrain tumors and caudal thalamic lesions may cause selective abnormalities of waves VI and VII. Similar changes in ABR may be found also in patients with vascular lesions (such as infarctions or hemorrhages) in the brainstem.

Starr and Achor (1975) first showed that the anatomical localization of brainstem tumors could be verified by ABR. In their study the ABR were abnormal in all four patients with tumors in this region. All components after wave III were absent in three patients, and latencies of waves II and III were prolonged in a patient with a brainstem glioma.

Stockard and Rossiter (1977) correlated ABR with clinical findings in over 100 patients with neurological disorders and showed a close relationship between the location of the pathology and certain ABR abnormalities. For instance, wave III was prolonged bilaterally in three patients with bilateral infarcts in the caudal pontine tegmentum. In three patients with vascular lesions of the mid or rostral pons, IPL of waves I to III were normal, but latencies of waves III to V were prolonged. These same findings appeared also in a patient with a tumor involving the upper two-thirds of the pons. Selective latency changes of wave VI were

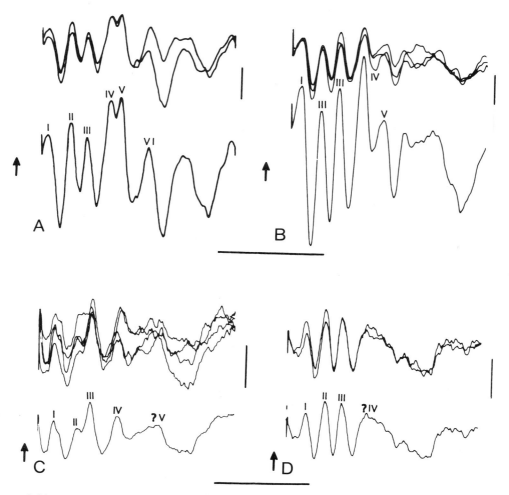

Figure 4.14.   ABR abnormalities in patients with multiple sclerosis. Recordings *A* and *B* are from the same patient, 2 months apart, and there is prolonged latency of wave V as well as decreased amplitude of wave V. Recordings *C* and *D* are from two different patients, showing absence of wave V in patient C and absence of waves IV and V in patient D. (Positive up.) (From Chiappa KH, Harrison JL, Brooks EB, Young RR: Brainstem auditory evoked responses in 200 patients with multiple sclerosis. *Ann Neurol* 7:135–143, 1980.)

found in two patients with rostral midbrain and caudal thalamic tumors. However, it is important to point out that while ABR abnormalities reflect disturbances of the neural pathways, they do not reveal the anatomical cause of the disturbance.

Fisher et al (1982) evaluated 25 patients with vascular lesions involving the brainstem. Patients with Wallenberg's syndrome (four cases), locked-in syndrome (four cases), transient vertebrobasilar ischemic attacks (TIA) (eight cases), and posterior fossa angiomas (four cases) showed no abnormalities in ABR morphology or latency. Tumors of the posterior fossa with vascular involvement, such as meningiomas (eight cases) and cerebellar tumors (five cases), on the other hand, caused varying degrees of abnormalities in the ABR, depending upon the size of the tumor and its relationship to the auditory pathways. However, the tumors had already been diagnosed by computerized to-

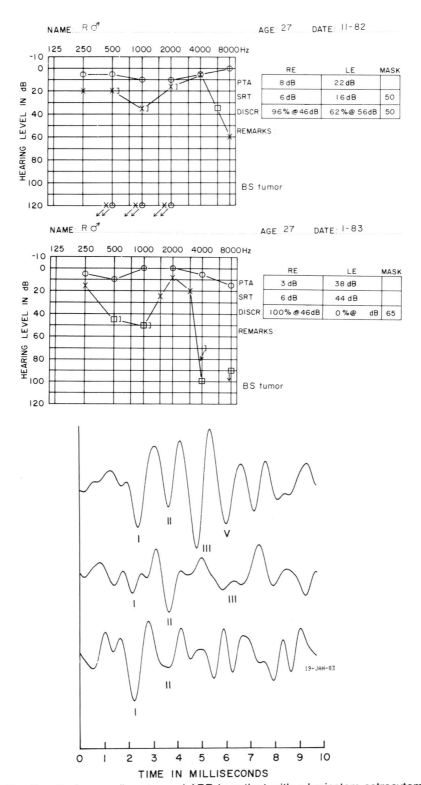

Figure 4.15. Results from audiometry and ABR in patient with a brainstem astrocytoma involving the left pontine region. The patient's hearing deteriorated over a period of 2 months, and there also was involvement of N V and N VIII on the left side. Upper tracing of ABR is recorded from the right side and shows normal latencies and amplitudes. Lower two tracings are from left side, tested 2 months apart. In midtracing wave III is present but with a delay of 2 msec, while in bottom tracing wave II is broad. No later waves can be detected.

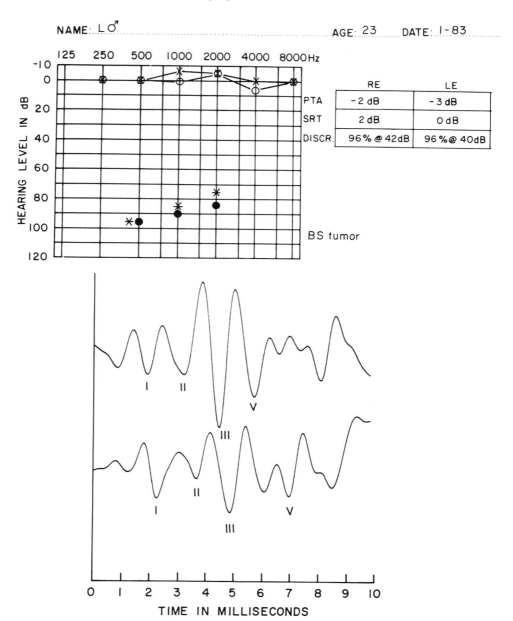

Figure 4.16. Results from audiometry and ABR in a patient with a glioma involving the left cerebellar peduncle and bottom of the fourth ventricle on the left side. Lower tracing of ABR is from the left side showing a moderate latency change of wave III but with more than 1 msec delay of wave V.

mography, and the ABR only added information regarding involvement of the brainstem in a few cases.

ABR in Intoxication, Coma, and Brain Death

ABR have proven to be very useful in the evaluation of patients in coma. Starr and

Achor (1975) tested 51 patients who were comatose due to intoxication, metabolic disorders, or trauma. They found that the structural changes which occurred in the auditory pathways of the brainstem as a result of trauma or reduced circulation caused abnormal amplitudes and latencies of the ABR, whereas in patients in coma induced by intoxication or metabolic disturbances the ABR was normal, even when the coma was severe enough to simulate clinical brain death.

Head Trauma

Uziel and Benezech (1978) correlated ABR with clinical examination in 20 comatose patients, of whom 75% were in coma due to trauma. They were able to show a relationship between the clinical level of function and ABR abnormalities. Patients with cortical or subcortical lesions (ten patients) all had normal ABR. Those with high brainstem lesions had abnormalities only of wave V, while those with midbrain lesions had no electrical activity following wave III and patients with low pontine lesions had no electrical activity beyond wave I.

Similar findings were obtained by Seales et al (1979) using ABR to evaluate patients who were comatose due to blunt head trauma. Seventeen patients were tested and all had specific signs of brainstem damage and/or generalized neurological cephalic findings. The ABR was classified as abnormal if the latency of a wave was prolonged by more than 2 SDs from normal values, or if there was reduced amplitude of wave V or of all waves. The ABR was of significant prognostic value within the first 3 to 6 days after the injury. Three patients who had no ABR died, and abnormal ABR preceded death in another two patients. In 12 patients who recovered follow-up tests were normal.

Therefore, ABR in patients with head trauma can be of diagnostic value and assist the physician in monitoring the patient. Seales et al (1979) also emphasized that the repetition rate of the stimulus had to be slow, usually less than 10/sec, in order to obtain reproducible test results in patients with severe head injuries. In fact, in almost every patient the repetition rate had to be reduced to 4/sec or 1/sec to get interpretable results.

Brain Death

Starr (1976) used ABR to evaluate 27 patients who fulfilled the criteria of brain death. He found ABR absent in 16 patients and only wave I present with prolonged latencies in 11 patients. During serial recordings in four patients who suffered acute anoxia, ABR deteriorated simultaneously with

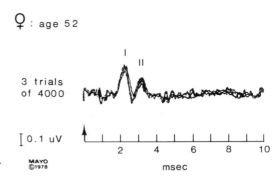

Figure 4.17. ABR recordings in a patient with brain death. Only waves I and II are present. Postmortem changes showed complete necrosis of pons and medulla including cochlear nucleus. (Positive up.) (From Stockard JJ, Stockard JE, Sharbrough FW: Brain stem auditory evoked responses in clinical neurology—methodology, interpretations, clinical applications. In Aminoff MJ (ed): *Electrodiagnosis in Clinical Neurology*. New York, Churchill-Livingstone, 1980, pp 370–413.)

clinical deterioration. In patients close to anoxia the ABR was normal, but subsequently waves IV and V decreased in amplitude and increased in latency. In time, the later waves disappeared, until finally only wave I was present with prolonged latency. These findings provide evidence that damage to the brainstem occurs gradually and in a rostral-caudal direction. Deaf patients (acute or nonacute) and patients with preexisting brainstem lesions, such as multiple sclerosis and tumors, as well as technical artifacts, may have similar ABR when recording at bedside in intensive care units. Figure 4.17 shows an example of ABR in a patient with brain death. Only waves I and II are present, consistent with preserved function of only the eighth nerve.

CONCLUSIONS

Measuring auditory brainstem responses (ABR) has proved to be a sensitive, noninvasive test of the function of the eighth nerve and its central connection in the brainstem. ABR can provide diagnostic information about a large number of neurological deficits, including lesions of the audiovestibular nerve, such as tumors or vascular compression, and intrinsic brainstem lesions, such as tumors, infarcts, and multiple sclerosis. ABR have been shown to contribute also to the diagnosis of coma due to intoxication, metabolic disorders, traumatic head injuries, and brain death. In addition, ABR may assist in the establishment of a prognosis for patients with such disorders.

References

Chiappa KH, Harrison JL, Brooks EB, Young RR: Brainstem auditory evoked responses in 200 patients with multiple sclerosis. *Ann Neurol* 7:135–143, 1980.

Clemis JD, McGee T: Brain stem electric response audiometry in the differential diagnosis of acoustic tumors. *Laryngoscope* 89:31–42, 1979.

Coats AC: On electrocochleographic electrode design. *J Acoust Soc Am* 56:708–711, 1974.

Coats AC, Martin MCH: Human auditory nerve action potentials and brain stem evoked responses. Effects of audiogram shape and lesion location. *Arch Otolaryngol* 103:605–622, 1977.

Dawson WW, Doddington HW: Phase distortion of biological signals: extraction of signal from noise without phase error. *Electroencephalogr Clin Neurophysiol* 34:207–211, 1973.

Doyle DJ, Hyde ML: Bessel filtering of brain stem auditory evoked potentials. *Electroencephalogr Clin Neurophysiol* 51:446–448, 1981a.

Doyle DJ, Hyde ML: Analogue and digital filtering of auditory brainstem responses. *Scand Audiol* 10:81–89, 1981b.

Eggermont JJ, Don M, Brackmann DE: Electrocochleography and auditory brainstem electric responses in patients with pontine angle tumors. *Ann Otol Rhinol Laryngol* (Suppl 75) 89:1–19, 1980.

Fisher C, Mauguiere F, Echallier JF, Courjon J: Contribution of brainstem auditory evoked potentials to diagnosis of tumors and vascular diseases. *Adv Neurol* 32:177–185, 1982.

Gardner JW: Concerning the mechanism of trigeminal neuralgia and hemifacial spasm. *J Neurosurg* 19:947–958, 1962.

Gardner JW, Sava GA: Hemifacial spasm. A reversible pathological state. *J Neurosurg* 19:240–247, 1972.

Glasscock MC, Jackson C, Josey A, Rickens J, Wiet R: Brainstem evoked response audiometry in clinical practice. *Laryngoscope* 89:1021–1034, 1979.

Hausler R, Levine RA: Brain stem auditory evoked potentials are related to interaural time discrimination in patients with multiple sclerosis. *Brain Res* 191:589–594, 1980.

Hyde ML, Blair RL: The auditory brainstem responses in neurotology: perspectives and problems. *J Otolaryngol* 10:117–125, 1981.

Jannetta PJ: Microsurgical exploration and decompression of the facial nerve in hemifacial spasm. *Curr Top Surg Res* 2:217–220, 1970.

Jannetta PJ: Hemifacial spasm. In Samii M, Jannetta PJ (eds): *The Cranial Nerves.* New York, Springer-Verlag, 1981a, pp 484–493.

Jannetta PJ: Neurovascular cross-compression of the eighth cranial nerve in patients with vertigo and tinnitus. In Samii M, Jannetta PJ (eds): *The Cranial Nerves.* New York, Springer-Verlag, 1981b, pp 552–555.

Jannetta PJ: Treatment of trigeminal neuralgia by micro-operative decompression. In Youmans J (ed): *Surgical Neurology.* Philadelphia, WB Saunders, 1982a, vol 6, pp 3589–3603.

Jannetta PJ: Cranial rhizopathies. In Youmans J (ed): *Surgical Neurology,* Philadelphia, WB Saunders, 1982b, vol 6, pp 3771–3884.

Jannetta PJ, Møller MB, Møller AR: Disabling positional vertigo. *N Engl J Med* 310:1700–1705, 1984.

Josey AF, Jackson CG, Glasscock ME: Brainstem evoked response audiometry in confirmed eighth nerve tumors. *Am J Otolaryngol* 1:285–290, 1980.

Kinney SE, Nodar RH: Brainstem auditory evoked potentials for detection of retrocochlear pathology. *Ann Otol Rhinol Laryngol* 89:291–295, 1980.

Mazzoni A, Hansen CC: Surgical anatomy of the arteries of the internal auditory canal. *Arch Otolaryngol* 91:128–135, 1970.

Møller AR: A digital filter for brain stem evoked responses. *Am J Otolaryngol* 1:372–377, 1980.

Møller AR: Improving brain stem auditory evoked potential recordings by digital filtering. *Ear Hear* 4:108–113, 1983.

Møller AR: Physiology of the ascending auditory pathway with special reference to the auditory brainstem responses (ABR). In Pinheiro ML, Musiek FE (eds): *Assessment of Central Auditory Dysfunction: Foundations and Clinical Correlates.* Baltimore, Williams & Wilkins, 1985.

Møller AR, Jannetta PJ: Evoked potentials from the inferior colliculus in man. *Electroencephalogr Clin Neurophysiol* 53:612–620, 1982a.

Møller AR, Jannetta PJ: Auditory evoked potentials recorded intracranially from the brainstem in man. *J Exp Neurol* 78:144–157, 1982b.

Møller AR, Jannetta PJ: Monitoring auditory functions during cranial nerve microvascular decompression operations by direct recording from the eighth nerve. *J Neurosurg* 59:493–499, 1983.

Møller AR, Jannetta PJ, Bennett M, Møller MB: Intracranially recorded responses from the human auditory nerve: new insights into the origin of brainstem evoked potentials (BSEPs). *Electroencephalogr Clin Neurophysiol* 52:18–27, 1981a.

Møller AR, Jannetta PJ, Møller MB: Neural generators of brainstem evoked potentials. Results from human intracranial recordings. *Ann Otol Rhinol Laryngol* 90:591–596, 1981b.

Møller AR, Jannetta PJ, Møller MB: Intracranially recorded auditory nerve response in man: new interpretations of BSER. *Arch Otolaryngol* 108:77–82, 1982a.

Møller AR, Møller MB, Millner D: A computer system for auditory evoked responses. In Shriver BD, Walker TH, Grams RR, Sprague RH (eds): *Proceedings of the Fourteenth Hawaii International Conference on System Sciences,* Honolulu, Jan 1981. North Hollywood, CA, Western Periodicals Company, 1981c.

Møller MB, Møller AR: Brainstem auditory evoked potentials in patients with cerebellopontine angle tumors. *Ann Otol Rhinol Laryngol* 92:645–650, 1983.

Møller MB, Møller AR, Jannetta PJ: Brainstem auditory evoked potentials in patients with hemifacial spasm. *Laryngoscope* 92:848–852, 1982b.

Musiek FE, Kibbe K, Rackliffe L, Weider D: Auditory brainstem response I–V amplitude ratio in normal, cochlear and retrocochlear ears. *Ear Hear* 5:52–55, 1984.

Musiek FE, Kibbe K, Strojny L: ABR Results in the Ear Opposite Large Cerebellopontine Angle Lesions. A paper presented at the American Speech-Language and Hearing Assn Convention, Cincinnati, Nov 19, 1983.

Nodar RH, Kinney SE: The contralateral effects of large tumors on brain stem auditory evoked potentials. *Laryngoscope* 90:1762–1768, 1980.

Ouaknine GE: Microsurgical anatomy of the arterial loops in the pontocerebellar angle and the internal acoustic meatus. In Samii M, Jannetta PJ (eds): *The Cranial Nerves.* New York, Springer-Verlag, 1981, pp 378–390.

Rosenhall U: Brain stem electrical responses in cerebello-pontine angle tumours. *J Laryngol Otol* 95:931–940, 1981.

Rosenhamer HJ: Observations on electric brain-stem responses in retrocochlear hearing loss. A preliminary report. *Scand Audiol* 6:179–196, 1977.

Salah S, Bock FW, Perneczky A, Koos WT, Tschabitscher M: Vascular anatomy of the cerebello-pontine angle. In Koos WT, Bock FW, Spetzler RF (eds): *Microneurosurgery.* New York, Thieme-Stratton, 1978, pp 70–71.

Seales DM, Rossiter VS, Weinstein ME: Brainstem auditory evoked responses in patients comatose as a result of blunt head trauma. *J Trauma* 19:347–353, 1979.

Selters WA, Brackmann DE: Acoustic tumor detection with brain stem electric response audiometry. *Arch Otolaryngol* 103:181–187, 1977.

Selters WA, Brackman DE: Brainstem electric response audiometry in acoustic tumor detection. *Diagnosis.* In House WF, Luetje CM (eds): *Acoustic Tumors.* Baltimore, University Park Press, 1979, vol 1, pp 225–235.

Shanon E, Gold S, Himelfarb MZ: Auditory brain stem responses in cerebellopontine angle tumors. *Laryngoscope* 91:254–259, 1981.

Starr A: Auditory brain-stem responses in brain death.

Brain 99:543–554, 1976.

Starr A, Achor JL: Auditory brain stem responses in neurological disease. *Arch Neurol* 32:761–768, 1975.

Stockard JJ, Rossiter VS: Clinical and pathologic correlates of brain stem auditory response abnormalities. *Neurology* 27:316–325, 1977.

Stockard JJ, Sharbrough FW: Unique contributions of the short latency auditory and somatosensory evoked potentials to neurologic diagnosis. *Clinical Uses of Cerebral, Brainstem and Spinal Somatosensory Evoked Potentials.* In Desmedt JE (ed): *Progress in Clinical Neurophysiology.* Basel, Switzerland, Karger, 1978, vol 7.

Stockard, JJ, Stockard JE, Sharbrough FW: Detection and localization of occult lesions with brain stem auditory responses. *Mayo Clin. Proc.* 52:761–769, 1977.

Stockard JJ, Stockard JE, Sharbrough FW: Nonpathologic factors influencing brainstem auditory evoked potentials. *Am J EEG Technol* 18:177–209, 1978.

Stockard JJ, Stockard JE, Sharbrough FW: Brain stem auditory evoked responses in clinical neurology—methodology, interpretations, clinical applications. In Aminoff MJ (ed): *Electrodiagnosis in Clinical Neurology.* New York, Churchill-Livingstone, 1980, pp 370–413.

Sunderland S: The arterial relations of the internal auditory meatus. *Brain* 68:23–27, 1945.

Thomsen J, Terkildsen K, Osterhammel P: Auditory brain stem responses in patients with acoustic neuromas. *Scand Audiol* 7:179–183, 1978.

Thornton ARD: Interpretation of cochlear nerve and brain stem responses. In Naunton RF, Fernandez C (eds): *Evoked Electrical Activity in the Auditory Nervous System.* New York, Academic Press, 1978, pp 429–442.

Uziel A, Benezech J: Auditory brain-stem responses in comatose patients: relationship with brain-stem reflexes and levels of coma. *Electroencephalogr Clin Neurophysiol* 45:515–524, 1978.

Zappulla RA, Karmel BZ, Greenblatt E: Prediction of cerebellopontine angle tumors based on discriminant analysis of brain stem auditory evoked responses. *Neurosurgery* 9:542–547, 1981.

CHAPTER 5

Physiology of the Cerebral Auditory System

JAMES O. PICKLES, Ph.D.

Dr. Pickles explains the essentials of functional organization of cerebral cortex with its tonotopicity and isofrequency strips. He describes single neuron responses, binaural dominance, callosal connections, feature detectors, analysis of sound localization, and the importance of frequency- and amplitude-modulated stimuli for the brain. Behavioral studies in animals illustrate frequency and pattern discrimination and sound localization, and the importance of ear selection and selective attention is pointed out.

THE ORGANIZATION OF THE AUDITORY CORTEX

One of the problems faced by the early electrophysiologists was the multiple representation of auditory stimuli in the cortex. Analysis of the different cortical areas has for very many years, therefore, been an essential prerequisite for the understanding of cortical function. The picture that has emerged is that of a central, or "core" area, surrounded by a "belt" area. The belt itself consists of several subareas, each of which may have its own special functions. Within these areas, or at least within some of them, two further schemes of organization have been described, based on the tonotopic representation of stimulus frequency and the direction in space of the stimulus source. A recent review of the organization of the auditory cortex has been given by Imig and Morel (1983), and of its function by Pickles (1982).

Core and Belt Organization

The anatomy of the primate cortex has been described in Chapter 2 on the anatomy of the auditory system. However, since many of the experimental analyses of cortical function have been undertaken in the cat, the organization of cat cortex will be described here.

Rose (1949), on cytoarchitectonic grounds, described the primary auditory cortex (AI), surrounded by secondary cortex (AII). He also described a further area on the posterior ectosylvian gyrus (Ep) (Fig. 5.1*A*). Auditory evoked potentials could be recorded from these areas, and Woolsey (1960) showed that these cortical areas were surrounded by additional areas from which auditory evoked potentials also could be recorded (Fig. 5.1*B*). While AI receives a heavy projection from the core area of the medial geniculate body (MGB), the surrounding area receives its projections from the belt area of the MGB (Niimi and Matsuoka, 1979). The belt also receives projections from other thalamic groups, particularly the posterior group of thalamic nuclei. The auditory cortex, therefore, seems to continue the core and belt organization of the lower auditory nuclei. The belt area is less specifically auditory than the core area, and it has a greater proportion of multisensory input. Moreover, in the cortex the ratio of belt to core is relatively greater than in lower auditory nuclei such as the inferior colliculus.

Tonotopic Organization

The tonotopic organization of the auditory cortex has attracted a great deal of attention, not only because of its possible functional significance, but because it has been one of the tools by which the multiple cortical areas have been defined.

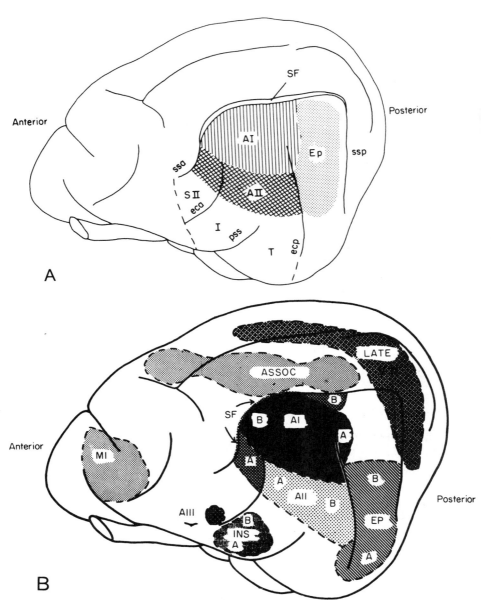

Figure 5.1. (A) The divisions of the cat's auditory cortex described by Rose (1949) are shown shaded, together with other areas now recognized. Cortical areas: *AI*, primary cortex; *AII*, secondary cortex; *Ep*, posterior ectosylvian gyrus; *SII*, second somatosensory area; *I*, insular area; *T*, temporal area; *SF*, suprasylvian fringe area, buried in the upper surface of the Sylvian sulcus. Sulci: *ssa* and *ssp*, anterior and posterior suprasylvian sulci; *eca* and *ecp*, anterior and posterior ectosylvian sulci; *pss*, pseudosylvian sulcus. (Modified from Rose, JE: The cellular structure of the auditory region of the cat. *J Comp Neurol* 91:409–439, 1949). (B) Woolsey (1960) determined cortical areas in the cat by gross evoked potentials. Where areas are organized tonotopically, the representation of the high-frequency base of the cochlea (*B*) and the low-frequency apex (*A*) is indicated. *MI*, precentral motor area. AIII lies in SII. Other abbreviations as in *A*. (Modified from Woolsey CN: Organization of the cortical auditory system: a review and a synthesis. In Rasmussen GL, Windle WF (eds): *Neural Mechanisms of the Auditory and Vestibular Systems*. Springfield, IL, Charles C Thomas, 1960, p 165.)

Tonotopicity is seen in all lower stages of the auditory system and refers to the representation of stimulus frequency in spatially ordered sets of neurons. Woolsey's map in Figure 5.1*B* indicates that in certain of the cortical areas, evoked potentials could be evoked preferentially by electrical stimulation of the base of the cochlea (*B*) or the apex (*A*). Based on the fact that the base of the cochlea is stimulated predominantly by sounds of high frequency, and the apex by sounds of low frequency, his figure indicates a tonotopic organization for some of the cortical areas. Using evoked potentials in the dog, Tunturi (1952) showed that between these two extremes there was a complete representation of stimulus frequencies, with areas having the same best frequency lying in strips at right angles to the line of frequency progression (Fig. 5.2).

Tonotopicity determined by evoked potentials may indicate a tonotopicity related only to the afferent input, rather than to a tonotopicity in the cortical cells themselves. However, tonotopicity also has been shown at the single cell level (e.g., Merzenich et al, 1975; Reale and Imig, 1980; and Fig. 5.3). In AI, where cells are sufficiently sharply tuned for best frequencies to be definable, the tonotopic organization and isofrequency strips described above have been found. Reale and Imig (1980) used the tonotopic progression of single cells to provide a more

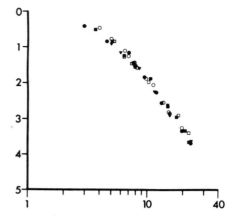

Figure 5.3. Best frequencies of single neurons in a cat's auditory cortex are plotted in relation to distance across the cortex. The neurons were located on five parallel lines across the cortex, and different symbols are used for each line. Abscissa, neuron best frequency in kHz. Ordinate, distance across cortex in mm. (From Merzenich MM, Knight PL, Roth GL: Representation of cochlea within primary auditory cortex in the cat. *J Neurophysiol* 38:231–249, 1975.)

detailed parcellation of the different cortical areas than had been possible with gross evoked potentials. They agreed with Woolsey (1960) on the position and organization of AI, although their AI did not stretch as far rostrally. The rostral part of Woolsey's AI was, they suggested in agreement with Knight (1977), part of a further field (the anterior auditory field) with its own tonotopic organization. This included the anterior part of the suprasylvian fringe (SF) of Figure 5.1*B*. They divided Ep (Fig. 5.1*A*) into two fields, each with its own tonotopic organization. They called the lower part the ventroposterior field. The region above that was a separate tonotopically organized area, which they called the posterior field. In AII, by contrast, it was difficult to describe any clear tonotopicity, since cells often had tuning curves with multiple best frequencies. When single best frequencies could be defined, no clear frequency progression could be seen (Reale and Imig, 1980).

Attempts have been made to associate tonotopicity with a columnar organization of discrete frequency-specific columns (see also Chapter 2). However, in spite of careful analyses, no discrete frequency-specific columns have been found, in the sense of all the cells in one column having the same best frequency, with definite jumps in best fre-

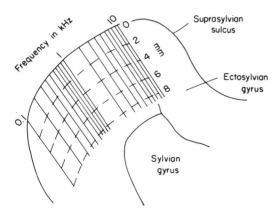

Figure 5.2. Isofrequency strips in the dog auditory cortex according to Tunturi (1952). (From Tunturi AR: A difference in the representation of auditory signals for the left and right ears in the iso-frequency contours of the right middle ectosylvian auditory cortex of the dog. *Am J Physiol* 168:712–727, 1952.)

quency as an electrode leaves one column and enters an adjacent one (e.g., Abeles and Goldstein, 1970). Instead, Abeles and Goldstein (1970) showed that, while neurons close together indeed had similar best frequencies, frequency separation increased smoothly rather than discretely with distance across the cortex. Cells separated horizontally tended to be no further apart in best frequency than cells situated a similar distance apart vertically. The anatomical columns of cells described by Sousa-Pinto (1973) in auditory cortex were, it was suggested, too small to be discrete frequency-specific columns, since the separation of the columns was less than the lateral spread of the incoming axonal arborization.

Although tonotopicity has been useful in working out the anatomical organization of the cortex, its functional significance is still obscure. Given that the organ of Corti is tonotopically organized, tonotopicity may reflect only an efficient packing of the fibers of the auditory nerve and all succeeding stages of the auditory pathway. On the other hand, it can be argued that tonotopicity promotes the interaction of neurons having adjacent best frequencies. It may, therefore, be a sign of a system in which interactions, such as lateral inhibition between stimuli of adjacent frequencies, are important.

Binaural Dominance and Callosal Connections

In the analysis of binaural dominance, there has been greater success in finding specific cortical columns than there has been in the analysis of tonotopicity. Imig and Adrian (1977) showed that in AI, cells in which the ipsilateral ear was dominant were separate from cells in which inhibitory responses from the contralateral ear were dominant. These different categories of cells were located in discrete radial columns. In a surface view, the columns of the two types of cells formed patches wandering over the surface of the cortex, the patches being aligned approximately orthogonal to the isofrequency lines (Fig. 5.4). Within AI, therefore, the cortex seems to be organized in both directions. In one direction, the cortex appears to be organized according to frequency. In the other direction, it seems to

be organized in terms of binaural dominance, and perhaps, therefore, in terms of stimulus location in space. As a result of this analysis, we might expect a single point on the cortex to respond to sounds of a specific frequency emerging from a specific location.

The demonstration of binaural dominance columns has been tied in with the demonstration of bands of callosal afferents in the dominance columns. Since the main input to the auditory cortex crosses in the brainstem, some of the input from the ipsilateral ear can be expected to arrive indirectly, via the contralateral cortex and callosal fibers. Imig and Brugge (1978) demonstrated callosal connections by the injection of tritiated proline into the contralateral AI. The callosal afferents were concentrated into patches, or *callosal columns* in the terminology of Jones and associates (1975). Exploration of the cortex with microelectrodes running nearly parallel with the cortical surface showed a neat and close relationship between the binaural dominance columns and the callosal columns.

Imig and Brugge (1978) also showed some consistency in the organization of the callosal afferents in the cat, in that each cortex contained two prominent elongated callosal columns, running approximately orthogonal to the isofrequency strips, and crossing several frequency octaves. Ventral to these two columns, similar columns were still present, though less prominent and less obviously orthogonal to the isofrequency strips.

THE RESPONSES OF SINGLE NEURONS

Patterns of Response

The difficulties faced by electrophysiologists investigating the responses of cells in the auditory cortex include the suppressing effect of anesthetic, the great variety of response types, the inconsistency and lability of the responses, and the dependence of the responses on the state of the animal.

Erulkar and associates (1956), using a variety of anesthetics, found that 34% of units were completely unresponsive to sound, and that a further 52% were driven so inconsistently that analysis was not possible. The anesthetics used were sodium pentobarbi-

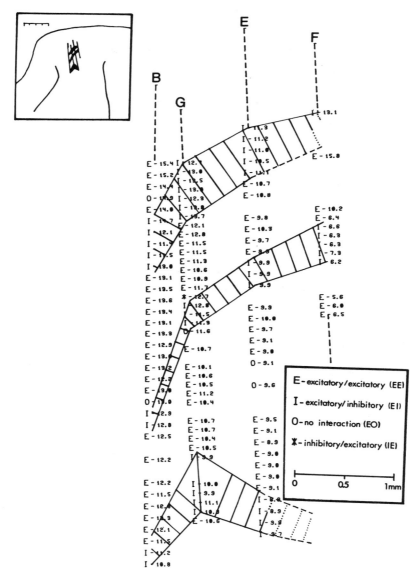

Figure 5.4. Cells excited by both ears (E cells) and cells excited by ipsilateral stimuli and inhibited by contralateral ones (I cells) are segregated into separate columns in the cortex. The columns run approximately orthogonal to the isofrequency lines (cell CFs are shown on the electrode tracks, which can be seen to be nearly parallel to the isofrequency lines). *Inset*, position of tracks on cortex. (From Middlebrooks JC, Dykes RW, Merzenich MM: Binaural response-specific bands in primary auditory cortex (AI) of the cat: topographical organization orthogonal to isofrequency contours. *Brain Res* 181:31–48, 1980.)

tone, pentothal, paraldehyde, chloral hydrate, and chloralose, but the proportions of responsive units did not seem to depend on the type of anesthetic used, but merely on its depth. In unanesthetized and freely moving cats the proportion of responsive cells was somewhat higher (77% according to Evans and Whitfield (1964)), but here too lability of response often made complete characterization impossible, particularly when dealing with neurons responsive only to complex stimuli. Therefore, reliable categorization of neural response types, in relation to position in the cortical core or belt or position within the different belt areas, has been difficult. Moreover, since one cannot reliably describe the complexity in the responses measured by different investigators, it has not been possible to determine a clear hierarchy of neuronal response types in the higher stages of the auditory system.

One seemingly reliable and novel feature of cortical responses is the existence of "multipeaked" units, i.e., units having tuning curves with more than one clear dip (Fig. 5.5; Oonishi and Katsuki, 1965). Where such units have inhibitory sidebands, the response to an excitatory tone in one frequency range can be inhibited only by stimuli in the same frequency range (Abeles and Goldstein, 1972). Other units have very broad tuning curves, and their inhibitory range of frequencies varies with the frequency of the excitatory tone. Some of these properties can be explained by the convergence onto single units of the projections of cells with different best frequencies, where each of the projecting cells has inhibitory sidebands.

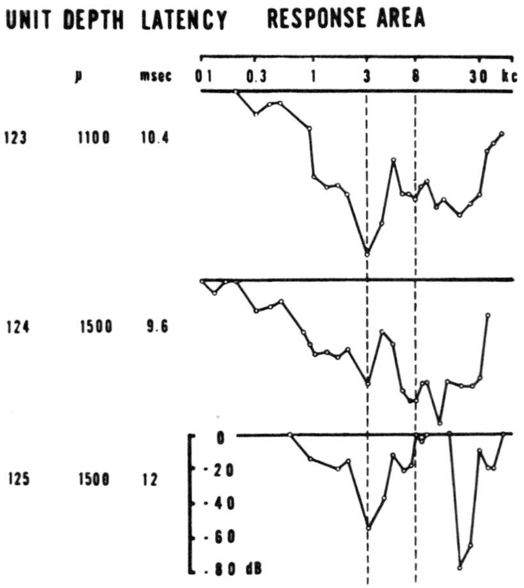

UNIT DEPTH LATENCY   RESPONSE AREA

Figure 5.5. Broad and multipeaked units are seen in the auditory cortex, as well as a single peaked tuning curve. (From Oonishi S, Katsuki Y: Functional organization and integrative mechanism on the auditory cortex of the cat. *Jpn J Physiol* 15:342–365, 1965.)

In their temporal responses many of the cortical cells show patterns similar to those seen in the lower stages of the auditory system. For cells which responded in a determinate way, Abeles and Goldstein (1972) described "through" (i.e., sustained), "on," "off," and "on-off" responses (Fig. 5.6). As in the lower stages of the auditory system, the temporal response pattern of cortical cells could vary with the stimulus frequency. It is not certain that such responses are any more complex than those seen in lower auditory neural centers.

The rate-intensity functions of many cortical neurons are sharply nonmonotonic, with the firing rate sometimes being reduced to the spontaneous level for stimuli 10 dB on either side of the optimum. In other auditory centers nonmonotonic responses are often caused by the dominance of inhibitory sidebands at the higher intensities.

The Analysis of Sound Location

The analysis of binaural dominance columns has shown the importance of binaural interactions in the function of the auditory cortex. This suggests that a correlate of binaural interactions, namely sound localization, might be important in cortical function (see Chapter 10). In the detection of the position of sound sources, two dominant cues are used. The sound waves from a source on one side of the head will be more intense in one ear than the other. Since diffraction around the head is less at high frequencies and absorption of sound by air greater, such a cue will be most important for stimuli of high frequency. On the other hand, the sound wave will reach the nearer ear first. Thus, a time difference also may be used as a cue.

Some neurons have been reported as giving optimum responses for specific intensity differences between the two ears (Brugge and Merzenich, 1973) and so will presumably give their maximum response to sound arising from a particular direction. We would expect such intensity differences to be extracted by inhibitory interactions between the two ears. The binaural dominance columns (Imig and Brugge, 1978) were analyzed in terms of these interactions, and it might have been expected that these columns would relate to sound location ex-

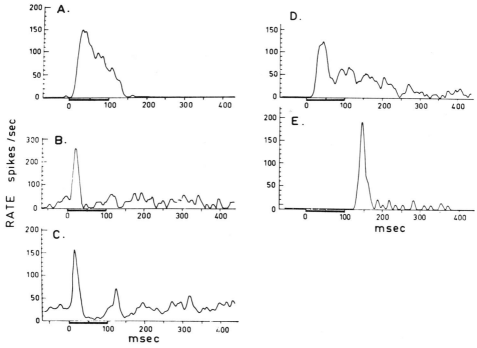

Figure 5.6. The temporal patterns of response seen in the auditory cortex. *A*, Through. *B*, On. *C*, On-off. *D*, Through. *E*, Off. (From Abeles M, Goldstein MH: Responses of single units in the primary auditory cortex of the cat to tones and to tone pairs. *Brain Res* 42:337–352, 1972.)

tracted on the basis of intensity differences. Also, it might have been expected that they would be most important for high-frequency stimuli. Indeed, it has been noted that in the cat, binaural dominance columns are less prominent in the low-frequency part of AI (Imig and Brugge, 1978), although Imig and Brugge (1978) reported a degree of callosal input still present, in contrast to some previous reports (Diamond et al, 1968). However, it should be noted that intensity differences between the two ears are initially extracted at the superior olive (Tsuchitani and Boudreau, 1969), where the first stage of sound localization occurs. Therefore, it is likely that localization on an intensity basis will have been performed before the signal arrives at the cortex. The additional interactions which occur at the cortical level are likely to be related either to refining the localization extracted earlier, or to functions more complex than simple sound localization. Some hypotheses will be discussed later in this chapter, in the context of behavioral experiments on the cortex.

Timing cues in sound localization can be

revealed in the activity of single cortical cells. One way this has been demonstrated is by presenting a sinusoidal stimulus to the two ears, varying the phase relationship between the two ears so that the stimulus at one ear was made to lead or lag behind the stimulus in the other. This type of experiment has revealed neurons which give their maximum response for specific time differences between the two ears (Benson and Teas, 1976). Figure 5.7*A* shows a cell in which the maximum response was given when the stimulus in the contralateral ear led by 200 to 300 μsec, and in which the preferred lead did not vary with stimulus frequency. Thus, this type of cell would respond maximally to a sound arising from a certain direction in space, irrespective of stimulus frequency. On the other hand, Figure 5.7*B* shows a cell in which the preferred time disparity did vary with stimulus frequency. In this type of cell, the preferred direction of the sound source also would vary with frequency. An analysis of such cells in terms of sound location may not always be appropriate, especially since different stimuli such as clicks and tones

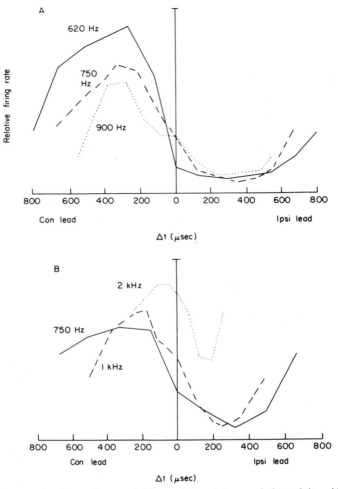

Figure 5.7. (A) The cyclic dependence of firing rate on interaural time delay. Here, the preferred time delay was independent of stimulus frequency. (B) In this cell, the preferred time delay was a function of stimulus frequency. (From Benson DA, Teas DC: Single unit study of binaural interaction in the auditory cortex of the chinchilla. *Brain Res* 103:313–338, 1976.)

may result in quite different preferred directions (Benson and Teas, 1976).

While experiments in which interaural timing and intensity disparities are varied may give information about the mechanisms by which sound localization is performed, it is also important to show that the localization of *real* sound sources in space is possible. In such experiments, a speaker is moved around the head of an animal or stimuli are presented through a set of speakers arranged in a circle, while the activity of a neuron is being recorded. In this type of experiment some cells indeed show selective responsive-

ness to direction, although in many cases the responsiveness has been found to be rather broadly tuned (Evans, 1968; Eisenman, 1974; Fig. 5.8). Generally, but not always, the direction giving the maximal response was independent of the type of stimulus and its intensity.

Cells specifically responsive to the direction of *movement* of a sound source have also been described (Sovijärvi and Hyvärinen, 1974). In response to stationary stimuli, these cells gave a complex on-off response, indicating particular sensitivity to multiple excitatory and inhibitory inputs to the cell.

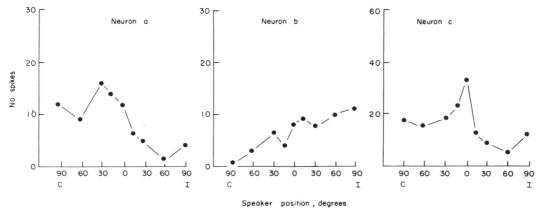

Figure 5.8. Three cortical neurons illustrating different degrees of directional selectivity. *C*, contralateral; *I*, ipsilateral. (From Eisenman LM: Neural encoding of sound location: an electrophysiological study in auditory cortex (AI) of the cat using free field stimuli. *Brain Res* 75:203–214, 1974.)

The Detection of Other Complex Features

Suga and associates (1979) have investigated multipeaked units in the bat auditory cortex. Although the earlier reports of multipeaked units in the cat cortex (Oonishi and Katsuki, 1965; Abeles and Goldstein, 1972) did not show any particular tendency for the peaks to be harmonically related, multiple peaks at harmonically related frequencies did seem to exist in the bat. Suga and associates showed that stimuli represented in the different peaks were mutually facilitatory. If two stimuli were presented together, the response was much greater than could be obtained by single stimuli, even at greater intensity. Therefore, such cells seem specialized for the detection of harmonic complexes.

Other apparently specific detectors have been shown for frequency- and amplitude-modulated stimuli. Whitfield and Evans (1965) described cells which were especially responsive to frequency-modulated tones in the unanesthetized, unrestrained cat (see Chapter 3). In some such cells, in particular those with complex temporal patterns of discharge, the response to frequency-modulated stimuli could not be predicted from the response to steady tones. While cells with these properties have been described even in the dorsal cochlear nucleus, in some ways the cortical cells showed a higher level of stimulus processing than cells in lower stages

of the auditory system. The effective range of frequency modulation, sometimes smaller than ±2.5% of stimulus frequency, was far smaller than generally effective at lower stages of the central auditory system. In some cases, cells responded to small frequency modulations, where the stimulus frequencies lay entirely within the response area determined with steady tones. In other cases, small sweeps all gave similar responses, irrespective of their position within the steady tone response area. In still other cases, responses to frequency-modulated stimuli were obtained for stimulus frequencies entirely *outside* the steady tone response area. This agreed with Whitfield and Evans' observation that modulated stimuli were in general the more effective stimuli for cortical cells. They also observed that some cells could be driven by frequency-modulated stimuli but not by steady tones at all. It is only these latter cells that could truly be called feature detectors for frequency modulation, since frequency-modulated stimuli were the only stimuli that could drive them.

These studies using frequency-modulated stimuli did not show differences between the different cortical areas. With respect to amplitude-modulated stimuli, however, a specific difference has been reported, i.e., the anterior auditory field, described earlier on the rostral edge of AI, has been reported to be more responsive to amplitude-modulated stimuli and to higher frequencies of modulation (Schreiner et al, 1983). In this region the best frequency of amplitude modulation seems to be related to the characteristic frequency of the cell, high characteristic frequencies being associated with the highest best frequencies for modulation (Schreiner et al, 1983).

While it appears that there is a degree of specificity for certain features in the auditory cortex, it is doubtful whether we can actually divide the cells into separate classes of specific feature detectors, as has been done with simple and complex cells in the visual system. Thus, while it has been shown that frequency-modulated tones are very effective stimuli for some cortical cells, it seems that these cells are situated in a continuum of cells responding to a range of features (Goldstein and Abeles, 1975). Moreover, the difficulty of classifying cells as specific feature detectors also makes it difficult to describe a hierarchy of detectors in the auditory system.

If we wanted to postulate a hierarchy of specific feature detectors, we might expect neurons at the highest levels of the system to respond only to stimuli of particular significance for the animal concerned. Attempts have been made to measure the responses of cortical cells to the vocalizations of the species or to other sounds of presumed biological significance. Such responses to animal calls were measured by Newman and Wollberg (1973) and Sovijärvi (1975). Ninety percent of the cortical cells investigated responded to one or more of the calls, and in some cases the responses to the calls could not be predicted from the responses to tones. It was suggested that the cells must have been responding to some of the more complex features of the calls, although evidence was not presented to show that animal calls in general were more effective stimuli than other complex sounds. Therefore, while the results suggest that complex sounds are indeed effective stimuli for cortical cells, we cannot presume that animal calls, or any other stimuli of presumed biological significance, when not incorporated in a behavioral task, form special classes specifically represented in the cortex.

Some of the difficulties of such experiments arise from the lability of the responses. Such lability was noted by Manley and Müller-Preuss (1978), who found that

50% of cells in AI and 62% of cells in AII spontaneously varied their response to a constant vocalization. Evans and Whitfield (1964) noted that the responses of many cells habituated rapidly. In such units, the novelty of the stimulus was an important factor. Moreover, the animal's attitude to the stimulus was sometimes important, since some cells responded only when the animal's attention was drawn to the source of the sound, perhaps by visual means; in some cases the response to sound disappeared when the animal shut its eyes. With such stimuli, it is obvious that the animal's behavioral relationship with the stimulus is an important factor governing the response. Therefore, it is possible that greater consistency in the function of cortical neurons might be obtained by controlling the level of arousal or by incorporating the stimuli in a behavioral task. This is demonstrated by the fact that a greater number of action potentials are found to auditory stimuli in the awake animal than in the drowsy or sleeping animal (Brugge and Merzenich, 1973; Pfingst et al, 1977). The stability of the response is enhanced by incorporating the stimulus in a reaction time task or a frequency discrimination task (Beaton and Miller, 1975). Selective attention can also increase responsiveness (Benson and Hienz, 1978).

BEHAVIORAL STUDIES OF THE AUDITORY CORTEX IN ANIMALS

Introduction

The auditory cortex has been investigated systematically by behavioral scientists for more than 40 yr. At many times during that period, it has seemed as though definitive descriptions of the function might be just around the corner. However, negative evidence on all unifying hypotheses has been produced, and we are still uncertain as to its overall function or functions.

Ablation of the auditory cortex does not lead to a complete loss of simple function as in the visual system. Indeed, it is often difficult to show any losses at all. For instance, absolute detection thresholds and differential intensity thresholds are little, if at all, affected (Kryter and Ades, 1943; Oesterreich et al, 1971). Therefore, research has concentrated on higher level functions.

Frequency Discrimination

An early experiment on frequency discrimination was performed by Allen (1945), who showed that the discrimination was lost after large lesions of the auditory cortex. He trained dogs to distinguish between the sounds produced by tapping a bell and by tapping a tin cup, a task which he presumed was accomplished on the basis of frequency rather than any other aspect of the stimulus. The result was supported a few years later by Meyer and Woolsey (1952), who trained cats in a rotating cage to sit still to a short series of 1 kHz tone pips, but to rotate the cage when the series was terminated by a tone pip at 1.1 kHz (Goldberg and Neff, 1961; Fig. 5.9A). The discrimination could be relearned if any portion of AI, AII, Ep, or I-T (Fig. 5.1A) remained but was lost if all areas were removed. Therefore, at the time it seemed as though the auditory cortex was needed for frequency discrimination. However, only a few years later Butler and associates (1957) showed that frequency discrimination was still possible with a different behavioral task. The cat was trained to cross a shuttle box when 1 kHz tone pips were interspersed in a continuous background of 800 Hz tone pips (Fig. 5.9B). Not only was performance intact after the lesion, but frequency discrimination limens were nearly as

good as before. A reason for the apparent conflict in results of the different studies was pointed out by Thompson (1960), who showed that it depended on the differences between the behavioral tasks. In the experiments in which deficits had been found, such as those of Allen (1945) and Meyer and Woolsey (1952), both the positive and negative stimuli were presented against a neutral background of silence. Therefore, the animals had to make responses to one stimulus, but withhold responses to the other. In the experiment in which no deficits were found, the negative stimulus was presented continuously, forming the neutral background. Thus, the animal simply had to respond to a change from the background. Thompson showed that the task was critical by training cats either with the negative stimulus presented continuously as a background or with the positive and negative stimuli presented on discrete trials against a silent background (Fig. 5.10). After complete auditory cortical lesions, cats were able to perform the first task but not the second. He also showed that the lesioned animals tended to make responses to all stimuli, whether positive or negative. He suggested that they suffered from an inability to withhold responses to irrelevant stimuli. His hypothesis suggested that the function of the auditory cortex was related more to motor than to sensory function.

While Thompson's hypothesis (1960) was intriguing, there are reasons why it did not

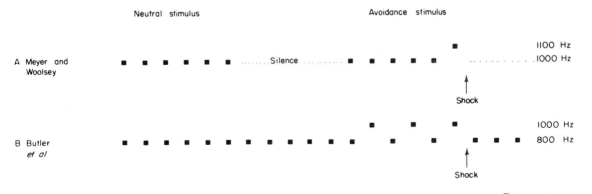

Figure 5.9. The sequences of stimuli used by Meyer and Woolsey (A) and Butler and associates (B). Lesions of the auditory cortex interfered with performance on task A but not task B. (From Pickles JO: *An Introduction to the Physiology of Hearing.* Copyright: Academic Press, Inc. (London) Ltd., 1982, p 341.)

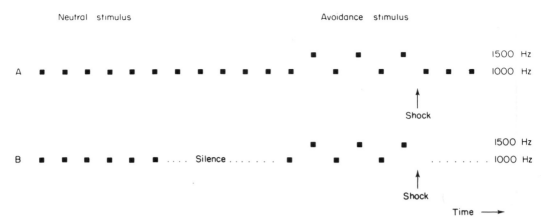

Figure 5.10. The two sequences of stimuli used by Thompson in tests of frequency discrimination. Cortical lesions interfered with performance on task *B* but not task *A*. (From Pickles JO: *An Introduction to the Physiology of Hearing.* Copyright: Academic Press Inc. (London) Ltd., 1982, p 341.)

provide a complete explanation. Firstly, although lesioned animals do tend to cross a shuttle box too often to irrelevant stimuli (i.e., make too many false-positive responses), Thompson's own data indicated that if, in training, the animals were given *countershock* for making false-positive responses, lesions reduced both false positives and correct crossings. Also other investigators have found that, if some form of punishment is given for false positives during the initial training, lesions similarly tend to reduce responses to the "no go" stimuli (Cranford et al, 1976a and 1976b). Therefore, other reasons must be sought to explain why cortical lesions uncouple stimulus and response only on certain tasks.

Neff (1960) suggested that, after cortical lesions, cats were able to respond only to the activation of new neural channels. In experiments by Allen and by Meyer and Woolsey, where both positive and negative stimuli were presented on discrete trials, this same hypothesis was valid, as both types of stimuli would activate new neural channels. Since a lesioned animal would not be able to tell which channels were activated, it would respond to both stimuli indiscriminately. On the other hand, in experiments where the positive stimulus involved a change from the background, the positive stimulus (but not the ongoing background) would have activated new neural channels, and a lesioned animal would be able to detect the stimulus. If Neff's hypothesis is stated in other words, lesioned animals are able only

to *detect* stimuli and cannot perform an absolute recognition task and *identify* them. The function of the cortex, therefore, might be that of classifying and identifying stimuli. This suggests that an intact auditory cortex might be necessary for providing the framework within which such classification can be done, or, in other words, that it is necessary for concept formation. This is a hypothesis to which we shall return, after considering other behavioral studies on the cortex.

Neff's hypothesis has been successful in predicting the results of many experiments. However, again there are some exceptions. Cranford and associates (1976a) showed that cats were able to perform an absolute recognition task after large cortical lesions. Cats were successfully trained to cross a shuttle box to a series of 800 Hz tone pips, and withhold responding to a 1200 Hz series, both stimuli being presented on discrete trials against a background of silence. Performance could be relearned after bilateral ablation of all auditory cortical areas. The cats, therefore, were able to perform satisfactorily on a task containing two elements which had been thought to make performance impossible, namely, an absolute frequency recognition task without a reference signal, and a go-no go task where they had to withhold responses to the negative signal presented against a silent background. One of the differences between this experiment and the previous ones occurred in the method of training. An absolute frequency recognition task is normally very difficult for cats; here the task was made easier by training them initially on a relative discrimination task, in which a reference signal was used at first. Then the cats were transferred to the absolute discrimination task by omitting the reference signal. The transfer was immediate; but in Thompson's (1960) experiment, for example, where some cats were initially trained on the absolute discrimination task, training was very slow. Perhaps when the task is easy, lesions have little effect, whereas if it is difficult, lesions may have a greater effect. The effect of lesions, therefore, may be related more to the complexity of the strategy used by the animal in solving the task than to the task itself.

The Involvement of the Time Dimension

In lesions of the auditory cortex it has been observed that subjects have had an impairment in discrimination of temporal patterns of auditory stimuli (see also Chapter 13). Thus, Diamond and Neff (1957) showed that cats with brain lesions were unable to relearn a pattern discrimination in which a change in the time-order of tone pips had to be detected (Fig. 5.11). The pattern could be relearned if any part of AI remained after the lesion, but could not be relearned after bilateral lesions of AI, AII, Ep, and insular-temporal cortex (I-T). I-T seemed to play an important part in the

initial establishment of the discrimination, since animals with only I-T lesions were unable to learn a pattern discrimination for the first time (Goldberg et al, 1957). I-T may have a supramodal role in pattern discriminations, since lesions have impaired visual and somatosensory as well as auditory pattern discrimination (Colativa, 1972, 1974; Colativa et al, 1974). There seems a correlate of this in man, since lesions of the temporal lobe impair the discrimination of temporal patterns of auditory stimuli (Milner, 1962; Karaseva, 1972) (see also Chapter 13). Lesions in AI or the belt area also upset the performance of cats, dogs, and monkeys on a task in which they had to indicate when two successive sounds were the same, but not when they were different (Cornwell, 1967; Chorazyna and Stepien, 1963; Stepien et al, 1960). Similar deficits have been found by Dewson and associates (1970) on a task in which monkeys had to reproduce a two-element pattern of tone and noise bursts on two panels. However, the deficit was not one of short-term memory alone, since forcing the monkeys to wait before making a response did not produce further deficits (Cowey and Weiskrantz, 1976).

Another example of a temporal task which resulted in deficits after cortical lesions is that of duration discrimination. Scharlock and associates (1965) trained cats to respond when the duration of tone pips increased

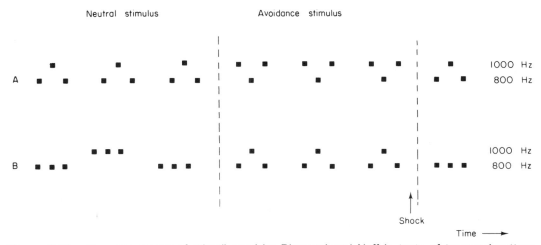

Figure 5.11. Two sequences of stimuli used by Diamond and Neff in tests of temporal pattern discrimination. Lesions of the auditory cortex interfered with performance on both of the tests. (From Pickles JO: *An Introduction to the Physiology of Hearing.* Copyright: Academic Press Inc. (London) Ltd., 1982, p 341).

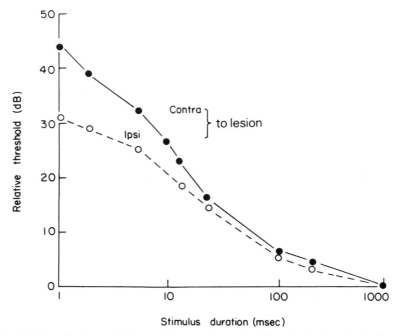

Figure 5.12.   Unilateral lesions of the auditory cortex raised thresholds for short stimuli, but not for long stimuli, in the contralateral ear. Before the lesion, thresholds for both ears followed the line shown here for the ear ipsilateral to the lesion. (From Abeles M, Goldstein MH: Responses of single units in the primary auditory cortex of the cat to tones and to tone pairs. *Brain Res* 42:337–352, 1972.)

from 1 sec to 4 sec. Lesions of AI, AII, Ep, somatosensory cortex (SII), and I-T made retraining impossible.

A very simple task which indicates an involvement of the time dimension in auditory cortical function is that of the detection of short stimuli (Gershuni et al, 1967; Baru and Karaseva, 1972). Unilateral lesions of the auditory cortex raised thresholds for very short (but not longer) stimuli in the contralateral ear (Fig. 5.12). Perhaps the cortex plays some part in extending the effect of brief stimuli. The subjects seemed to have a general difficulty with short stimuli, since frequency discrimination thresholds were also raised for short (but not long) stimuli (Gershuni et al, 1967; Cranford, 1979b).

Sound Localization

An important area of performance affected by lesions of the auditory cortex is that of sound localization. This agrees with electrophysiological and anatomical evidence which also points to sound localization as one of the functions of the cortex.

In such experiments, cats were trained to go to the source of a sound (Fig. 5.13). They were unable to perform correctly after bilateral ablation of all auditory areas of the cortex, including AI, AII, Ep, I-T, SII, and the suprasylvian gyrus (Neff, 1968; Strominger, 1969). Similar effects have been found in the monkey and in man (Wegener, 1973; Jerger et al, 1969). However, later experiments showed that, when a different type of response was used, lesioned animals were able to localize sounds after all. The deficit, therefore, must have had something other than a simple sensory basis. For instance, Ravizza and Masterton (1972) showed that when opossums had to indicate whether a sound came from a speaker on the left or the right, by either drinking or stopping drinking from a water spout, performance survived ablation of nearly the complete neocortex. Similar results have been obtained also from a "lateralization" task, in which stimuli of different interaural time delays or intensity differences were presented to the two ears through headphones (Cranford, 1979a). In man, such stimuli ap-

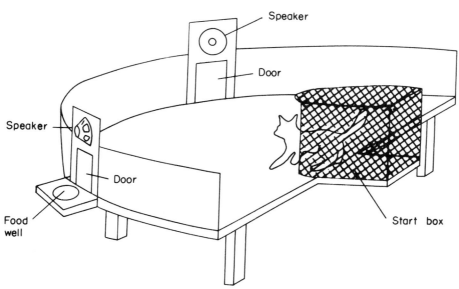

Figure 5.13.   The apparatus for a sound localization experiment. The cat is held in the start box. One speaker sounds, the cat is released and has to push open the door under the correct speaker for a food reward. In some experiments, the cat is released only when the stimulus has ended, so that the animal has to perform the localization when in the start box and cannot track its way to the speaker while it is sounding. (From Pickles JO: *An Introduction to the Physiology of Hearing.* Copyright: Academic Press Inc. (London) Ltd., 1982, p 341.)

pear to be coming from one side of the head or the other (see also Chapter 10). Lesioned cats were able to use such changes, which in man would be interpreted as changes in the apparent direction of the stimulus, as a signal to cross a shuttle box.

In the experiments in which performance survived ablation of the cortex, the direction of the stimulus was merely being used as a sign that a response was needed. The animals did not have to recognize the actual direction or relate it to the space around them. By contrast, in the experiments affected by lesions, the animals had to approach the source of the sound. Therefore, they had to recognize the spatial orientation of the stimulus. This suggests the possibility that we are not dealing with a deficit in detecting the direction of a sound source, but a deficit in either fitting the direction into auditory space or making a movement within that space.

An experiment of Heffner (1978) addressed this latter problem. He trained dogs to approach one of two goal boxes, on the basis of the rate of a brief train of clicks presented through a central speaker. After bilateral removal of AI and AII, the dogs

were able to use this cue to approach one goal box or the other. However, if the same stimuli were presented through one of two speakers over the goal boxes as a cue in a localization task, the animals failed. This suggests that neither making the motor response nor remembering the correct response nor attending to the stimulus were the critical factors. As suggested by Neff and associates (1975), "Perhaps, in the absence of auditory cortex, organization of a 'spatial world' based on acoustic information is no longer possible."

Current work on the auditory cortex suggests that it might have a role in forming a concept of auditory space. However, the analysis of frequency discrimination has taught us to be very cautious in suggesting such hypotheses. An example from a human patient who had unilateral damage to the temporal lobe illustrates this. The patient had deficits both in sound localization and in abnormal temporal integration for short stimuli (Jerger et al, 1969). Abnormal temporal integration of brief stimuli, if unilateral, could lead to a *distortion* of auditory space with the result that he might not be able to point to or walk to the source of a sound, while still being able to discriminate changes in its direction. This could erroneously be interpreted as a loss of the concept of auditory space.

Ear Selection and Selective Attention

The auditory cortex has been implicated in the process of selective attention, where it is necessary to pay attention to stimuli in one ear when stimuli are presented to the other ear at the same time. Kaas and associates (1967) trained cats to respond to changes in the pattern of tone pulses, when the elements of the pattern were presented separately to the two ears through headphones. Figure 5.14 illustrates the patterns used. Although the task can be solved on the basis of the summed binaural pattern, it is easier to solve it on the basis of one ear only, the ear in which the pattern changes from L-L-L-L (neutral stimulus) to L-H-L-H (warning stimulus). Transfer tests showed that this was, in fact, what the cats did. Unilateral ablation of the complete auditory cortex (AI, AII, Ep, SII, I-T) resulted in severe initial deficits, if the lesion was contralateral to the attending ear, but not if it was ipsilateral. This suggests that each auditory cortex governs responses to stimuli in the contralateral ear, when competing stimuli are present in the ipsilateral ear. These results also agree with electrophysiological and anatomical evidence supporting the dominance of the auditory projection to the contralateral hemisphere (see Chapters 2 and 3).

Cranford (1975) also showed the importance of the auditory cortex in selective attention to stimuli in the contralateral ear. He used a train of noise bursts as a masker in one ear, synchronized with tone pips in the opposite signal ear. Unilateral lesions of the cortex increased the effect of contralateral masking only when the lesion was contralateral to the signal ear. If the auditory cortex on the second side was ablated as well, the amount of contralateral masking needed returned to normal.

These experiments are similar to those that have been used in the analysis of interaural attention in man. For instance, a subject might be required to listen to a stimulus (such as a spoken text) in one ear, while a competing stimulus is presented to the other ear. Such tests also are affected by unilateral cortical damage (Berlin and McNeil, 1976) (see also Chapter 12).

POSSIBLE CONCLUSIONS AS TO THE FUNCTION OF AUDITORY CORTEX

Several hypotheses have been suggested for the function of the auditory cortex.

1. The auditory cortex may well have a role in the analysis of complex sounds. Electrophysiological experiments indicate that many neurons are driven only by complex sounds, although from such experiments it is difficult to decide the extent to which the cortical processing contributes to their analysis. Behavioral experiments in animals (Dewson, 1964; Dewson et al, 1969) as well as brain lesions in man, also suggest that the auditory cortex is needed for the processing of complex stimuli.

2. Thompson (1960) suggested that the auditory cortex was needed for the inhibition of inappropriate responses. However, this hypothesis is not valid in its simplest form, because, with certain methods of training, animals make too few rather than too many responses after cortical lesions (Cranford et al, 1976a and b). Some of the changes in behaviors studied may have been due to the lesion affecting the efficacy of the punishment employed.

3. Neff (1960) suggested that after lesions of the auditory cortex cats could detect stimuli, but could not identify them. However, with the appropriate method of training cats *can* identify stimuli absolutely (Cranford et al, 1976a and b; Cranford, 1979a and b).

4. The auditory cortex may be involved in interaural attention, each hemisphere selecting stimuli from the opposite ear input (Kaas et al, 1967; Cranford, 1975; Berlin and McNeil, 1976). There are suggestions

	Neutral stimulus	Avoidance stimulus
Attending ear	L −L −L −L −L −L	L −H−L −H−L −H−
Ignoring ear	−L −H−L −H−L −	−L −H−L −H−L −H
Binaural pattern	L L L H L L L H L L L	L L H H L L H H L L H H

Figure 5.14. The sequences of stimuli used by Kaas and associates (1967) in their test of interaural attention. The stimuli were presented to the two ears through headphones. Performance was upset by cortical lesions.

that such a hypothesis can be extended to the selection of sound sources in the contralateral half field of space in a situation in which the sound reaches both ears (Whitfield et al, 1972).

5. The auditory cortex may be necessary for fitting auditory stimuli into a temporal context, since discrimination of the duration of auditory stimuli (Gershuni et al, 1967) and discrimination of temporal patterns in auditory stimuli are affected by lesions of the auditory cortex (Diamond and Neff, 1957; Goldberg et al, 1957; Colativa, 1972, 1974; Colativa et al, 1974; Milner, 1962; Karaseva, 1972; Cornwell, 1967; Chorazyna and Stepien, 1963; Stepien et al, 1960; Dewson et al, 1970; Cowey and Weiskrantz, 1976). The cortex may also be necessary for prolonging the effect of short stimuli, since lesioned animals and brain-damaged man seem to have a general difficulty with short stimuli (Gershuni et al, 1967; Baru and Karaseva, 1972; and Cranford, 1979b).

6. It has been suggested that it is not possible to form the concept of auditory space (Neff, 1968; Neff et al, 1975), i.e., to fit the position of sound sources into a general schema, without an auditory cortex.

7. Whitfield (1979) suggested that the role of the cortex in forming the concept of auditory space was a reflection of its role in forming auditory concepts in general. For instance, if it is believed that the auditory cortex is necessary for the absolute identification of auditory stimuli (3 above), it is possible that it provides the framework within which the identification is accomplished.

8. Difficult tasks are more easily affected by cortical lesions than are simple tasks. In other words, it is not the difficulty of the task itself but the complexity of the strategy used by the animal in solving it that governs whether a deficit is found. This suggests that the strategy actually used by the animal or man, as well as the task itself, will have to be taken into account in assessing cortical function.

References

Abeles M, Goldstein MH: Functional architecture in cat primary auditory cortex: columnar organization and organization according to depth. *J Neurophysiol* 33:172–187, 1970.

Abeles M, Goldstein MH: Responses of single units in the primary auditory cortex of the cat to tones and to tone pairs. *Brain Res* 42:337–352, 1972.

Allen WF: Effect of destroying three localized cerebral cortical areas for sound on correct conditioned differential responses of the dog's foreleg. *Am J Physiol* 144:415–428, 1945.

Baru AV, Karaseva TA: *The Brain and Hearing*. New York, Consultants Bureau, 1972, p 116.

Beaton R, Miller JM: Single cell activity in the auditory cortex of the unanesthetised, behaving, monkey: correlation with stimulus-controlled behavior. *Brain Res* 100:543–562, 1975.

Benson DA, Hienz RD: Single unit activity in the auditory cortex of monkeys selectively attending left vs. right ear stimuli. *Brain Res* 159:307–320, 1978.

Benson DA, Teas DC: Single unit study of binaural interaction in the auditory cortex of the chinchilla. *Brain Res* 103:313–338, 1976.

Berlin CI, McNeil MR: Dichotic listening. In Laas NJ (ed): *Contemporary Issues in Experimental Phonetics*. New York, Academic Press, 1976, p 327.

Brugge JF, Merzenich MM: Responses of neurons in auditory cortex of the macaque monkey to monaural and binaural stimulation. *J Neurophysiol* 36:1138–1158, 1973.

Butler RA, Diamond IT, Neff WD: Role of auditory cortex in discrimination of changes in frequency. *J Neurophysiol* 20:108–120, 1957.

Chorazyna H, Stepien L: Effect of bilateral Sylvian gyrus ablations on auditory conditioning in dogs. *Bull Acad Pol Sci [Biol]* 11:43–45, 1963.

Colativa FB: Auditory cortical lesions and visual pattern discrimination in cat. *Brain Res* 39:437–447, 1972.

Colativa FB: Insular-temporal lesions and vibrotactile pattern discrimination in cats. *Physiol Behav* 12:215–218, 1974.

Colativa FB, Szeligo FV, Zimmer SD: Temporal pattern discrimination in cats with insular-temporal lesions. *Brain Res* 79:153–156, 1974.

Cornwell P: Loss of auditory pattern discrimination following insular-temporal lesions in cats. *J Comp Physiol Psychol* 63:165–168, 1967.

Cowey A, Weiskrantz L: Auditory sequence discrimination in *Macaca Mulatta*: the role of the superior temporal cortex. *Neuropsychologia* 14:1–10, 1976.

Cranford JL: Role of neocortex in binaural hearing in the cat. I. Contralateral masking. *Brain Res* 100:395–406, 1975.

Cranford JL: Auditory cortex lesions and interaural intensity and phase-angle discriminations in cats. *J Neurophysiol* 42:1518–1526, 1979a.

Cranford JL: Detection versus discrimination of brief tones by cats with auditory cortex lesions. *J Acoust Soc Am* 65:1573–1575, 1979b.

Cranford JL, Igarashi M, Stramler JH: Effect of auditory neocortex ablation on identification of click rates in cats. *Brain Res* 116:69–81, 1976a.

Cranford JL, Igarashi M, Stramler JH: Effect of auditory neocortex ablation on pitch perception in the cat. *J Neurophysiol* 39:143–152, 1976b.

Dewson JH: Speech sound discrimination by cats. *Science* 144:555–556, 1964.

Dewson JH, Cowey A, Weiskrantz L: Disruptions of auditory sequence discrimination by unilateral and bilateral cortical ablations of superior temporal gyrus in the monkey. *Exp Neurol* 28:529–548, 1970.

Dewson JH, Pribram KH, Lynch JC: Effects of ablations of temporal cortex upon speech sound discrimination in the monkey. *Exp Neurol* 24:579–591, 1969.

Diamond IT, Jones EG, Powell TPS: Interhemispheric fiber connections of the auditory cortex of the cat. *Brain Res* 11:177–193, 1968.

Diamond IT, Neff WD: Ablation of temporal cortex and discrimination of auditory patterns. *J Neurophysiol* 20:300–315, 1957.

Eisenman LM: Neural encoding of sound location: an electrophysiological study in auditory cortex (AI) of the cat using free field stimuli. *Brain Res* 75:203–214, 1974.

Erulkar SD, Rose JE, Davies PW: Single unit activity in the auditory cortex of the cat. *Bull Johns Hopkins Hosp* 99:55–86, 1956.

Evans EF: Cortical representation. In de Reuck AVS, Knight J (eds): *Hearing Mechanisms in Vertebrates.* London, Churchill, 1968, p 272.

Evans EF, Whitfield IC: Classification of unit responses in the auditory cortex of the unanaesthetised cat. *J Physiol* 171:476–493, 1964.

Gershuni GV, Baru AV, Karaseva TA: Role of auditory cortex in discrimination of acoustic stimuli. *Neurol Sci Trans* 1:370–382, 1967.

Goldberg JM, Diamond IT, Neff WD: Auditory discrimination after ablation of temporal and insular cortex in cat. *Fed Proc* 16:47, 1957.

Goldberg JM, Neff WD: Frequency discrimination after bilateral ablation of cortical auditory areas. *J Neurophysiol* 24:119–128, 1961.

Goldstein MH, Abeles M: Single unit activity of the auditory cortex. In Keidel WD, Neff WD (eds): *Handbook of Sensory Physiology.* Berlin, Springer-Verlag, 1975, vol 5/2, p 199.

Heffner HE: Effects of auditory cortex ablation on localization and discrimination of brief sounds. *J Neurophysiol* 41:963–976, 1978.

Imig TJ, Adrian HO: Binaural columns in the primary field (AI) of cat auditory cortex. *Brain Res* 138:241–257, 1977.

Imig TJ, Brugge JF: Sources and terminations of callosal axons related to binaural and frequency maps in primary auditory cortex of the cat. *J Comp Neurol* 182:637–660, 1978.

Imig TJ, Morel A: Organization of the thalamocortical auditory system in the cat. *Ann Rev Neurosci* 6:95–120, 1983.

Jerger J, Weikers NJ, Sharbrough FW, Jerger S: Bilateral lesions of the temporal lobe. *Acta Otolaryngol [Suppl] Stockh* 258:1–51, 1969.

Jones EG, Burton H, Porter R: Commissural and cortico-cortical 'columns' in the somatic sensory cortex of primates. *Science* 190:572–574, 1975.

Kaas J, Axelrod S, Diamond IT: An ablation study of the auditory cortex in the cat using binaural tonal patterns. *J Neurophysiol* 30:710–724, 1967.

Karaseva TA: The role of the temporal lobe in human auditory perception. *Neuropsychologia* 10:227–231, 1972.

Knight PL: Representation of the cochlea within the anterior auditory field (AAF) of the cat. *Brain Res* 130:447–467, 1977.

Kryter KD, Ades HW: Studies on the function of the higher acoustic centers in the cat. *Am J Psychol* 56:501–536, 1943.

Manley JA, Müller-Preuss P: Response variability of auditory cortex cells in the squirrel monkey to constant acoustic stimuli. *Exp Brain Res* 32:171–180, 1978.

Merzenich MM, Knight PL, Roth GL: Representation of cochlea within primary auditory cortex in the cat. *J Neurophysiol* 38:231–249, 1975.

Meyer DR, Woolsey CN: Effects of localized cortical destruction on auditory discriminative conditioning in cat. *J Neurophysiol* 15:149–162, 1952.

Middlebrooks JC, Dykes RW, Merzenich MM: Binaural response-specific bands in primary auditory cortex (AI) of the cat: topographical organization orthogonal to isofrequency contours. *Brain Res* 181:31–48, 1980.

Milner B: Laterality effects in audition. In Mountcastle VB (ed): *Interhemispheric Relations and Cerebral Dominance.* Baltimore, Johns Hopkins Press, 1962, p 177.

Neff WD: Role of the auditory cortex in sound discrimination. In Rasmussen GL, Windle WF (eds): *Neural Mechanisms of the Auditory and Vestibular Systems.* Springfield, IL, Charles C Thomas, 1960, p 211.

Neff WD: Localization and lateralization of sound in space. In de Reuck AVS, Knight J (eds): *Hearing Mechanisms in Vertebrates.* London, Churchill, 1968, p 207.

Neff WD, Diamond IT, Casseday JH: Behavioral studies of auditory discrimination: central nervous system. In Keidel WD, Neff WD (eds): *Handbook of Sensory Physiology.* Berlin, Springer-Verlag, 1975, vol 5/2, p 307.

Newman JD, Wollberg Z: Multiple coding of species-specific vocalizations in the auditory cortex of squirrel monkeys. *Brain Res* 54:287–304, 1973.

Niimi K, Matsuoka H: Thalamocortical organization of the auditory system in the cat studied by retrograde axonal transport of horseradish peroxidase. *Adv Anat Embryol Cell Biol* 57:1–56, 1979.

Oesterreich RE, Strominger NL, Neff WD: Neural structures mediating sound differential intensity discrimination in the cat. *Brain Res* 27:251–270, 1971.

Oonishi S, Katsuki Y: Functional organization and integrative mechanism on the auditory cortex of the cat. *Jpn J Physiol* 15:342–365, 1965.

Pfingst BE, O'Connor TA, Miller JM: Response plasticity of neurons in auditory cortex of the rhesus monkey. *Exp Brain Res* 29:393–404, 1977.

Pickles JO: *An Introduction to the Physiology of Hearing.* London, Academic Press, 1982, p 341.

Ravizza RJ, Masterton RB: Contribution of neocortex to sound localization in opossum (*Didelphis virginiana*). *J Neurophysiol* 35:344–356, 1972.

Reale RA, Imig TJ: Tonotopic organization in auditory cortex of the cat. *J Comp Neurol* 192:265–291, 1980.

Rose JE: The cellular structure of the auditory region of the cat. *J Comp Neurol* 91:409–439, 1949.

Scharlock DP, Neff WD, Strominger NL: Discrimination of tone duration after bilateral ablation of cortical auditory areas. *J Neurophysiol* 28:673–681, 1965.

Schreiner Chr, Urbas JV, Mehrgardt S: Temporal resolution of amplitude modulation and complex signals in the auditory cortex of the cat. In Klinke R, Hartmann R (eds): *Hearing—Physiological Bases and Psychophysics.* Berlin, Springer-Verlag, 1983, p 169.

Sousa-Pinto A: Structure of the first auditory cortex (AI) in the cat. I. Light microscopic observations on its organization. *Arch Ital Biol* 111:112–137, 1973.

Sovijärvi ARA: Detection of natural complex sounds in the primary auditory cortex of the cat. *Acta Physiol Scand* 93:318–335, 1975.

Sovijärvi ARA, Hyvärinen J: Auditory cortical neurons in the cat sensitive to the direction of sound source movement. *Brain Res* 73:455–471, 1974.

Stepien LS, Cordeau JP, Rasmussen T: The effect of temporal lobe and hippocampal lesions on auditory and visual recent memory in monkeys. *Brain* 83:470–489, 1960.

Strominger NL: Localization of sound in space after unilateral and bilateral ablation of auditory cortex. *Exp Neurol* 25:521–533, 1969.

Suga N, O'Neill WE, Manabe T: Harmonic-sensitive neurons in the auditory cortex of the mustache bat. *Science* 203:270–274, 1979.

Thompson RF: Function of auditory cortex of cat in frequency discrimination. *J Neurophysiol* 23:321–334, 1960.

Tsuchitani C, Boudreau JC: Stimulus level of dichotically presented tones and cat superior olive S-segment discharge. *J Acoust Soc Am* 46:979–988, 1969.

Tunturi AR: A difference in the representation of auditory signals for the left and right ears in the iso-frequency contours of the right middle ectosylvian auditory cortex of the dog. *Am J Physiol* 168:712–727, 1952.

Wegener JG: The sound localizing behavior of normal and brain-damaged monkeys. *J Aud Res* 13:191–219, 1973.

Whitfield IC: The object of the sensory cortex. *Brain Behav Evol* 16:129–154, 1979.

Whitfield IC, Cranford JL, Ravizza R, Diamond IT: Effects of unilateral ablation of auditory cortex in cat on complex sound localization. *J Neurophysiol* 35:718–731, 1972.

Whitfield IC, Evans EF: Response of auditory cortical neurons to stimuli of changing frequency. *J Neurophysiol* 28:655–672, 1965.

Woolsey CN: Organization of the cortical auditory system: a review and a synthesis. In Rasmussen GL, Windle WF (eds): *Neural Mechanisms of the Auditory and Vestibular Systems.* Springfield, IL, Charles C Thomas, 1960, p 165.

CHAPTER 6

Middle Latency (MLR) and Late Vertex Auditory Evoked Responses (LVAER) in Central Auditory Dysfunction

PAUL KILENY, Ph.D.

Dr. Kileny describes the middle latency and late vertex auditory responses with details on latency, electrode placement, generator sources, maturational changes, and the effect of barbiturates. He discusses the P-300 event-related potential and illustrates clinical usefulness of these electrical responses with case examples.

With the introduction of auditory brainstem responses into clinical practice, the interest in middle latency and late vertex auditory evoked responses (MLR and LVAER) and their clinical utilization declined. The relative ease with which brainstem responses could be acquired contributed significantly to this trend. A recent review article (Vivion, 1980) addressed itself solely to the early auditory evoked responses (auditory brainstem responses) (ABR), MLR, and frequency-following responses and completely excluded the late vertex auditory evoked responses because of limited current clinical use. While recognizing the various limitations imposed by the use of the late vertex auditory evoked responses, Picton et al (1977) stated that "they are the best evoked potential measurements available, if they can be reproducibly recorded," as their presence indicates the complete integrity of the auditory pathways in the central nervous system.

THE MIDDLE LATENCY RESPONSE (MLR)

The middle latency components of the auditory evoked response (MLR) occur within a time frame of 100 msec following the presentation of an effective auditory stimulus. Geisler et al (1957) were the first to describe the MLR as "an early response with an onset latency of about 20 msec" characterized by a vertex-positive peak (Pa) with a latency of about 30 msec. The scalp distribution of the MLR is widespread, but it is most prominent over frontocentral regions (Picton et al, 1974, Özdamar and Kraus, 1983). With monaural stimulation, the responses recorded between vertex (Cz) and ipsilateral or contralateral ear lobe (A1 or A2) were reported to be symmetrical (Peters and Mendel, 1974). The configuration of the recorded MLR depends on the characteristics (cutoff frequencies, filter slopes) of the EEG filter (Scherg, 1982, Sprague and Thornton, 1982, Kileny, 1983). Considerable distortion is introduced by high-pass filtering when utilizing relatively steep analog filters. Low-pass filtering affects peak latencies (i.e., the higher the setting, the earlier the latency of Pa) and the fine structure of the brainstem response complex. Figure 6.1*A* illustrates a typical adult MLR recorded with a filter setting of 5 to 1500 Hz (12 dB/oct slopes) and identifies its components. Pa is the most prominent and stable

MLR, Normal Adult, 60 dB HL Clicks

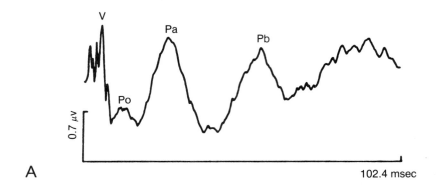

A   102.4 msec

MLR, 18 days, M, 60 dB HL Clicks

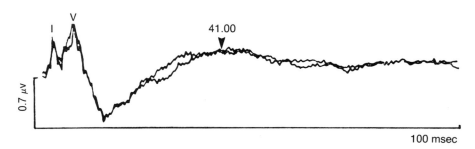

100 msec

F, 7 mo., 50 dB HL Clicks

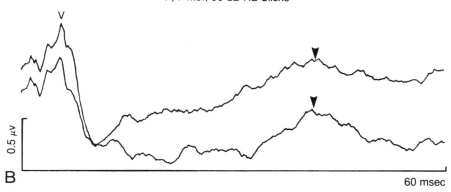

B   60 msec

Figure 6.1. (*A*) Normal adult middle latency auditory evoked responses elicited by 60 dB HL clicks presented at a rate of 10/sec. Electrode placement: midline forehead (below hairline), ipsilateral mastoid. Filter settings: 5 to 1500 Hz (12 dB/oct slope). (*B*) Middle latency auditory evoked responses from two normal hearing infants.

component in adults. When recorded with a lower low-pass cutoff frequency (i.e., 100 Hz), the brainstem response complex appears as the earliest broad positive peak of the response (Kileny, 1983). Between the brainstem complex and Pa, there often appears another smaller positive peak labeled here, Po (latency 12 to 15 msec). This peak is partially the result of the activation of the postauricular muscle reflex (Kileny, 1983).

It must be emphasized that while there is some overlapping of myogenic and neurogenic activity during the 100-msec latency range, the MLR is basically a neurogenic auditory response which remains unaffected following the administration of neuromuscular blocking agents (Harker et al, 1977; Kileny et al, 1983).

Until recently the notion that the infant and the adult MLR were identical, with some relatively negligible differences, was well-accepted (Mendelson and Salamy, 1981). However, the recent work of Scherg (1982) and Sprague and Thornton (1982) indicates that, in fact, the infant and the adult MLR differ significantly and that the earlier notion of similarity may have been partially the product of relatively steep analog filter distortions which significantly affected the infant MLR (Kileny, 1983). Figure 6.1*B* illustrates MLRs recorded from two normal hearing infants during sleep (aged 18 days and 14 days, respectively) obtained with the same recording and stimulus parameters utilized to obtain the adult response illustrated in Figure 6.1*A*. In both cases, the response is dominated by the early (brainstem) component and the following negative trough. Both sets of traces also exhibit broad, low amplitude positive peaks with midpoint latencies of approximately 40 msec. Neither of these infant traces exhibits as prominent a Pa component as the adult MLR illustrated in Figure 6.1*A*. Other infant responses exhibit only a slow return to the baseline following the negative trough (Sprague and Thornton, 1982; Kileny, 1983). Further developmental studies are needed to define the characteristics of the infant MLR both awake and asleep.

Controversy surrounds the identity of the generator sources of the MLR. Responses have been recorded from the exposed human cortex within the latency range associated with the scalp-recorded MLR (Heath and Galbraith, 1966; Celesia et al, 1968; Puletti and Celesia, 1970). These have been considered to be primary auditory responses and were elicited by both ipsilateral and contralateral auditory stimulation. Their cortical distribution was limited to the posterior part of the superior temporal gyrus and the parietal and frontal operculum. Cortical sensory responses recorded in this latency range are considered to be mediated by the specific lemniscal sensory pathways and specific thalamic nuclei (Brazier, 1972). Picton et al (1974) listed several possible neural generator sources: thalamus and association cortex in frontal, parietal, and temporal lobes. They ruled out a significant contribution from the primary auditory cortex, citing a study by Celesia and Puletti (1971) who failed to detect a temporal correspondence between the scalp-recorded MLR sequence and responses recorded from the exposed human primary auditory cortex. The results of a recent clinical study of patients with confirmed cortical lesions (Kraus et al, 1982) suggested, however, a bilateral temporal lobe contribution to the Pa component of the MLR. This study will be discussed further, later on in this chapter.

THE LATE VERTEX AER

Latency Characteristics

The late vertex auditory evoked response occurs within a poststimulus latency range of 50 to 500 msec, and it is considered to be generated by the frontal association and/or the primary auditory cortex (Picton et al, 1974). In waking adults it consists of a vertex-negative peak with a latency of 80 to 110 msec (N1) followed by a positive peak at 160 to 180 msec (P2). In sleep, P2 is delayed to approximately 200 msec, a prominent N2 appears at approximately 300 msec, and N1 is markedly diminished or disappears (Davis, 1976; Kevanishvili and Von Specht, 1979). The latencies of the waking LVAER components have been reported to be longer and more variable in infants and children of preschool age and to assume a more typical configuration in this age range during sedative-induced sleep. Under these conditions they were reported to be characterized by a prominent positive polarity peak with an approximate latency of 300 msec (Skinner and Atinoro, 1969).

Reference Electrode Sites

Wolpaw and Wood (1982) have demonstrated that some often utilized reference sites for late vertex AEP recording, such as the nose, ear, and mastoid processes, were located within the AEP field and were characterized by significant voltage gradients.

They found minimal voltage gradients over the lower neck. In order to avoid recording the results of potential field changes at both the active and reference electrode sites they recommended the use of the balanced sternovertebral reference of Stephenson and Gibbs (1951). This reference is both well outside the field of the AEP and also relatively free of EKG artifact in adults. However, in this author's experience the sternovertebral reference is contraindicated because it introduces large EKG artifacts in newborn infants.

Generator Sources

The N1 and P2 components are considered to be "nonspecific" components of the auditory evoked response mediated by the reticular formation. The cortex and scalp-recorded components occurring within this time frame correlate reasonably well and are diffusely distributed. Unlike the "specific" components, the nonspecific components are significantly affected by general anesthesia and habituate with repeated stimulation (Davis et al, 1966; Celesia et al, 1968). An extensive mapping study (Wood and Wolpaw, 1982) utilizing a noncephalic reference suggested that in adults the scalp-recorded neuroelectrical activity elicited by auditory stimulation occurring between 60 and 250 msec is generated by several generator sources, with their activity overlapping in time. These sources may include auditory structures located on both the superior and lateral cortical planes. A study of the distribution of auditory magnetic fields produced by the human brain and measured perpendicular to the scalp revealed a striking similarity between magnetic and electric evoked responses (Hari et al, 1980). This study also localized the magnetic equivalent of the neuroelectric N100 bilaterally at the superior surface of the temporal lobe at the primary auditory cortex.

Maturational Changes

The late vertex auditory evoked response undergoes maturational changes consisting of latency reductions and modifications of the amplitude ratios of the N1, P2, and N2 components. By 4 months of age, a complete maturation of the responses is reached according to Davis and Onishi (1969). Ohlrich et al (1978) studied the late vertex auditory evoked responses during sleep in 16 children from early infancy to 3 yr of age. They found an overall decrease of component latencies and increases of peak amplitudes with age. The latencies of P2 and N2 exhibited the least amount of intersubject variability across ages.

Figure 6.2 illustrates a late vertex AER (LVAER) elicited from a waking adult by 1000-Hz tone pips presented at 60 dB HL. The response consists of a typical P60 (P1)-

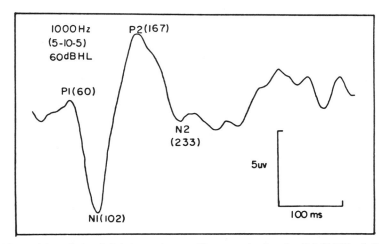

Figure 6.2. Normal (awake) adult late vertex auditory evoked potential (AEP) elicited by a 60 dB HL, 1000 Hz toneburst presented monaurally at a rate of 1.3/sec. Electrode placement: vertex-ipsilateral mastoid. In this and subsequent figures positive polarity of the response is plotted as an upward deflection. Filter setting: 1 to 30 Hz (12 dB/oct slope).

N102 (N1)-P167 (P2) (P and N designate positive and negative polarity peaks, respectively) peak sequence. Figure 6.3A illustrates LVAERs elicited from a sleeping 4-week-old infant by identical stimuli. Both replications (a and b) are characterized by a P65-N108-P219 peak sequence. The second replication (b) is identical to the first one (a) in the latency and polarity of its major peaks; however, its amplitude is reduced overall, and it is less "smooth" in appearance. Response "b" was obtained as the baby began showing signs of awakening and moving slightly. This may account for the difference between "a" and "b," in particular the addition of some high-frequency energy to "b" that gives it a slightly less smooth appearance resulting from previously absent myogenic activity. The difference between "a" and "b" also underlines an important aspect of late AER recording: the configuration of the late AER depends to a great extent upon the general state of the subject and one of its electrophysiological manifestations, the electroencephalogram (EEG). Therefore, in order to collect a replicable series of late AERs the individual samples must all originate from reasonably similar EEG background activities. In addition, if the neuroelectrical activity segments summed for a late AER originate from varying EEG backgrounds, one may fail to obtain a recognizable evoked potential pattern. This problem does not apply to the earlier brainstem auditory evoked responses, where one operates well outside the frequency spectrum range of the ongoing EEG. One way to overcome this problem in late AER work is to monitor the ongoing EEG at the recording sites used for AER recording by means of an oscilloscope or a strip chart recorder.

Figure 6.3B illustrates replicated LVAERs elicited from a sleeping 3-day-old newborn baby by 60 dB HL, 1000-Hz tonebursts. The major peaks in this response are P72-N144-P258. It is interesting to note the differences between the responses illustrated in Figures 6.2, 6.3A, and 6.3B. The major difference between the response elicited from the waking adult and that of the sleeping 4-week-old infant is the latency of P2 (167 msec vs 219 msec). This difference may be the consequence of both maturation and difference in state. The responses obtained from the 3-day-old (6.3B) were essentially a replica of the responses obtained from the 4-week-old, with an overall delay of 40 msec.

Effect of Barbiturates

While it is recognized that the cortical auditory evoked potential undergoes modifications following the administration of barbiturates, it is not completely abolished except under deep anesthesia. Barbiturates may induce the following modifications: increased or attenuated peak amplitudes, changes in peak latencies, and the disappearance of some components or all components with deep anesthesia (Kiang et al, 1961; Pradhan and Galambos, 1963; Teas and Kiang, 1964; Borbely and Hall, 1970). Teas and Kiang (1964) found that localized lesions to the auditory cortex of cats affected the early components of the auditory evoked response complex. The later components were more likely to be affected by the state of the animal (i.e., sleep or barbiturate anesthesia).

P-300: AN EVENT-RELATED POTENTIAL

Additional so-called "cognitive" components beyond P2 may be elicited by stimulus paradigms that necessitate more than passive listening. Thus, a P300 (or P3) component may be elicited by low probability (target) stimuli presented against a background of higher probability nontarget stimuli. This paradigm may be combined with a task requiring the subject to keep a mental record of, or to respond to, the low probability target stimuli. The P300 is not stimulus-modality-specific, as it can be elicited across different sensory modalities. It is also an "endogenous" potential, i.e., it may be elicited by stimuli that are missing from a sequence, if the absence of a stimulus is task-significant (Tueting, 1978). Roth (1978) advocated the use of the term "late positive waves" (LPW) to refer to a series of positive waves following P2 related to the detection of low probability target stimuli. Roth distinguished several components within the LPW: (1) P3a, the earliest component, sometimes merged with P2 or appeared as an independent peak as late as 300 msec. It was elicited by rare target stimuli unrelated to a task. (2) P3b (latency 300 to 400 msec)

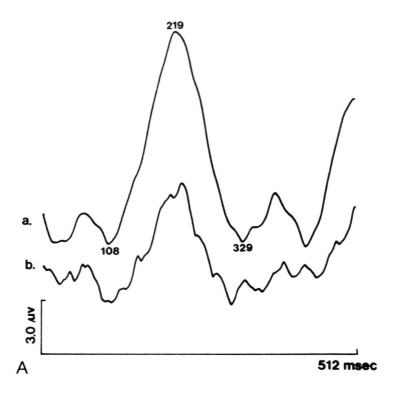

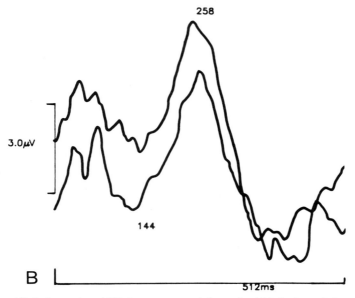

Figure 6.3. (*A*) Late vertex AEP from a normal 4-week-old infant. *a*, Asleep. *b*, In the process of waking. N1-108 msec; P2-219 msec; N2-329 msec. (*B*) Late vertex AEP from a 3-day-old infant.

was elicited by rare task-relevant stimuli. (3) A "positive missing stimulus potential" (mean latency 465 msec) was elicited when the targets consisted of low probability omitted stimuli. The latency of P3 was reported to decrease with age between 6 and 15 yr and to increase with advancing age in adults (Goodin et al, 1978; Pfefferbaum et al, 1980). The amplitude of the N2-P3 component was reported to decrease with age by Goodin et al (1978). Figure 6.4 illustrates auditory ERP complexes elicited from an 18-yr-old (*A*) and a 58-yr-old subject (*B*). These responses were elicited by 1500 Hz target stimuli (20%) presented in a background of frequent (80%) 1000 Hz nontarget stimuli. The subjects, both with no history

of neurological disease, were asked to keep a mental record of the target stimuli and report their number at the end of the session. The event-related potentials (ERPs) elicited by the nontarget stimuli (frequent, 1000 Hz) are characterized for both the 18-yr-old (Fig. 6.4*A*) and the 58-yr-old (Fig. 6.4*B*) subjects by N1 and P2 components. The latency of P2 is relatively delayed for the younger subject, at 207 msec. This may be due to the presence of a small P3 component blended with P2 in the response elicited by the nontarget stimuli. The response elicited by the target stimuli (rare) is characterized by well-resolved N1, P2 (latency 165 msec), and P3 component peaks. As indicated by Goodin et al (1978) and Pfefferbaum et al (1980),

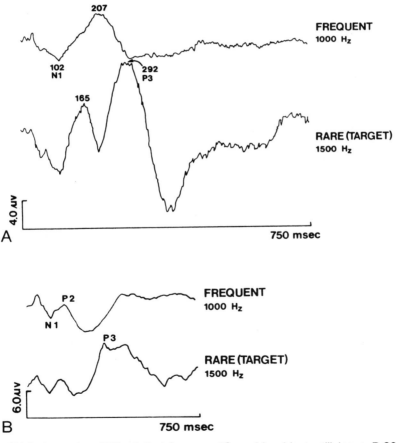

Figure 6.4. (*A*) Late vertex AEP elicited from an 18-yr-old subject utilizing a P-300 (cognitive) paradigm. Top trace consists of N1-102 msec and P2-207 msec components and was elicited by the frequent nontarget stimuli. Bottom trace, elicited by the rare target stimuli, consists of N1, P2, N2, and P3 components. Both target and nontarget stimuli were presented at 60 dB HL and were gated with rise-fall times of 9 msec and a plateau of 20 msec. Electrode placement: vertex-linked mastoids. Filters: 1 to 100 Hz (*B*) Late vertex AEP elicited from a normal 58-yr-old subject utilizing a P-300 paradigm. Stimulus and recording parameters as in *A*.

P3 was delayed in the older subject with respect to the younger subject (348 msec measured at the leading edge of the P3 peak).

CLINICAL APPLICATIONS OF MLR AND LVAER

Several recent studies have investigated the clinical applications of the later (MLR, LVAER) components of the auditory evoked response.

Based on a study of neurologically impaired, multiply handicapped children (some with **hypsarrhythmic** EEGs) Cohen and Rapin (1978) regarded the early (brainstem) and the late auditory evoked potentials as "complementary methods." In some of the cases described by these authors there were major discrepancies between the early brainstem (reflecting normal peripheral auditory thresholds) and late cortical (absent or elicited at high suprathreshold levels only) auditory evoked responses.

MLR

There have been conflicting reports in the literature concerning the effects of temporal lobe lesions on the MLR. Parving et al (1980) reported on a patient with auditory agnosia and documented bilateral temporal lobe lesions who exhibited normal MLRs (Pa latency = 30 msec). On the other hand, Özdamar et al (1982) reported on a patient who also presented with bilateral temporal lobe lesions, inconsistent awareness of sound, and impaired pure tone sensitivity whose MLRs were abnormal (Pa was missing bilaterally). Based on their respective results, the two groups of investigators arrived at opposite conclusions regarding the role of the primary auditory cortex in the generation of the MLR. In another case study (Michel et al, 1980), bilateral lesions involving the supratemporal planes resulted in an absence of LVAERs. The MLRs were not elicited in this study.

Kraus et al (1982) studied the effects of temporal lobe lesions on the MLR in 24 patients. They found that a unilateral temporal lobe lesion diminished the amplitude of the vertex-recorded Pa without affecting its latency. Pa was more significantly reduced or absent, however, over the involved

hemisphere. They concluded that the vertex-recorded MLR reflects contributions from symmetrical bilateral generators. Under normal circumstances, their electrical activity is summed at the vertex. With a unilateral lesion, the vertex response will be diminished due to a reduction of the contribution originating from the affected side.

Two of our patients (Kileny and Berry, 1983) had confirmed bilateral temporal lobe lesions. (1) A 33-month-old male had bilateral temporal lobe infarcts secondary to a severe **anoxic** episode (accidental suffocation) at 6 months of age. (2) A 7-month-old male infant with convulsive disorder, irritability, and spastic quadriplegia secondary to severe birth asphyxia had **cystic** changes in the temporal regions and dilated lateral and third ventricles. Both patients exhibited normal ABRs elicited by 60 and 20 dB HL clicks. In the first case, MLRs were absent at initial testing at 11 months of age. At 33 months, some partially replicable activity was detected in the Pa latency range. Maturation may have been a significant factor in this case. In the second case the MLRs were not impaired.

LVAER

A recent report (Kileny and Berry, 1983) dealt with 15 patients aged 6 weeks to 15 yr with evidence of neurological involvement (12 were aged 8 to 20 months at initial evaluation). Hypoxia or anoxia were primary factors in 13 patients. Age-appropriate behavioral audiological testing resulted in either no response whatsoever to a variety of auditory stimuli or in elevated threshold estimates in these patients. However, the auditory brainstem responses indicated normal bilateral peripheral auditory sensitivity in all but two cases, where slight or mild peripheral hearing impairments were found. Waves I through V were present in all cases. In 11 of these 15 patients the late vertex auditory evoked response (LVAER) was absent. In the remaining four the LVAER had an abnormal configuration (i.e., a reversal of polarity). In all cases the LVAER was elicited by supra-ABR-threshold stimuli. In each one of the 15 patients CT scan and/or EEG results were abnormal. However, it must be pointed out that in spite of the common auditory evoked response configuration, the specific EEG and CT scan diagnoses differed widely among the 15 patients. Knight et al (1980) found that the amplitude of the N1 component of the LVAER was reduced consistently with well-defined and well-documented unilateral temporoparietal lesions. Such accurate lesion localization did not occur in our patients. One fairly homogenous subgroup consisted of four patients in whom a generalized cortical atrophy was diagnosed on CT scan, and the LVAER was absent. In general, improvements in LVAER correlated well with behavioral responses to auditory stimuli.

P-300

The P3 component of the auditory (or other sensory modality) ERP originates from nonmodality-specific unknown neural generators. It is an electrophysiological manifestation of strategies employed by the central nervous system informing us about an individual's attentive abilities. Because of the nature of this electrophysiological response, we cannot expect it to provide the kind of direct, no nonsense information provided by the earlier evoked potentials, such as the ABR. A comparison of P3 in the target and the nontarget channel could provide information about an individual's potential to disregard irrelevant competing information, or, in other words, his selective attention capabilities. Thus, a reduced or delayed P3 elicited by the target stimuli may suggest deficiencies of later stages of processing (Hillyard et al, 1978). So far the clinical observations of P3 have been limited to a great extent to psychopathology and aging. Thus Roth et al (1981) found that P3 was of normal latency but reduced amplitude in schizophrenia. Squires et al (1982) found delayed P3 latencies in patients with dementia of various etiologies. At the same time, P3 latency was within normal limits in nondemented patients with various neurological impairments and in nondemented psychiatric patients.

CASE STUDIES

Case 1

A 71-yr-old lady suddenly developed speech difficulties during a bridge game 5 days prior to admission to the hospital. Previous history included hypertensive retinopathy and two myocardial infarcts that occurred approximately 7 yr prior to her present ailment. A neurological examination revealed slightly increased reflexes on the right side, Babinski-type plantar responses, some right arm drift, and an unsteady gait. Fine coordination was intact bilaterally. Results of a CT scan, augmented brain scan, and angiographic studies were all compatible with a deeply located left temporal-frontal infarction.

Psychological and language-speech evaluations revealed impairments of recent and short-term memory, mild mixed aphasia, and mild word finding difficulties. An audiological evaluation indicated a bilateral high-frequency mild to moderate hearing loss, with excellent speech discrimination scores bilaterally.

Figure 6.5 illustrates middle latency auditory evoked responses elicited by left ear stimulation and recorded simultaneously from four scalp locations from this patient (left-hand column) and for comparison, responses elicited by the same paradigm from a normal control subject (right-hand column). The following active electrode locations, all in the central coronal plane, were utilized (International 10–20 system, Jasper, 1958): right parietal, just above the sylvian fissure (C6), vertex (CZ), left parietal above the sylvian fissure (C5), and left temporal below the sylvian fissure (T3). All leads were referenced to linked ear lobes, and the ground electrode was attached to the forehead. As suggested by Kraus et al (1982), the ABR was present at all leads, and Pa was largest at the vertex and quite symmetrical above the right and the left sylvian fissures (C6 and C5) in the normal subject. It is of interest to note that the response obtained from the subsylvian electrode (T3) was diminished in amplitude with respect to the C5 (suprasylvian) response, unlike in the earlier mentioned case of the late vertex response (Vaughan and Ritter, 1970). The MLRs elicited from the patient may be summarized as follows. The brainstem response and a prominent Po (probably significant postauricular muscle response contribution) are present at all four leads. Although somewhat blended together with Po, Pa is well-defined at the vertex. Pa is reduced in amplitude at all other leads, especially those over the left hemisphere. The response obtained from the left subsylvian lead (T3) exhibited the most reduced Pa (Pa amplitudes measured relative to Na suggested by Kraus et al (1982)). The MLRs obtained from this case confirm the Kraus et al (1982) observations that the Pa peak of the MLR is most significantly diminished when recorded over the affected hemisphere. While Kraus et al (1982) did not record below the sylvian fissure, in this author's experience, and as indicated by this case, a recording site

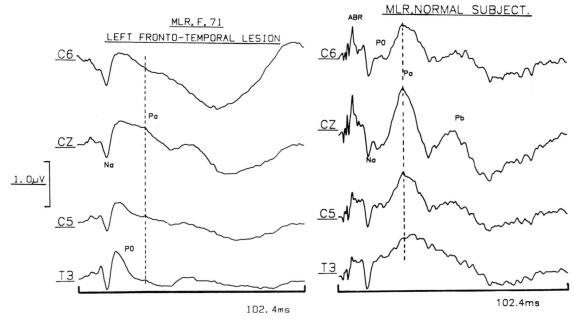

Figure 6.5. MLRs recorded simultaneously at four electrode locations (detail in text) from a neurologically normal control subject (*right*) and a 71-yr-old patient with a deep left frontotemporal lesion (case 1). 60 dB HL clicks presented to the left ear at a rate of 10/sec for both cases.

below the sylvian fissure (i.e., T3) may be even more sensitive to MLR alterations induced by unilateral lesions involving the temporal lobe.

Case 2

A 35-yr-old man was admitted to the hospital because of headaches and the onset of left hemiparesis. The patient had a 15-yr history of right-sided migraine headaches. A CT scan of the brain performed on the day of admission identified a cerebral infarction involving the right hemisphere. A cerebral angiography done 3 days later identified the presence of multiple cerebrovascular anomalies: the right cerebral artery and the posterior parietal and angular vessels were absent. Collateral circulation was established through the posterior cerebral vessels. A congenital absence of the left posteroinferior cerebellar artery was also noted. Edema affecting the right temporoparietal region and a slight shift of midline structures from right to left were noted on a CT scan done 2 weeks following admission.

A routine audiological evaluation indicated normal pure tone thresholds bilaterally up to 2000 Hz and a symmetrical bilateral mild high-frequency hearing loss affecting the frequency range of 4000 to 8000 Hz. Speech discrimination scores were excellent bilaterally (100%). A speech language assessment performed 6 weeks following admission revealed normal receptive and expres-

sive language skills and an absence of speech motor problems.

Figure 6.6 illustrates middle latency auditory evoked responses elicited by right ear stimulation

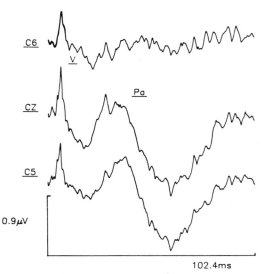

Figure 6.6. MLRs recorded simultaneously at three electrode locations from a 35-yr-old patient with a right temporoparietal lesion. 60 dB HL clicks presented to the right ear at a rate of 10/sec (case 2).

and recorded simultaneously from three scalp locations: right parietal, just above the sylvian fissure (C6), vertex (CZ), and left parietal (C5). As in the case illustrated in Figure 6.5, all leads were referenced to linked ear lobes. A prominent wave V was recorded at all electrode locations. Po did not resolve at any of the electrode locations. Pa was absent on the right side (C6) and was well-defined both at the vertex (CZ) and on the left side. This case further confirms the observations published by Kraus et al (1982): an absence or amplitude reduction of Pa over the hemisphere with an affected temporal lobe with a well-defined Pa at vertex and over the contralateral hemisphere. It is noteworthy that this patient presented with no communicative handicap as noted by himself and as indicated by the results of speech, language, and hearing assessments. Thus, unlike case 1 (left temporal-frontal infarction), in case 2 (right temporal-parietal infarction) the MLR impairment was not associated with a communicative handicap. The unilateral absence or impairment of MLR component Pa in both cases, along with the results of the series described by Kraus et al (1982), establish a connection between the adult human temporal lobe and Pa.

Case 3

The following is the case of a female patient first seen at 6 months of age. She was born at term by cesarean section because of cephalopelvic disproportion. Birth weight was 2730 g, with Apgar scores of 3 and 7. An absence of voluntary respiration during the neonatal period necessitated artificial ventilation and oxygen. At 4 months of age she was admitted to the hospital with seizures. The EEG was characterized by spikes in right posterior and central temporal areas. A CT scan revealed ventricular enlargement and a prominence of the sylvian and interhemispheric fissures, suggesting cerebral atrophy. The seizures persisted in spite of administration of phenobarbital and Dilantin. General language level was between 0 to 3 months.

Figure 6.7 illustrates brainstem responses from the left ear (A) elicited by broadband clicks (17.1/sec) at 60, 40, and 20 dB HL. Identical brainstem responses indicating normal peripheral hearing sensitivity with peak and interpeak latencies within normal limits were also elicited from the right ear. The late vertex responses, elicited by 1000 Hz tone bursts presented at 60 dB HL (Fig. 6.7B), were judged to be absent: the two stimulus runs exhibited no specific recognizable pattern, did not replicate, and were not significantly different from the silent control run (C).

Case 4

Figure 6.8 illustrates the late vertex auditory evoked responses obtained at 17 months of age

from a female patient who was born to a hypoparathyroid and diabetic mother who was on insulin during her pregnancy. The child was born with multiple congenital anomalies, including a hypoplastic mandible and cleft palate. She was diagnosed as presenting with a caudal regression syndrome. In addition, she had numerous episodes of asphyxia. A CT scan performed at 6 weeks of age revealed slightly enlarged ventricles. An EEG done at 3 months of age (while the patient was on phenobarbital and Dilantin) was considered to be normal. She was referred to audiology at 11 months of age, at which time there were no consistent responses to sound, with the exception of a possible orientation response to white noise presented at 85 dB HL. The tympanograms suggested some middle ear involvement. Auditory evoked potential studies performed at this time revealed the following: brainstem responses were within normal limits with 30 dB HL unfiltered click thresholds bilaterally, whereas the LVAERs had an unusual configuration characterized by replicable positive polarity peaks at a poststimulus latency of 80 msec. This patient was seen again at 17 months of age. She was still unable to suck or swallow and was fed through a nasogastric tube. The foster mother reported some vocalization, very inconsistent responses to sound, and no attempt whatsoever at imitation. The patient startled to voice at 65 dB HL and responded inconsistently in the sound field during visual reinforcement audiometry to warble tones at 30 dB HL. Tympanograms were within normal limits bilaterally. The LVAERs were again characterized by a replicable positive polarity peak, with a latency of 101 msec as illustrated in Figure 6.8.

A reversal of polarity of the late vertex auditory evoked response was described as occurring when the active electrode was moved from above to below the sylvian fissure (Vaughan and Ritter, 1970). The explanation of this phenomenon is that above and below the sylvian fissure the electrode is charged by opposite poles of the dipole which consists of the primary auditory cortical projection in the superior surface of the temporal lobe. If one accepts this explanation, the polarity inversion in some of our patients could be due to topographical or morphological changes in the generator of the LVAER; hence, our vertex electrode may record from the opposite pole of a dipole instead of the standard, expected one. Another explanation for this response configuration is that it could be the result of an immature generator: similar LVAERs have been recorded from premature infants (Barnet et al, 1975).

Case 5

Figure 6.9 illustrates auditory evoked potential data from a 53-yr-old male with anoxic enceph-

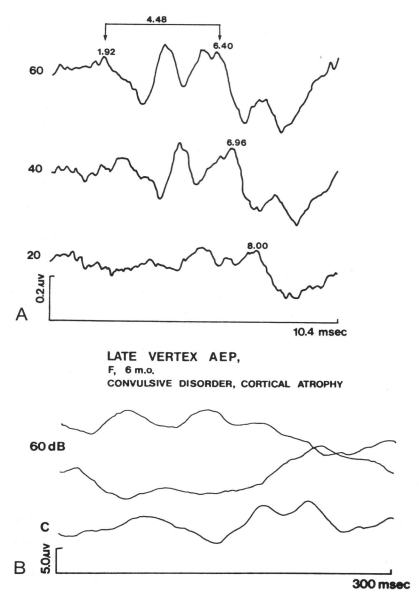

Figure 6.7. Brainstem responses elicited by 60-, 40-, and 20 dB HL clicks (*A*) and late vertex AEP (*B*) elicited by 60 dB HL 1000 Hz tonebursts from a 6-month-old female with convulsive disorder and cortical atrophy (case 3). Electrode placement: vertex-ear lobe. (From Kileny P, Robertson C: Neurological aspects of infant hearing assessment. *J Otolaryngol* 14(Suppl. 14):34, 1985.)

alopathy secondary to cardiac arrest. The patient was in a coma for 5 weeks with an extremely guarded prognosis. He came out of coma with signs of Wernicke-type aphasia and profound oral apraxia. There was still evidence of severe dysphasia following several weeks of intensive speech-language therapy. Brainstem responses were elicited by unfiltered clicks presented monaurally. The responses elicited from the right and

left ears (Fig. 6.9*A*, responses from the left) were symmetrical and exhibited a normal configuration, with an I–V interpeak interval of 4.32 msec. Figure 6.9*B* illustrates auditory ERPs elicited by 1500 Hz target stimuli (20%) presented binaurally in a background of 1000 Hz tonebursts (80%) (rise-fall times 9.9 msec, plateau 20 msec, 60 dB, HL). This response is characterized by an N1 component (120 msec), a P2 component (177

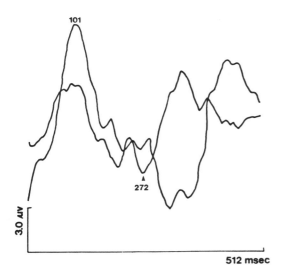

LATE VERTEX AEP,
F, 17 m.o.
MULTIPLE CONGENITAL ANOMALIES

101

272

3.0 µV

512 msec

Figure 6.8. Unusual configuration late vertex AEP from a 17-month-old female patient with caudal regression syndrome and a history of numerous asphyxial episodes (case 4). Electrode placement: vertex-mastoid.

msec), and a relatively small P3 component (377 msec). In fact, P3 is nearly absent in one of the two replications (see *target* traces). It is interesting to note that, in spite of being quite disoriented, this pleasant and cooperative patient performed the task, consisting of keeping a mental record of the target stimuli, with reasonable accuracy: for the first run (the one characterized by the smaller P3) he reported 77 target stimuli when in reality a total of 105 (five traces rejected due to artifacts) were presented. For the second run, he reported 101 target stimuli for a total of 117 presented. Let us compare these responses to those obtained from a normal subject of similar age (Fig. 6.4*B*). The normal subject's response to the target stimuli (*target*) is characterized by a large P3 and a smaller P2 component, while in the case of the patient there is a small P3 and a relatively larger P2. Whereas in the case of the normal subject P3 is virtually absent for the frequent nontarget stimuli, in the case of the patient, the very small P3 in one of the target traces is equivalent to the P3 component of the nontarget (frequent) traces. Both in the normal subject and in the patient the latency of P3 is within the normal range for the 6th decade as reported by Squires et al (1982). The N2–P3 amplitude was reduced in our patient with respect to the norm in the 6th decade (4.0 and 7.0 vs 10.00) (Goodin et al, 1978).

The results of the evoked potential studies in this patient may be summarized as follows: (1) With the exception of a possible slight prolongation of the I–V interpeak interval (4.32 msec is still within the accepted normal range), the auditory brainstem responses were within normal limits. (2) All the components of the late auditory evoked response were present, including P3. However, there were some subtle deviations: N1 was slightly delayed; P2 dominated the response elicited by the cognitive paradigm; P3 was relatively small and was not much enhanced in response to the target stimuli in comparison to the nontarget stimuli (this may suggest difficulty in disregarding irrelevant competing information). More studies involving brain-injured patients are needed to elucidate the possible diagnostic and prognostic significance of these subtle deviations.

Conclusions

Several conclusions may be drawn from this chapter. First, the battery approach in auditory evoked potential work with children and infants with proven or suspected brain lesions provides meaningful information about the status of their auditory function. It is risky to equate functional hearing abilities with ABR results in neurologically impaired patients: such practice may provide misleading results. In those cases, as recommended by Cohen and Rapin (1978), a careful investigation with a complete evoked response battery is warranted. The ABR serves to rule out a peripheral hearing loss. The LVAER and the MLR elicited by suprathreshold stimuli assess the integrity of the higher auditory centers.

Inasmuch as the brainstem components of the auditory evoked response reflect neuroelectrical activation of the peripheral portion of the auditory pathway, the ABR alone may provide misleading results when dealing with cases with possible central lesions. While at the moment there is not much we can offer the patient with central auditory dysfunction, a different course of intervention would be indicated in those cases than in cases with a peripheral hearing impairment. There are benefits in the use of auditory evoked responses beyond the ABR (MLR and LVAER) in patients with positively proven or suspected diffuse or localized brain lesions. The ABR alone may not provide sufficient diagnostic information in these cases. The presence of MLRs and

ABR

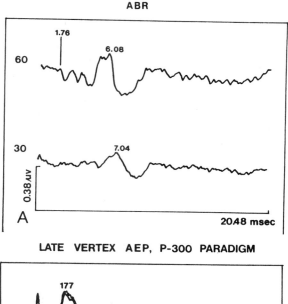

LATE VERTEX AEP, P-300 PARADIGM

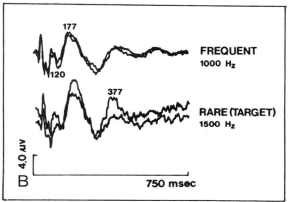

Figure 6.9. Auditory brainstem responses (*A*) and late vertex auditory evoked responses (*B*) elicited by a P-300 paradigm from a 53-yr-old male with anoxic encephalopathy secondary to cardiac arrest (case 4). Electrode placement: vertex-mastoid (linked mastoids for the P-300 paradigm) (case 5).

LVAERs in addition to normal ABR thresholds would provide strong evidence of normal peripheral and central auditory function. In our experience, if the LVAER is utilized strictly as a suprathreshold device, its status will correlate well with central dysfunction (Kileny and Berry, 1983).

In the future the auditory evoked response battery, including the cognitive components such as P3, may be used to monitor progress in patients with CNS impairment following various habilitative interventions. More information may be derived with multiple electrode measurements. As the imaging techniques become more and more sophisticated, there may be better correspondence between specific sites of lesions and the results of evoked potential studies.

References

Barnet AB, Ohlrich ES, Weiss IP, Shanks B: Auditory evoked potentials during sleep in normal children from ten days to three years of age. *Electroencephalogr Clin Neurophysiol* 39:29–41, 1975.

Borbely AA, Hall RD: Effects of pentobarbitone and chlorpromazine on acoustically evoked potentials in the rat. *Neuropharmacology* 9:575–586, 1970.

Brazier MAB: the neurophysiological background of anesthesia. Springfield, IL, Charles C Thomas, 1972, ch 5, pp 82–117.

Celesia GG, Broughton RJ, Rasmussen TH, Branch C: Auditory evoked responses from the exposed human cortex. *Electroencephalogr Clin Neurophysiol* 24:458–466, 1968.

Celesia GG, Puletti F: Auditory input to the human cortex during drowsiness and surgical anesthesia. *Electroencephalogr Clin Neurophysiol* 31:603–609, 1971.

Cohen MM, Rapin I: Evoked potential audiometry in neurologically impaired children. In Naunton R, Zerlin S, (eds): *Evoked Electrical Activity in the Auditory Nervous System.* New York, Academic Press, 1978, pp 551–572.

Davis H: Principles of electric response audiometry. *Ann Otol Rhinol Laryngol* 28(suppl):1–96, 1976.

Davis H, Mast T, Yoshie N, Zerlin S: The slow response of the human cortex to auditory stimuli: recovery process. *Electroencephalogr Clin Neurophysiol* 21: 105–113, 1966.

Davis H, Onishi S: Maturation of auditory evoked potentials. Int Audiol 8:24–33, 1969.

Geisler CD, Frishkopf LS, Brown RM: The 'early' response to clicks in awake subjects. *Quarterly Progress Report, Research Laboratory of Electronics, MIT*, July 15, 1957, pp 144–148.

Goodin DS, Squires KC, Henderson BH, Starr A: Age-related variations in evoked potentials to auditory stimuli in normal human subjects. *Electroencephalogr Clin Neurophysiol* 44:447–458, 1978.

Hari R, Aittoniemi K, Järvinen M-L, Katila T, Varpula T: Auditory evoked transient and sustained magnetic fields of the human brain. *Exp Brain Res* 40:237–240, 1980.

Harker LA, Hosick E, Voots RJ, Mendel MI: Influence of succinylcholine on middle component auditory evoked potentials. *Arch Otolaryngol*, 103:133–137, 1977.

Heath RG, Galbraith GC: Sensory evoked responses recorded simultaneously from human cortex and scalp. *Nature* 212:1535–1537, 1966.

Hillyard SA, Picton TW, Regan D: Sensation, perception and attention: analysis using ERPs. In Callaway E, Tueting P, Koslow SH (eds): *Event-Related Brain Potentials in Man.* New York, Academic Press, 1978, pp 223–322.

Jasper HH: The ten twenty electrode system of the International Federation. *Electroencephalogr Clin Neurophysiol* 10:371–375, 1958.

Kevanishvili Z Sh, Von Specht H: Human slow auditory evoked potentials during natural and drug-induced sleep. *Electroencephalogr Clin Neurophysiol* 47:280–288, 1979.

Kiang NYS, Neame JH, Clark LF: Evoked cortical activity from auditory cortex in anesthetized and unanesthetized cats. *Science* 13:1927–1928, 1961.

Kileny P: Auditory evoked middle latency responses: current issues. *Semin Hear* 4:403–413, 1983.

Kileny P, Berry DA: Selective impairment of late vertex and middle latency auditory evoked responses in multiply handicapped infants and children. In Mencher G, Gerber S (eds): *The Multiply Handicapped Hearing Impaired Child,* New York, Grune & Stratton, 1983, pp 233–258.

Kileny P, Dobson D, Gelfand ET: Middle-latency auditory evoked responses during open-heart surgery with hypothermia. *Electroencephalogr Clin Neurophysiol* 55:268–276, 1983.

Kileny P, Robertson CMT: Neurological aspects of infant hearing assessment. *J. Otolaryngol* 14(Suppl 14):34, 1985.

Knight RT, Hillyard SA, Woods DL, Neville HJ: The effects of frontal and temporal-parietal lesions on the auditory evoked potential in man. *Electroencephalogr Clin Neurophysiol* 50:112–124, 1980.

Kraus N, Özdamar Ö, Hier D, Stein L: Auditory middle latency responses (MLRs) in patients with cortical lesions. *Electroencephalogr Clin Neurophysiol* 54: 275–287, 1982.

Mendelson T, Salamy A: Maturational effects on the middle components of the averaged electroencephalic response. *J Speech Hearing Res* 46:140–144, 1981.

Michel F, Peronnet F, Schott B: A case of cortical deafness: clinical and electro-physiological data. *Brain Lang* 10:367–377, 1980.

Ohlrich ES, Barnett AB, Weiss IP, Shanks BL: Auditory evoked potential development in early childhood: a longitudinal study. *Electroencephalogr Clin Neurophysiol* 44:411–423, 1978.

Özdamar Ö, Kraus N: Auditory middle-latency responses in humans. *Audiology* 13:195–204, 1983.

Özdamar Ö, Kraus N, Curry F: Auditory brainstem and middle latency responses in a patient with cortical deafness. *Electroencephalogr Clin Neurophysiol* 53:224–230, 1982.

Parving A, Solomon G, Elberling C, Larsen B, Lassen NA: Middle components of the auditory evoked response in bilateral temporal lobe lesions. *Scand Audiol* 9:161–167, 1980.

Peters JF, Mendel MI: Early components of the averaged electroencephalic response to monaural and binaural stimulation. *Audiology* 13:195–204, 1974.

Pfefferbaum A, Ford JM, Roth WT, Kopell BS: Age-related changes in auditory event-related potentials. *Electroencephalogr Clin Neurophysiol* 49:266–276, 1980.

Picton TW, Hillyard SA, Kraus HI, Galambos R: Human auditory evoked potentials. I. Evaluation of components. *Electroencephalogr Clin Neurophysiol* 36:179–190, 1974.

Picton TW, Woods DL, Baribeau-Braun J, Healey TL: Evoked potential audiometry. *J Otolaryngol* 6:90–119, 1977.

Pradhan SN, Galambos R: Some effects of anesthetics on the evoked responses in the auditory cortex of cats. *J Pharmacol Exp Ther* 139:97–106, 1963.

Puletti F, Celesia GG: Functional properties of the primary cortical auditory area in man. *J Neurosurg* 32:244–247, 1970.

Roth WT: How many late positive waves are there? In Otto DA (ed): *Multidisciplinary Perspectives in Event-Related Brain Potential Research.* Washington, DC, US Environmental Protection Agency, 1978, pp 170–172.

Roth W, Pfefferbaum A, Kelly A, Berger P, Kopel B: Auditory event related potentials in schizophrenia and depression. *Psychiatry Res* 4:199–212, 1981.

Scherg M: Distortion of the middle latency auditory response produced by analog filtering. *Scand Audiol* 11:57–60, 1982.

Skinner P, Atinoro F: Auditory evoked responses in normal hearing adults and children before and during sedation. *J Speech Hear Res* 12:394–401, 1969.

Sprague BH, Thornton A: Clinical utility and limitations of middle-latency auditory-evoked potentials. Toronto. American Speech-Language-Hearing Association, 1982.

Squires KC, Chippendale TJ, Wrege KS, Goodin DS, Starr A: Electrophysiological assessment of mental function in aging and dementia. In *Aging in the 1980's: Psychological Issues.* Washington, DC, American Psychological Association, 1982, pp 125–134.

Stephenson WA, Gibbs FA: A balanced non-cephalic reference electrode. *Electroencephalogr Clin Neurophysiol* 3:237–240, 1951.

Teas DC, Kiang NYS: Evoked responses from the auditory cortex. *Exp Neurol* 10: 91–119,1964.

Tueting P: Event-related potentials cognitive events and information processing: a summary of issues and discussion. In Otto DA (ed): *Multidisciplinary Perspectives in Event-Related Brain Potential Research.* Washington, DC, US Environmental Protection Agency, 1978, pp 159–169.

Vaughan HG, Ritter W: The sources of auditory evoked responses recorded from the human scalp. *Electroencephalogr Clin Neurophysiol* 28:360–367, 1970.

Vivion MC: Clinical status of evoked response audiometry. *Laryngoscope* 90:437–447, 1980.

Wolpaw JR, Wood CC: Scalp distribution of human auditory evoked potentials. I. Evaluation of reference electrode sites. *Electroencephalogr Clin Neurophysiol* 54:15–24, 1982.

Wood CC, Wolpaw JR: Scalp distribution of human auditory evoked potentials. II. Evidence for overlapping sources and involvement of auditory cortex. *Electroencephalogr Clin Neurophysiol* 54:25–38, 1982.

CHAPTER 7

The Acoustic Reflex in Central Auditory Dysfunction

JAMES W. HALL, III, Ph.D.

This chapter by Dr. Hall discusses the principles and methodology of acoustic reflex measurements and the factors that influence them. He then describes the acoustic reflex in nerve VIII and intraaxial and extraaxial brainstem pathologies with case examples.

Clinical application of acoustic impedance (immittance) audiometry was first comprehensively described by Metz in 1946. Subsequently, tympanometry and measurement of static compliance and the acoustic reflex became integrated into an effective test battery for objective assessment of middle ear function (Hall and Jerger, 1982; Jerger, 1970; Jerger et al, 1974a). Measurement of the **acoustic stapedial reflex**, however, provided a sensitive index of auditory function extending far beyond the middle ear, contributing significantly to the versatility of immittance audiometry. The neurodiagnostic value of acoustic reflex measurements have, for over a decade, been repeatedly documented. They are clinically useful in the prediction of sensorineural hearing impairment (Hall, 1980; Hall and Koval, 1982; Jerger et al, 1974b; Margolis and Fox, 1977; Niemeyer and Sesterhenn, 1974), the differentiation of cochlear vs retrocochlear auditory dysfunction (Anderson et al, 1969; Jerger et al, 1974c; Sanders et al, 1974; and others), and the identification and localization of brainstem auditory pathology (Borg, 1973; Griesen and Rasmussen, 1970; Jerger and Jerger, 1977; and others).

This final diagnostic application—the acoustic reflex in central auditory dysfunction—is the topic of the present chapter. In contrast to the substantial published clinical experiences with acoustic reflexes in peripheral (middle ear and sensorineural) impairment, there is only a modest number of reports documenting acoustic reflex abnormalities in patients with confirmed **central auditory nervous system** lesions. The neuroanatomy, neurophysiology, and neuropharmacology of the acoustic reflex in man is not adequately described. Also, there are only preliminary studies of the distinctive influence of central auditory system pathology on the major **acoustic reflex** parameters—**threshold, latency, decay, and amplitude.** Furthermore, effects of subject characteristics, such as age and sex, remain poorly understood and rather controversial, and yet they seem to be important in the clinical interpretation of acoustic reflex findings. Finally, there is only a limited number of comprehensive clinical reports of acoustic reflex measurements in patients with neoplastic, vascular, or demyelinating central neuropathies. The purpose of this chapter is to review current knowledge of the acoustic reflex in central auditory dysfunction, illustrating the above noted issues with case studies and original data. Recent detailed descriptions of acoustic reflex measurement procedures are available elsewhere (Hall and Jerger, 1982; Jerger and Northern, 1980; Lilly, 1973). The chapter concludes with a discussion of promising new research directions.

PRINCIPLES OF ACOUSTIC REFLEX MEASUREMENT

Anatomy

Fifty years ago, Lorente de Nó (1933a, b, and 1935) conducted comprehensive neuroanatomical investigations of the acoustic stapedial reflex. Yet, the *anatomy* of the acoustic reflex arc is still not completely known. Available information is based on experimental studies in animals and clinical correlation of acoustic reflex abnormalities with sites of neuropathology (Borg, 1973; Brask, 1978). The peripheral components of the arc, both afferent and efferent, are reasonably well-described. Structure and function of the afferent portion—the *middle ear system*, the *cochlea*, and the *eighth (acoustic) cranial nerve*—are presented elsewhere in this volume (Chapter 2). The efferent portion consists of the *seventh (facial) cranial nerve*, the *stapedius muscle and tendon*, and *the stapes*. The motor division of the facial nerve courses from its caudal pontine brainstem nucleus to the muscles of the face. After exiting the internal auditory canal at the stylomastoid foramen, it gives off a short branch of largely myelinated fibers (perhaps 10% of the entire motor division) to the stapedius muscle (Foley and DuBois, 1953). Interestingly, a greater number of fibers appear to innervate the right middle ear muscles than the left, at least in cat (Foley and DuBois, 1953; Lyon, 1975). The stapedius is the smallest skeletal muscle in mammals. Animal studies in cat, rat, rabbit, guinea pig, and chicken have shown that it consists of two types of fast, twitch fibers, and a morphologically slow fiber component (Anniko and Wroblewski, 1981; Borg et al, 1979; Burgener and Mayr, 1980; Erulkar et al, 1964; Fernand and Hess, 1969; Hirayama and Daly, 1974). Also, there are both multiply and singly innervated muscle fibers (Fernand and Hess, 1969; Tieg and Dahl, 1972). The stapedius muscle is largely enclosed within a bony canal in the posterior tympanic wall and runs parallel but anterior/interior to facial nerve. In some persons, the muscle and nerve are in the same bony compartment. The stapedius muscle tendon emerges at the pyramidal eminence in the tympanic cavity (middle ear) to attach on the posterior aspect of the neck of the stapes.

The central components of the acoustic reflex arc—mediating activity between the afferent portion on one side and both left and right efferent portions—are not completely described in animal, and poorly understood in man. Borg's (1973) often cited report of a comprehensive anatomic and physiologic investigation of the reflex pathways in rabbit is suggested for further reading. (A discussion of brainstem anatomy in general is presented in Chapter 2 of this volume.) There are direct and indirect arcs. The direct pathways are most studied and appear to consist of a 3- or 4 neuron chain, including (1) sensory neurons of the eighth cranial nerve, i.e., primary afferents, (2) neurons from the *ventral cochlear nucleus* terminating in the vicinity of the ipsilateral motor facial nerve nucleus and in the ipsilateral and contralateral *medial superior olive* (MSO), (3) neurons from in or around the MSO and terminating on the ipsilateral or contralateral *region near the motor nucleus of the facial nerve*, and (4) motor neurons of the facial nerve, i.e., the final efferents, arising from the area of the facial nerve motor nucleus and terminating on fiber(s) of the ipsilateral stapedius muscle. Thus, there are ipsilateral and contralateral acoustic reflex pathways, with the former involving afferent, brainstem intermediate and efferent structures on the same side, and the latter involving afferents on one side, neurons which cross the caudal pontine brainstem midline, presumably via the trapezoid body, and efferent neurons on the opposite side. These pathways and synapses are often depicted schematically in the literature (Brask, 1978; Clemis and Sarno, 1980; Djupesland, 1980; Jerger, 1980; Jerger et al, 1980; Møller, 1983). However, the components of the central reflex arc, especially in man, are not clearly defined, and such diagrams are probably a gross, and not entirely accurate, oversimplification of a complex temporal and spatial interaction of brainstem auditory structures.

One of the least understood features of the *direct* central acoustic reflex arc is the origin of the facial nerve efferents that innervate the stapedius muscle. Borg (1973) and others (Papez, 1927) offered evidence from lesioning and retrograde degeneration experiments suggesting that the motor neurons (third or fourth neuron of the reflex pathway) originate from the medial and/or lateral region of the nucleus of the seventh cranial nerve. In contrast, studies with horseradish peroxidase (HRP) retrograde transport techniques in monkey and cat (Lyon, 1978; Stach et al, 1983; Strominger et al, 1980) showed motor neurons predominately in an area that was clearly outside of the medial or lateral neuronal groups of facial nerve nucleus, and in close proximity to the lateral or medial superior olive. Further investigation on this component of the acoustic reflex with current neuroanatomic methodology is continuing.

An *indirect* acoustic reflex pathway clearly exists, although very little is known of its components in man or experimental animal. Borg (1973) speculated that this slower, polysynaptic pathway might involve the extrapyramidal motor system or the *reticular formation* (RF). The extreme sensitivity of the acoustic reflex to the influence of barbiturates, discussed and illustrated later in this chapter, supports the concept of an alternate, RF-mediated, pathway which may, in fact, predominate in man. Also, there are other, documented interactions between the traditional auditory structures and the RF (Brodal, 1981; Rasmussen, 1946). Furthermore, the short and long latency components of the acoustically elicited stapedius muscle EMG show differential sensitivity to state of arousal and higher CNS influences (Baust and Berlucchi, 1964; Salomon, 1966), much like the two temporal components of the corneal or blink response (Brodal, 1981), a cranial nerve five-to-seven reflex arc. The possible contribution of auditory cortical areas to acoustic reflex activity has been suggested in recent clinical reports (Downs and Crum, 1980; Jerger, 1980) and is the topic of ongoing experimental study (B Stach, personal communication, 1983).

Physiology

There are numerous recently published accounts detailing the physical and functional basis of the acoustic reflex (Jerger and Northern, 1980), and only a brief description will be presented here. Contraction of the stapedius muscle in response to high intensity sound has been repeatedly demonstrated in man for over 50 yr (Jepson, 1951; Lüscher, 1929; Metz, 1946). The reflex is bilateral or consensual; that is, a sound presented to one ear produces contraction of the stapedius muscle on the same side

(ipsilaterally) *and* on the opposite side (contralaterally). Clinically, contraction of the stapedius muscle can easily be detected by measuring the reflex-related change in middle ear acoustic immittance (primarily reduced mobility) close to the plane of the tympanic membrane (Jerger and Northern, 1980; Lilly, 1973; Møller, 1972). Other methods of acoustic reflex measurement, suitable in experimental preparations, include mechanical transduction of ossicular movements or direct EMG of the stapedius muscle (Møller, 1972).

Normal stapedial reflex activity in response to acoustic stimulation requires integrity of the afferent, brainstem, and efferent pathways. Clinical correlations among neurotologic pathophysiologies and acoustic reflex patterns will be discussed and illustrated later in this chapter. It is important to keep in mind, however, that although the diagnostic objective may be evaluation of neurotologic status, it is first necessary to rule out the influence of obvious middle ear and cochlear involvement in acoustic reflex abnormalities (Hall and Jerger, 1982; Jerger et al, 1974a and b). That is, to elicit normal acoustic reflex activity, a sound of 70 to 90 dB sound pressure level (SPL) must first reach the cochlea, then be transduced bioelectrically, and adequately transmitted via the eighth cranial nerve to the ventral cochlear nucleus. The contralateral or ipsilateral acoustic reflex cannot be measured, even with the probe in a normal ear, if the sound intensity reaching the cochlea of the stimulus ear is attenuated to less than 70 to 90 dB SPL by conductive impairment. And an ipsilaterally elicited acoustic reflex is rarely observed even in an ear with a minimal (5 to 10 dB) conductive component (Jerger et al, 1974a). Likewise, acoustic stimulation of an ear with severe cochlear impairment (60 to 70 dB) or mild eighth nerve auditory impairment (0 to 40 dB) is unlikely to produce measurable acoustic reflex activity, although middle ear functioning is normal (Jerger and Jerger, 1974c).

The actual *physiologic basis* of the stapedial acoustic reflex remains unclear. The role of middle ear function in acoustic reflex measurements, at both the afferent and efferent extremes of arc, is well-described (Møller, 1972). However, the sensorineural and brainstem physiologic substrate of the acoustic reflex is largely conjecture. In normal hearers, at least, the acoustic reflex appears to be dependent in some way on loudness summation, i.e., the perception of a sufficiently loud sound. This conclusion is supported, indirectly, by documented relationships between critical bandwidth estimations made by both acoustic reflex and psychophysical methods (Block and Wiley, 1979; Djupesland and Zwislocki, 1973; Flottorp et al, 1971; Popelka et al, 1976), although there are serious discrepancies in findings among studies (Margolis and Popelka, 1975). Acoustic reflex activity also seems to be closely related to temporal summation of acoustic energy, an interaction of stimulus duration and intensity (Djupesland et al, 1973; Gelfand et al, 1981; Jerger et al, 1977; Woodford et al, 1975; and others). These acoustic reflex phenomena have particular relevance to the present chapter as they are, presumably, mediated in the central auditory nervous system (Boudreau, 1965; Zwislocki, 1969).

More precise understanding of the neurophysiology of the acoustic reflex would significantly enhance its clinical exploitation. There are a host of unanswered questions: for example, aside from the vaguely defined role of loudness sensation, what neurophysiologic processes underly acoustic reflex threshold, latency, and amplitude parameters? Which types of auditory brainstem neurons mediate the acoustic reflex vs, for example, the auditory brainstem response or complex speech signals? Is there binaural neural interaction in acoustic reflex measurement, as suggested by the larger magnitude response to simultaneous diotic stimulation than to typical monaural stimulation (Møller, 1962; Reker, 1977)? Do central auditory structures rostral to the pons modulate (either excite or inhibit) acoustic reflex activity? What are the differences in the neural bases of the acoustic reflex among man and experimental animal materials (e.g., cat, rabbit, guinea pig, monkey)? In view of the now proven clinical value of acoustic reflex measurements, it is likely that these basic questions, and many others, will be the subject of further investigations.

Methodology

Twenty-five years ago, Møller (1958, 1961, 1962) described measurement of the acoustic reflex with specially constructed *experimental* instrumentation. In recent years, a number of investigators have also designed reflex-measuring systems that offer some distinct advantages over commercially available equipment, especially in the assessment of central auditory functioning. A popular approach is the use of laboratory devices for stimulus generation and manipulation (eg., gating, shaping, timing) with reliance on commercially available meters for measurement of immittance (Gelfand et al, 1981; Popelka et al, 1976; Thompson et al, 1980; Wilson, 1979). This arrangement permits virtually unlimited selection of stimulus parameters and assures that immittance changes will be validly measured and reported in acceptable units, such as acoustic admittance (millimhos) or as equivalent compliance in cubic centimeters. There are, however, four main limitations to this approach: (1) only one or two probe tone frequencies (220 and 660 Hz) are usually available; (2) accurate measurement of reflex temporal characteristics, such as latency, is confounded by time constraints inherent in the instruments (Mangham et al, 1982; Niswander and Ruth, 1979); (3) the wide variety of stimuli are presented via a standard contralateral earphone/cushion. Ipsilateral reflexes must be activated with the limited stimuli available on the commercial immittance meter; and (4) the type of acoustic transducer, and its coupling to the ear, differ substantially for contra- vs ipsilateral acoustic reflexes. This final limitation is extremely important in the assessment of central auditory functioning with acoustic reflexes.

Møller's original studies employed apparatus that circumvented the above noted drawbacks. The main concepts of this instrumentation have, within the past 5 yr, been revived, updated, and clinically documented by Jerger and colleagues (Hall, 1982a, b and, c; Hayes and Jerger, 1983; Jerger and Hayes, 1983; Jerger et al, 1978b). As illustrated in Figure 7.1, this system has unique and clinically attractive features: (1) Ipsilateral and contralateral reflex stimuli are presented by

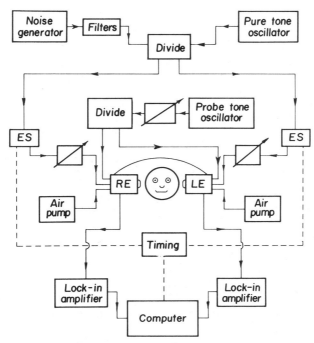

Figure 7.1. Specially constructed apparatus for equivalent measurement of ipsilateral and contralateral acoustic reflexes. Components include matched probe assemblies for presenting acoustic stimulus and detecting reflex-related changes in acoustic immittance, and minicomputer for averaging acoustic reflex activity.

identical, acoustically matched probe assemblies. Stimuli for the ipsilateral and contralateral modes can be calibrated equivalently and presented simultaneously under identical conditions. Reflex findings for the two stimulus modes, therefore, can be directly and confidently compared. (2) A wide variety of stimuli characteristics and probe tone frequencies can be selected with laboratory stimulus generators. (3) Changes in probe tone intensity are detected with the aid of a lock-in amplifier, eliminating the need for the filter components of standard immittance bridges which introduce, in part, the troublesome time constants. (4) Acoustic reflex activity for a sequence of stimuli is computer-averaged under each presentation condition (right and left, contra- and ipsilateral).

Factors Influencing Acoustic Reflex Measurements

Response Parameters. Four main acoustic reflex parameters—threshold, amplitude,

latency, and decay are described in the literature.

The acoustic reflex threshold is commonly defined as the lowest sound intensity level in dB (hearing level relative to audiometric dB (HL)) or SPL producing a reliable change in middle ear immittance as measured near the plane of the tympanic membrane. Clinically, acoustic reflex activity is usually detected by visual monitoring of a meter, although most commercial instruments offer an X-Y plotter or strip chart for graphically recording reflex-elicited changes in immittance. Using 5 dB increments, reflex threshold levels of 90 to 95 dB SPL for tonal stimuli and 70 to 80 dB for broadband noise are expected in normal hearers, with standard deviations of approximately 5 dB (tones) and 10 dB (noise), respectively (Jerger et al, 1972; Wilson and McBride, 1978). Adherence to the preferred threshold determination procedures used in pure tone audiometry is not necessary in reflex threshold measurement, and there are no differences in reflex thresholds obtained with ascending vs descending intensity techniques (Lilly and Franzen, 1970; Peterson and Lidén, 1972).

Metz (1951) first reported that the magnitude (amplitude) of acoustic immittance change increased directly as the intensity of the stimulus was increased. His observation, made on a single subject with a relatively primitive immittance measuring device, introduced a reflex parameter which, it now appears, has considerable clinical value in assessment of peripheral and central auditory functioning (Borg, 1973; Brask, 1978; Hall, 1982a, b, and c: Hayes and Jerger, 1983; Jerger et al, 1978b; Mangham and Miller, 1979). Acoustic reflex amplitude, often referred to as reflex growth, is calculated by comparison of the acoustic immittance of the middle ear (measured as described above) before acoustic stimulation (at rest) with the acoustic immittance during acoustic stimulation (reflexive). Reflex amplitude has been reported in a variety of units, including decibels (Jerger et al, 1978b; Peterson and Lidén, 1972; Silman and Gelfand, 1981), percent of maximum amplitude (Borg, 1973; Møller, 1961, 1962); acoustic ohms (Hung and Dallos, 1972), microvolts (Bosatra et al, 1975), millimhos (Thompson et al, 1980; Wilson and McBride, 1978), absolute cubic centimeters (milliliters) (Beedle and Harford, 1973), and mathematically derived cubic centimeters (Hall, 1982a, b, and c). These differences in the reflex recording units have contributed to discrepancies in amplitude findings among investigations and the variability often attributed to reflex amplitude measures (Wilson, 1979). In clinical studies of patients varying in age and middle ear status, it is important, when recording and interpreting reflex amplitude in any unit, to take into account the pronounced influences of static or resting immittance (Wilson, 1979) in the probe ear.

Latency is the time interval between stimulus presentation and some index of reflex-related immittance change. This statement is necessarily vague, since a major problem in calculating latency is difficulty in consistently defining the actual onset of reflex activity. The three acoustic reflex temporal characteristics most often cited as criteria for onset are: (1) any change from baseline in acoustic immittance (increase or decrease);

(2) the points at which immittance first increases from baseline; and (3) some predefined percentage of the maximum reflex amplitude (Borg, 1982b; Clemis and Sarno, 1980; Hall and Jerger, 1976; Jerger and Hayes, 1983; Mangham et al, 1980; Norris et al, 1974). Precise myographic measurements of reflex latency in man, made by Perlman and Case (1939), showed a time interval of approximately 10 msec between tonal stimulation of one ear and action potentials in the contralateral stapedius muscle. The latency of stapedius muscle contraction, when detected with laboratory instrumentation as changes in acoustic immittance, is on the order of 25 to 35 msec at high stimulus intensities and 150 msec near threshold (Metz, 1951; Møller, 1958). Latency values obtained with commercially available immittance measuring devices are, in fact, only relative, as they are invariably affected by the temporal distortion produced by filter components (Clemis and Sarno, 1980; Hall and Jerger, 1976; Mangham et al, 1980, 1982; McPherson and Thompson, 1977; Niswander and Ruth, 1979). The clinical utility of acoustic reflex latency is further compromised by its confounding relationship with stimulus intensity and absolute reflex amplitude (Borg, 1982b; Hung and Dallos, 1972; Jerger and Hayes, 1983). Nonetheless, temporal reflex characteristics have been successfully correlated with sensorineural and brainstem lesions experimentally (Borg, 1982a), and, with careful application, may yet have clinical value (see Borg, 1976 for review of this topic).

Acoustic reflex *decay* has long held an important place in the audiologic test battery as a screening procedure for retrocochlear dysfunction (Anderson et al, 1969). The test is generally administered by presenting the acoustic stimulus for 10 sec at an intensity level 10 dB greater than the reflex threshold level (10 dB SL). The reflex-related immittance change is recorded and then analyzed for evidence of a decrease in amplitude of 50% or more over the time course. Slight decay is not uncommon in cochlea-impaired ears, and, infrequently, decay is also found in normal ears (Alberti, 1978; Habener and Snyder, 1974), but, as illustrated in a subsequent section, significant decay is a strong audiometric sign of retrocochlear (eighth nerve or brainstem) pathology (Anderson et al, 1969; Jerger et al, 1974c; Olsen et al, 1981).

Stimulus Parameters. Meaningful interpretation of acoustic reflex findings in central auditory pathology requires an awareness of a broad range of stimulus effects on threshold, amplitude, latency, and decay parameters. (The following review is by no means exhaustive, and the reader is encouraged to consult original sources for details). These four reflex parameters are differentially influenced by the *mode of stimulus presentation—ipsilateral vs contralateral.* Investigations with clinical instrumentation have shown no significant difference between threshold levels for ipsilaterally vs contralaterally stimulated reflexes (Laukli and Mair, 1980). Equivalence in calibration of the standard earphone (contralateral transducer) and miniature (ipsilateral) transducer, which is sealed within the ear canal, is, of course, a problem in such studies and in clinical practice. Also troublesome are acoustic and eardrum artifacts with reflex measurements, especially in the ipsilateral mode (Danaher and Pickett, 1974; Kunoz, 1977; Leis and Lutman, 1979). Investigations with experimental, dual probe systems suggest that ipsilateral measurements yield more sensitive threshold levels than contralateral measurements, although the differences, on the average, do not exceed 5 dB, vary as a function of stimulus frequency, and are not consistently observed for all subjects (Hall et al, 1982a and b; Jerger et al, 1978b; Møller, 1962). Reflex amplitude, in contrast, is almost always larger for ipsilateral than contralateral stimulation, even with matched, dual probe acoustic transducers (Hall, 1982a, b, and c; Jerger et al, 1978b; Møller, 1962), and it is larger still for binaural stimulation (Møller, 1962; Reker and Baumgarten, 1981). Likewise, latency is relatively shorter in the ipsilateral mode. There are no comprehensive studies of the interaction of stimulus presentation mode with reflex decay. Alberti's (1978) findings suggest that, in normal ears at least, excessive decay is less common with ipsilateral stimulation. Borg and Ødman (1979), however, reported no ipsi- vs contralateral differences in decay for normal hearers.

Stimulus *frequency* is an important factor in all reflex measurements, and the result of basic investigations offer valuable guidelines for selection of test frequency in clinical assessments. First, reflex threshold and amplitude measures vary as a function of stimulus *bandwidth.* The effect of bandwidth on reflex threshold is particularly well-studied and, in fact, forms the basis for a variety of hearing loss prediction methods (see Hall, 1980 for details). There is universal agreement that acoustic reflex threshold levels improve when the activating stimulus exceeds a critical bandwidth, resulting in a difference of up to 20 dB for pure tones vs Gaussian noise stimuli (Djupesland and Zwislocki, 1973; Flottorp et al, 1971; Popelka et al, 1976). Acoustic reflex amplitude is greater for noise than tonal stimuli (Hall, 1982b; Møller, 1962; Silman et al, 1978; Wilson and McBride, 1978). The prevalence of spuriously abnormal acoustic reflex decay findings increases directly with frequency (Alberti, 1978; Jerger et al, 1974c), with up to 25% of a normal population yielding a false-positive (for retrocochlear lesion) outcome at 4000 Hz. Reflex latency appears to be comparable for very brief duration (25 msec) stimuli of differing frequencies (Møller, 1962), but may be longer for low than high frequencies for durations of 200 msec or more (Hung and Dallos, 1972; Møller, 1958; Ruth and Niswander, 1976). Increased variability of reflex threshold and latency parameters for higher frequency stimuli can confuse this relationship (Djupesland et al, 1973).

As noted earlier in this chapter, stimulus *duration* affects acoustic reflex parameters. Threshold levels increase as the stimulus is shortened to less than 200 msec but are independent of changes in stimulus durations exceeding 200 msec (Djupesland and Zwislocki, 1973). Rate of acoustic reflex amplitude growth also varies with stimulus duration when studied with specially constructed apparatus having minimal time constant characteristics (Jerger et al, 1977). As an aside, slope and maximum reflex growth also seem to be dependent on probe tone frequency (e.g., 220 vs 660 Hz) in normal hearers. This relationship, not unexpected (Møller, 1983), requires further study (Sprague et al, 1981). In summary, then, basic studies suggest that the clinical value, validity, and feasibility of combined ipsilateral *and* contralateral reflex measurements (threshold, amplitude, latency, and decay) are generally enhanced with the use of pure tone stimuli of adequate duration (200 msec) in the midaudiometric frequency region (500 through 2000 Hz).

Subject Characteristics. The influences of *age* and *sex* pervade virtually all aspects of auditory function, including pure tone sensitivity (Bunch, 1929), speech understanding (Pestalozza and Shore, 1955; Hall, 1983), auditory brainstem response (Jerger and Hall, 1980), and measures of static middle ear immittance (Hall, 1979). Pronounced age and sex effects on acoustic reflex parameters, then, are not surprising. Age differentially influences acoustic reflex thresholds for tonal vs noise stimuli in children and adults (Jerger et al, 1972; Jerger et al, 1978a; Hall and Weaver, 1979). In general, reflex thresholds for tonal stimuli appear to remain stable or to improve slightly, with advancing age, while noise-elicited threshold levels may show an increase. Sex is apparently not a factor. The exact interactions among age, reflex thresholds, and stimulus bandwidth, however, are not clear and, indeed, continue to be a rather controversial issue (Handler and Margolis, 1977; Jerger et al, 1978a; Jerger, 1979; Silman, 1979a and b; Thompson et al, 1980). Aging profoundly influences acoustic reflex amplitude (Hall, 1982a; Silman and Gelfand, 1981; Wilson, 1981). Hall (1982a) found that over the range of 20 through 80 yr, maximum reflex amplitude decreased by an average of 56%. These age-related amplitude changes are usually more pronounced for uncrossed (ipsilateral) than crossed acoustic reflexes (Gersdorff, 1978; Hall, 1982a). The basis for the age effect is unknown, although reasonable neurophysiologic explanations have been offered (Hall, 1982a; Wilson, 1981). There is, in addition, an interaction between age and sex. In younger subjects (20 to 30 yr), males and females show equivalent acoustic reflex amplitude values, while in subjects aged 60 to 80 yr, average maximum amplitude in males is less than 75% of female amplitude (Hall, 1982a). Again, no definitive cause for the age-sex interaction has been demonstrated. There are no comprehensive published investigations of

acoustic reflex latency on decay measures as a function of age and sex.

Peripheral Auditory Status. Middle ear and sensorineural status are very important factors in the interpretation of acoustic reflex findings in central auditory dysfunction. As noted earlier in this chapter, the acoustic reflex is characteristically not observed by immittance measuring techniques with the probe in an ear with clinically significant *middle ear pathology* (Jerger et al, 1974a; and many others). However, even relatively minor middle ear dysfunction, such as high static compliance or slight (−50 to −100 mm water) negative middle ear pressure, may contribute to abnormally raised acoustic reflex threshold levels (Hall and Weaver, 1979). The clinical implications of middle ear status and acoustic reflex amplitude measurements are profound (Hall, 1982b; Wilson, 1979). For example, in patients with clinically minor negative pressure or static compliance aberrations reflex amplitude is, on the average, only one-third of the amplitude in control subjects (Hall, 1982b; Jerger et al, 1978b), even when there is no evidence of middle ear impairment by pure tone audiometry. Successful clinical application of reflex amplitude measurements in patients with such subtle acoustic immittance aberrations requires careful documentation of middle ear status by history, otologic examination, and immittance audiometry. Also, the pattern of uncrossed and crossed reflex amplitude findings must be examined closely. Normal and bilaterally equal uncrossed amplitudes argue against a spurious middle ear effect. However, reflex amplitude abnormalities with a common probe (measurement) ear suggest confounding middle ear pathology. Again, the possible deleterious influence of middle ear abnormalities on reflex latency and decay has, to my knowledge, not been studied.

There are demonstrated interactions among acoustic reflex findings, stimulus bandwidth, and sensorineural hearing sensitivity loss. For *cochlear hearing impairments*, reflex threshold levels for tonal activators may show slight improvement in patients with mild to moderate (up to 45 dB HTL) deficits, in comparison to normal hearers, and then gradually worsen with increased loss (Hall and Weaver, 1979). Reflex activity often cannot be elicited with maximum acoustic tonal stimulus intensity levels (110 to 125 dB) in hearing impairment exceeding 70 dB HTL (Jerger and Jerger, 1974). Reflex threshold levels for noise stimuli, on the other hand, increase rather systematically with cochlear hearing impairment (Hall and Weaver, 1979). Eighth nerve auditory dysfunction, even with mild sensitivity loss, is associated with grossly elevated or unmeasurable, acoustic reflex threshold levels for tone or noise stimuli (Anderson et al, 1969; Jerger et al, 1974c; Jerger and Jerger, 1974).

Reports of acoustic reflex amplitude in sensorineural hearing loss are conflicting. Some investigators found decreased amplitude for contralateral stimuli in sensorineural (cochlear) hearing loss (Beedle and Harford, 1973; Peterson and Lidén, 1972; Sprague et al, 1981; Thompson et al, 1980; Wilson, 1981) but did not assess ipsilaterally stimulated reflex amplitude. Others reported varied findings for contralateral amplitude measures (Silman et al, 1978; Silman and Gelfand, 1981). Complicating interpretation of the outcome of these studies are the combined influences of age and stimulus frequency. In systematic investigations of simultaneously stimulated crossed and uncrossed reflex amplitude, Hall (1982b and c) and Jerger et al (1978b) described the relationship of amplitude, stimulus, and age. In young adult subjects (20 to 30 yr), amplitude was generally equivalent in normal vs sensorineurally impaired ears. In older subjects (60 to 80 yr), in contrast, reflex amplitude was significantly depressed for a noise band stimulus, but not a tonal stimulus (4000 Hz), when compared with a normal hearing age-matched control group (Hall, 1982b). As illustrated in the next section and demonstrated by others (Hayes and Jerger, 1983; Mangham and Miller, 1979), *neural auditory dysfunction* characteristically produces greatly reduced acoustic reflex amplitude values. Latency is apparently prolonged abnormally in retrocochlear (vs cochlear or normal) ears (Mangham and Miller, 1979; Mangham et al, 1980; Clemis and Sarno, 1980), although the validity of these conclusions has recently been questioned (Jerger and Hayes, 1983). Of all the reflex parameters, decay has been most extensively studied and clinically applied in sensorineural hearing loss. A number of studies have shown that excessive (greater than 50%) reflex decay provides early and yet strong evidence of retrocochlear auditory pathology (Anderson et al, 1969; Jerger et al, 1974c; Johnson, 1977; and others), even in patients with normal reflex threshold findings.

Drugs. CNS-acting drugs may influence acoustic reflex activity. Elevated threshold levels and decreased amplitudes were found with blood *alcohol* (*ethanol*) concentrations of 0.07 to 0.13% (Borg and Møller, 1967; Cohill and Greenberg, 1977; Robinette and Brey, 1978). Ipsi- and contralateral reflexes were influenced similarly, although the effects varied substantially among subjects. CNS depressants, particularly barbiturates, also suppress acoustic reflex activity (Borg and Møller, 1967, 1975; Bosatra et al, 1975; Giacomelli and Mozzo, 1964; Richards et al, 1975; Robinette et al, 1974; Thompson et al, 1984; Wersäll, 1958). The magnitude of the effect is dependent on the type of drug (e.g., pento-, pheno-, or secobarbital), the dosage, and the subject material (man vs experimental animals, such as cat, rabbit, and monkey). There is evidence that the effect is greater for the contralaterally stimulated reflex (vs ipsilateral) (Borg and Møller, 1967). Ketamine, an anesthetic agent acting on the CNS in a different manner than the barbiturates, also exerts a strong suppressive influence on reflex activity, even at low, preanesthetic doses (e.g., 5 mg/kg) (Thompson et al, 1984).

The pronounced influence of barbiturates on clinical measurements of acoustic reflex activity is illustrated in Figure 7.2, and related to neurologic status and auditory evoked response findings in Table 7.1. Data were obtained serially, by the author, from a 38-yr-old male during withdrawal from induced barbiturate coma. Barbiturates (pentobarbital, Nembutal) were administered therapeutically in management of intracranial pressure due to brain swelling secondary to an acute hypertensive cerebral insult. Acoustic reflex activity was not observed with barbiturate blood levels of 3.62 down to 1.50 mg/dl (Fig. 7.2) and was not consistently normal until there were no detectable barbiturates in the blood. Emergence of measurable acoustic reflex activity followed the reappearance of neurologic signs (pupillary response and corneal reflex) and the auditory middle latency evoked response. The auditory brainstem response, in contrast, was reliably recorded and consistently normal appearing throughout barbiturate coma. The acoustic reflex, then, is highly sensitive to the CNS depressant effect of barbiturates, more so than other electrophysiologic auditory measures and clinical

neurologic brainstem responses. These data provide further evidence that the acoustic reflex arc in man includes important indirect pathways and perhaps, as suggested by Borg (Borg, 1973; Borg and Møller, 1967, 1975), includes reticular formation components.

CENTRAL AUDITORY DYSFUNCTION

Acoustic reflex measurements have clinically proven value in the identification and

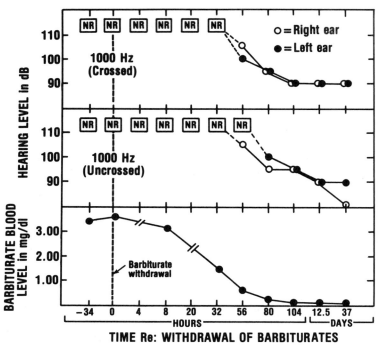

Figure 7.2. Acoustic reflex threshold levels in relation to barbiturate blood levels in a 38-yr-old male subject. Neurologic data and other auditory findings are provided in Table 7.1.

Table 7.1
Correlation of Acoustic Reflex Findings with Neurologic Signs and Auditory Evoked Responses for a 38-yr-old Male during Emergence from Barbiturate Coma[a]

Time postbarbiturate withdrawal (hr)	−34	0	4	8	20	32	56	80	104	300
Barbiturate blood level (mg/dl)	3.34	3.62	NA[b]	3.09	NA	1.50	0.57	0.18	0	0
Pupil reactivity	−	−	+/−	−	+/−	+	+	+	+	+
Corneal reflex	−	−	−	−	+/−	+/−	+/−	+	+	+
Auditory evoked response										
Brainstem	+	+	+	+	+	+	+	+	+	+
Middle latency	−	−	−	+/−	+/−	+/−	+/−	+	+	+
Acoustic reflex	−	−	−	−	−	−	+/−	+/−	+	+

[a] +, normal response; +/−, abnormal response; −, no response.
[b] Data not available.

localization of central auditory pathology. At least three factors contribute to their usefulness in diagnostic audiology. They are: (1) recognition of the patterns of acoustic reflex findings associated with different sites of lesions; (2) an understanding of the relationship among outcomes for acoustic reflex measurements, diagnostic speech audiometry, and the auditory brainstem response; and (3) routine use of reflex measures as a part of a basic audiology test battery. In this section, literature on the clinical application of acoustic reflexes in central auditory nervous system pathology is reviewed. Characteristic patterns of findings are illustrated and correlated with other diagnostic audiometric results in a series of case studies.

A dominant diagnostic role of acoustic reflexes is in the differentiation of cochlear vs retrocochlear lesions. As a result of their neuroaudiologic sensitivity and time effectiveness (Jerger and Jerger, 1983), acoustic reflex threshold and decay are widely used as primary measures of eighth nerve functional integrity (Anderson et al, 1969; Freyss and Casteran, 1979; Hirsch and Anderson, 1980a and b; Jerger and Jerger, 1974a; Jerger et al, 1974c; Jerger et al, 1975; Johnson, 1977; Lidén and Korsan-Bengtsen, 1973; Olsen et al, 1975, 1981; Sanders et al, 1974; Sheehy and Inzer, 1976; Sterkers et al, 1980; Thomsen and Terkildsen, 1975). Analysis of latency and amplitude parameters has further contributed to this diagnostic application of the acoustic reflex (Clemis and Sarno, 1980; Jerger and Hayes, 1983; McPherson and Thompson, 1977; Mangham et al, 1980).

Auditory abnormalities in intracanalicular eighth nerve lesions are ipsilateral, affecting peripheral afferent function exclusively, and are, therefore, not within the scope of this chapter. Lesions arising from within the region of the cerebellopontine (CP) angle or extending into this region from the internal auditory canal are termed extrinsic, or extraaxial, brainstem lesions. This dichotomy is, in part, artificial, distinguished in some patients only by millimeters in lesion location and size or months in time of progression. In clinical audiometry, it is usually not possible to differentiate prospectively between pure eighth nerve lesions and extrinsic brainstem lesions. Unfortunately, many clinical reports on auditory findings, including acoustic reflexes, in brainstem pathology do not even clearly define their patients on the basis of **intrinsic brainstem** vs. **extrinsic brainstem**/retrocochlear **pathology** (see Jerger and Jerger, 1975a). The following section, then, is a discussion of acoustic reflex findings in patients with brainstem level central auditory dysfunction in general. Every attempt, however, will be made to distinguish patterns of findings associated with intrinsic vs extrinsic brainstem sites of lesions.

Intrinsic (Intraaxial) vs Extrinsic (Extraaxial) Brainstem Pathology

Griesen and Rasmussen (1970) first reported clinical evidence of **contralateral (crossed) acoustic reflex** abnormalities in brainstem pathology. Their observations were subsequently confirmed repeatedly with clinical and experimental investigations (Alberti et al, 1977; Borg, 1971, 1973, 1977, 1982a; Bosatra, 1977; Bosatra and Russolo, 1976; Bosatra et al, 1975; Brask, 1978; Colletti, 1975; Hannley et al, 1983; Hayes and Jerger, 1983; Jerger and Jerger, 1974b; Jerger and Jerger, 1981; Jerger et al, 1979; Jerger, 1980; Lehnhardt, 1973, Lehnhardt et al, 1982; Lidén and Korsan-Bengtsen, 1973; Nagafuchi, 1982; Russolo and Poli, 1983; Steinberger and Lehnhardt, 1972; Stephens and Thornton, 1976). Three factors have contributed importantly to the continued interest and success in this application of acoustic reflexes.

First, Borg's (1973, 1982a) correlations of acoustic reflex abnormalities with carefully defined experimental lesions of brainstem auditory nuclei and pathways in rabbits provided much needed basic neuroanatomic information for meaningful interpretation of clinical reflex findings. For example, lesions in the ventral cochlear nucleus (but not the dorsal nucleus) in the vicinity of the eighth nerve root produced elevated reflex threshold levels and excessive reflex decay with ipsilateral stimulation. These findings would seem to be indistinguishable from pure eighth nerve dysfunction. In contrast, trapezoid body lesions spare ipsilateral reflex activity. They may cause only modest increases in crossed reflex thresholds, with no decay, yet produce pronounced latency and amplitude abnormalities. Subsequent total transection of the intermediate and dorsal stria, on the other hand, created no additional deficits. The medial portion of the superior olivary complex (SOC) is a major structure on both crossed and uncrossed reflex anatomy. Further experimental study of the neuropathologic correlates of acoustic reflex abnormalities will, no doubt, significantly enhance their clinical value.

Second, since the mid-1970s, it has been clinically feasible to measure contralateral *and* **ipsilateral (uncrossed) acoustic reflexes**, with commercially available instrumentation. Analysis and interpretation of the pattern of reflex findings for the four possible measurement conditions (ipsi- and contrastimulus X right and left ears) permits confident differentiation among afferent (sensorineural), efferent (middle ear or facial nerve), and central (brainstem) auditory dysfunction and substantially increases the specificity of reflex data. Clinical correlates of acoustic reflex patterns are described in detail in recent publications (Jerger, 1980; Jerger and Jerger, 1977; Jerger and Jerger, 1981; Jerger et al, 1980), and are illustrated in the following case studies.

Third, measurement of acoustic reflex amplitude, decay, and latency parameters has supplemented threshold information and has heightened sensitivity of acoustic reflexes to brainstem pathology. Amplitude decrements for crossed acoustic reflexes may be found in experimental and clinical brainstem auditory lesions, which do not influence reflex threshold levels (Borg, 1973; Bosatra et al, 1975; Brask, 1978; Hayes and Jerger, 1983). Similarly, there are clinical reports of excessive decay of acoustic reflex amplitude in intraaxial brainstem pathology, in the absence of eighth nerve involvement and reflex threshold abnormalities (Borg, 1982a; Hannley et al, 1983; Jerger and Jerger, 1977; Stephens and Thornton, 1976), although this is certainly not an invariable sign of brainstem dysfunction (Russolo and Poli, 1983). Abnormally prolonged acoustic reflex latency also appears to be associated with brainstem pathology (Borg, 1973, 1982a; Bosatra et al, 1975; Colletti, 1975; Jerger and Jerger, 1977; McCandless and Harmer, 1975). Recent study of this phenomenon, however, suggests that reduced reflex amplitude may account for the apparently increased latency values (Jerger

and Hayes, 1983). In short, suprathreshold measures have added a new dimension to acoustic reflex application in the identification and localization of brainstem auditory pathology.

CASE STUDIES

Case 1

Cerebellopontine angle tumor. The patient was a 7-yr-old female whose chief complaint was an awkward and stumbling gait and difficulty in self-feeding. Physical examination indicated cerebellar ataxia and 6th and 7th cranial nerve paresis on the left. CT scan showed a mass in the posterior fossa on the left, with questionable compression of the anterior-lateral aspect of the 4th ventricle on the left. Electroencephalography was normal. Clinical impression was a left cerebellopontine angle tumor. This diagnosis was later confirmed surgically.

As shown in Figure 7.3, pure tone sensitivity was generally within normal limits and symmetric, with the exception of thresholds at 8000 Hz on the right and 250 Hz on the left. Performance intensity (PI) functions for kindergarten phonetically balanced word lists showed good maximum scores bilaterally, but borderline-normal rollover (20%) on the right ear, and a dramatic decrease in performance with increased intensity above 40 dB on the left. Tympanometry and static compliance values were normal. Acoustic reflex measurement yielded the "inverted L" pattern of abnormalities (see Jerger and Jerger, 1977, 1981), with only the right uncrossed reflexes observed. ABR findings are also illustrated in Figure 7.3. Each wave form is the averaged response to 2000 clicks at 85 dB HL. With right ear stimulation, there is a distinct wave I, II, and III, and no later waves. Only wave I was observed with left ear stimulation.

Acoustic tumors in young children are not common. Yet, even basic audiologic findings in case 1 provided powerful evidence of retrocochlear dysfunction, thus confirming the neurologic impression. Furthermore, the pattern of audiologic findings suggested that the tumor was large and not within a primarily eighth nerve site. That is, the left ear results of normal hearing sensitivity and PB max and a well-formed ABR wave I component with normal latency argued for relatively preserved eighth nerve function. The "L"-shaped acoustic reflex pattern, the contralateral (right-sided) abnormalities for ABR, and, to a lesser extent, PI-PB, coupled

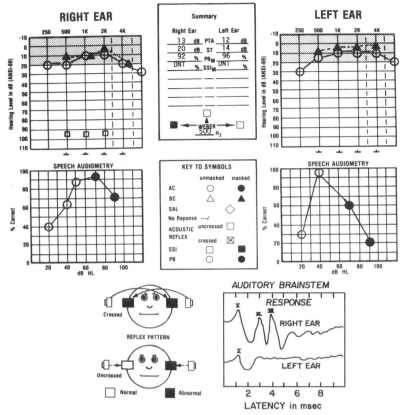

Figure 7.3. Audiometric findings for case 1, a 7-yr-old female with a left cerebellopontine angle tumor. Note evidence of bilateral brainstem dysfunction by acoustic reflex and auditory brainstem response measures.

with the highly significant PI-PB rollover and the absence of an ABR, except wave I on the left, are consistent with a tumor producing a direct effect on pontine auditory brainstem structures, plus contralateral brainstem compression.

Case 2

Vertebral basilar artery transient ischemic attacks. A 49-yr-old female was admitted to the hospital with a 26-yr history of hypertension, treated with multiple drugs, and recent difficulty in hearing with the telephone at the left ear and in understanding speech in crowds. Chief complaints included vertigo, nausea, and tinnitus. On admission in the emergency room blood pressure was 220/140. Rotatory and lateral nystagmus on right lateral gaze was noted. Initial medical impression was vertebral basilar transient ischemic attacks, although peripheral vestibular disease was also considered.

Audiometric findings, obtained 5 days after hospital admission, are shown in Figure 7.4. Hearing sensitivity was within normal limits (*shaded region*), with the exception of a mild notching deficit in the 4000 Hz region on the left. A slight rising configuration, however, was apparent. There was no air-bone difference in pure tone thresholds. Speech audiometry performance for word (PB) recognition and synthetic sentence identification (SSI) tasks was excellent bilaterally. Immittance audiometry yielded normally shaped tympanograms (type A) in each ear, with static compliance values in the low-normal range. Acoustic reflexes were observed under all stimulus conditions, but crossed reflex thresholds for lower frequencies were elevated relative to uncrossed. There was no reflex decay. This horizonal pattern of reflex threshold aberrations is displayed pictorially in the lower portion of the record form.

The single audiometric abnormality for case 2 was a discrepancy between crossed

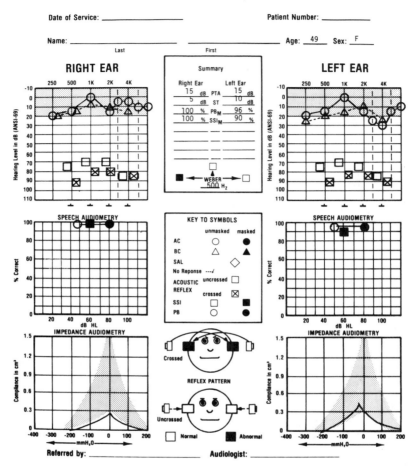

Figure 7.4. Audiometric findings for case 2, a 49-yr-old female with acute hypertension and vertebral basilar transient ischemic attacks. Note discrepancy in crossed vs uncrossed reflex thresholds for 500 and 1000 Hz stimuli.

and uncrossed reflex thresholds. Differential medical diagnosis was not clear-cut, with symptoms characteristic of Ménière's disease, but also not inconsistent with brain stem vascular insufficiency. Crossed acoustic reflex abnormalities in CNS vascular disease at the brainstem level were observed by Bosatra and colleagues (1975). Their patients also presented with complaints of vertigo and both clinical and electronystagmogram (ENG) evidence of spontaneous nystagmus. The reflex pattern in case 2 argues against a purely peripheral labyrinthine dis-

ease. The slightly rising configuration is, of course, consistent with the diagnosis of Ménière's disease but not unexpected in central auditory system involvement (Hayes and Jerger, 1979a). This case illustrates the possible utility of acoustic reflexes as a functional correlate of vascular status. Additionally, it illustrates the frequent independence in outcome for different measures of auditory functioning, such as the acoustic reflex vs SSI, and the clinical value of *routinely* administering multiple tests of peripheral and central auditory status.

Case 3

Caudal brainstem stroke. A 57-yr-old male was admitted to the hospital with a history of diabetes mellitus, glaucoma, and hypertension, status postcerebrovascular accident in 1963 with slight residual deficit. Chief complaint was loss of balance and falling to the right, worsening over the past 3 days. Associated symptoms were tinnitus and decreased hearing on the left, hoarseness, and numbness of the right face (fifth cranial nerve). Blood pressure was 190/106. Physical examination on admission was significant for decreased tone and slightly decreased strength on the right, decreased pin prick sensation on left leg, cerebellar signs of dysmetria right, with a wide-based gait, upbeat nystagmus with lateral and rotatary components on lateral gaze, and right vocal cord paralysis. There was a sluggish corneal reflex and central facial deficit on the right and a spastic gag reflex. Diagnosis was right posterior inferior cerebellar artery (PICA) infarction, with medullary and pontine brainstem involvement.

Auditory findings are displayed in Figure 7.5. There was a mild sensorineural hearing impairment in both ears, with a greater deficit for frequencies above 1000 Hz, particularly on the left. Audiometric Weber at 500 Hz was lateralized to the right ear. Maximum speech audiometry performance for word (PB) recognition and synthetic sentence identification (SSI) was excellent on the right and good on the left ear. Excessive rollover (Jerger and Hayes, 1977) was present on the SSI task for the right ear (30%) and left ear (70%). Immittance audiometry showed normal tympanograms and static compliance bilaterally. Acous-

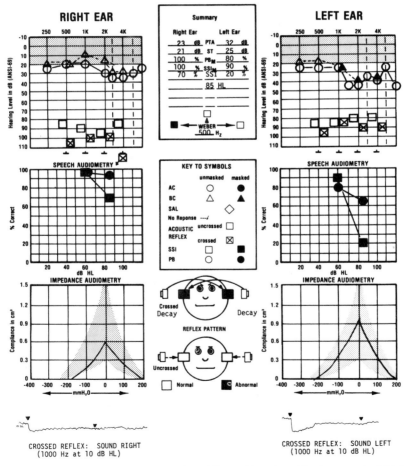

Figure 7.5. Audiometric findings for case 3, a 57-yr-old male with documented history of caudal brainstem stroke. Note excessive decay of crossed acoustic reflex amplitude bilaterally and rollover in speech audiometry for synthetic sentence identification.

tic reflexes were generally observed. There was, however, no measurable reflex for the contralateral condition at 4000 Hz on the right and somewhat elevated low-frequency threshold levels. Notably, abnormal crossed acoustic reflex decay was recorded in both ears (see tracings in bottom portion of Fig. 7.5).

There was abnormal crossed acoustic reflex decay bilaterally and also grossly elevated right to left crossed reflex threshold levels. SSI performance, however, was relatively poorer for the left ear. Consistent with the previous two cases, and with expectations, findings for an incomplete audiologic assessment (pure tone audiometry and word recognition at 40 dB SL) showed no signs of central auditory dysfunction. Yet, the patient clearly had neurologic signs and hearing complaints. Routine application of acoustic reflex and SSI measures were of value in confirming and localizing the source of these clinical deficits.

Case 4

Rostral brainstem stroke. A 58-yr-old female was admitted to the hospital with the chief complaint of a "burning" sensation on the right side of her face and body of 3 weeks duration. Soon after the onset of this sensation, she noted blurred vision and rapid movements of the right eye. There was a longstanding history of hypertension, medically controlled. Physical examination revealed intermittent lateral (left beating) nystagmus in the right eye, decreased sensation on the right face, and suggestion of right-sided motor weakness. Medical impression was a hypertensive vascular insult in the rostral pontine-midbrain region.

Audiometric findings are displayed in Figure 7.6. Pure tone testing showed a mild, symmetric high-frequency sensitivity impairment bilaterally. Maximum speech audiometry performance was excellent (92 to 96%) for word (PB) recognition but poor bilaterally (50%) for SSI materials. Significant rollover in SSI performance was observed for each ear. Performance deficits on the SSI-ICM at varying message to competition ratios

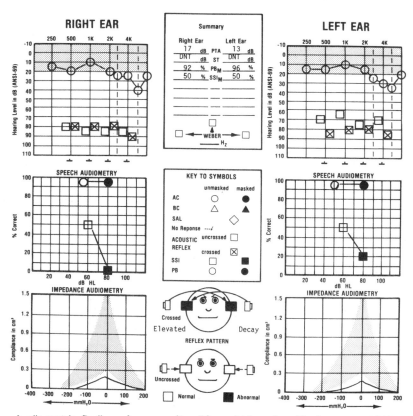

Figure 7.6. Audiometric findings for case 4, a 58-yr-old female with documented history of rostral brainstem stroke. Note "horizontal" pattern of acoustic reflex abnormalities (elevated threshold levels and excessive amplitude decay) and depressed performance for synthetic sentence identification.

(not shown) confirmed this finding. Immittance audiometry demonstrated tympanograms that were normally shaped but somewhat shallow. Acoustic reflexes were present in all four measurement conditions. However, crossed reflexes with stimulus-left were elevated relative to the left uncrossed condition, and excessive reflex decay (greater than 50% in 10 sec) was recorded for the crossed stimulus-right condition. In combination, these reflex abnormalities yielded the horizontal pattern, as shown in the lower center portion of Figure 7.6. The ABR was normal for left ear stimulation, but for the right ear the wave I to V latency interval was abnormally prolonged. The auditory middle latency response appeared normal bilaterally.

In this case, neurologic evidence contributed to the diagnosis of a brainstem (pontine-midbrain) vascular insult, and both acoustic reflex and SSI outcome provided evidence of bilateral central auditory system involvement. Reflex abnormalities were in the characteristic horizontal pattern (Jerger and Jerger, 1977), yet were varied for the left (elevated threshold) vs right (excessive decay) ears. Both of these deficits have long been associated with intrinsic brainstem pathology (Bosatra et al, 1975; Griesen and Rasmussen, 1970; Jerger J and Jerger S, 1974a and b, 1975; Jerger S and Jerger J, 1975a, 1977). The differential effect of the brainstem lesion on the two reflex parameters is, however, intriguing.

In combination, cases 2, 3, and 4 illustrate the sensitivity of acoustic reflex measurements to varying degrees of vascular brainstem impairment, ranging from transient ischemic attacks to stroke. This apparent influence of ischemic pathophysiology on reflex activity is clinically exciting and worthy of basic investigation.

Multiple Sclerosis

By definition, neuropathy in multiple sclerosis (MS), a disseminating demyelinating disease, may have both peripheral and central nervous system components. Consequently, there are clinical reports of eighth nerve and brainstem auditory dysfunction in MS. Studies of acoustic reflex patterns in MS are no exception (Bosatra et al, 1975; Colletti, 1975; Hannley et al, 1983; Hayes and Jerger, 1983; Jerger and Jerger, 1977; Lehnhardt et al, 1982; McCandless and Harmer, 1975; Russolo and Poli, 1983).

Indeed, a major clinical contribution of acoustic reflex measurements in this population is the early confirmation of peripheral *and/or* central nervous system involvement, and the rather precise localization of brainstem lesions. In addition to these neuroanatomic variations, MS may produce diverse types of reflex abnormalities, including elevated threshold levels (Colletti, 1975; Bosatra et al, 1975; Hannley et al, 1983; Hess, 1979; Jerger et al, 1979; Lehnhardt et al, 1982; Russolo and Poli, 1983), excessive decay (Hannley et al, 1983; Jerger and Jerger, 1977; McCandless and Harmer, 1975), prolonged latency (Bosatra et al, 1975; Colletti, 1975), and reduced amplitude (Hayes and Jerger, 1983).

Case 5

Multiple Sclerosis. The patient was a 24-yr-old female with a 3 yr history of multiple sclerosis. She was referred by the Neurology Service to Audiology for auditory brainstem response assessment. Symptoms included other sensory deficits and abnormal visual evoked responses.

Auditory findings, including ABR data, are shown in Figure 7.7. There was a mild, unilateral sensorineural hearing impairment for the left ear on this test date. Two years before, a complete audiologic assessment, including diagnostic testing (SISI, tone decay, Békésy audiometry, SSI-ICM, SSI-CCM, time compressed speech) failed to reveal any evidence of eighth nerve or central auditory dysfunction, and hearing sensitivity at that time was normal in each ear (PTAs of 3 dB on right and 5 dB on left). As shown in Figure 7.7 speech audiometry performance at this test date was excellent on the right. On the left, maximum SSI scores were depressed relative to word (PB) recognition scores, and there was abnormal rollover for both speech materials. Tympanograms and static compliance values were normal. Acoustic reflexes were observed bilaterally, but thresholds were elevated for all activating stimuli presented to the left ear. In addition, there was excessive decay of crossed acoustic reflexes for both ears, resulting in the "inverted L" pattern (Jerger and Jerger, 1977, 1981) depicted in the lower portion of Figure 7.7. The auditory brainstem response with left ear stimulation was grossly abnormal, with the wave I component prolonged in latency and poorly formed and an excessive wave I to V latency interval (brainstem transmission time). With right ear stimulation, the ABR was reasonably normal in appearance, although the wave V component was delayed in latency, variable in morphology, and noticeably reduced in amplitude (vs waves I, II, III, and IV).

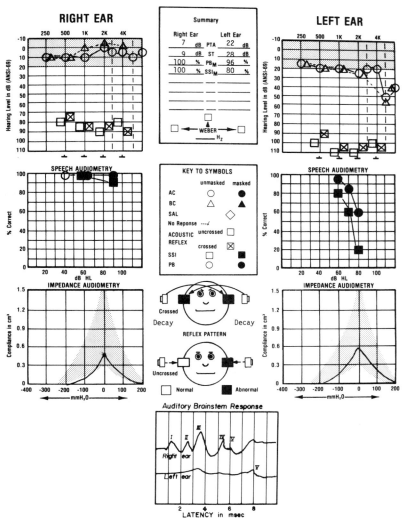

Figure 7.7. Audiometric findings for case 5, a 24-yr-old female with multiple sclerosis. Note "inverted L" pattern for acoustic reflex findings, unilateral (left) rollover for speech materials, and primarily left ear auditory brainstem response abnormalities.

Acoustic reflex amplitude data for case 5 are plotted as a function of stimulus (1000 Hz) intensity in Figure 7.8. The right uncrossed reflex alone shows normal, systematic amplitude growth with increasing intensity. For the crossed reflex with stimulus-right, the amplitude function is relatively flattened. Strikingly, both crossed and uncrossed reflex amplitude values with stimulus-left are grossly depressed, even at highest intensity levels. This pattern of reflex amplitude abnormalities is a graphic extension of the threshold aberrations noted above and cannot be explained by middle ear afferent or efferent dysfunction.

The audiometric outcome for case 5 is entirely consistent with previously reported findings in MS. The acoustic reflex pattern, however, contributes uniquely to the localization of the lesions. Pure tone and speech audiometry argue for unilateral (left-sided) involvement. Abnormal crossed reflex decay and decreased amplitude in both ears are evidence of bilateral brainstem lesions. This pattern is confirmed by ABR audiometry. Once again, these rather clear-cut clinical audiometric deficits would have gone unnoticed with a simple, routine hearing evaluation consisting of pure tone audiometry

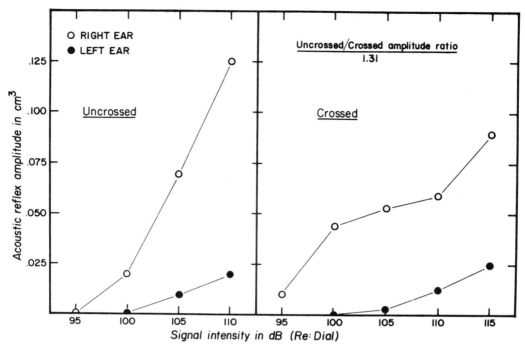

Figure 7.8. Acoustic reflex amplitude as a function of intensity for case 5. Systematic reflex amplitude growth is apparent only in the right ear, uncrossed condition.

and word recognition at a comfortable listening level.

Facial Nerve Dysfunction

By virtue of its efferent anatomy and physiology, the acoustic stapedius reflex is clinically useful in localizing and quantifying seventh (facial) cranial nerve dysfunction (Alford et al, 1973; Citron and Adour, 1978; Draskovich and Szekély, 1984; Koike et al, 1977; Matzui, 1981; Ruth et al, 1978). Unequivocally normal acoustic reflex activity in facial nerve palsy implies that the lesion is distal (peripheral) to the facial nerve branch innervating the stapedius muscle. Absence of measurable acoustic reflexes is a sign of gross facial nerve dysfunction proximal (central) to the stapedial branch. Of primary interest clinically are elevations of acoustic reflex threshold levels, abnormal decay, or a reduced reflex amplitude. These reflex parameters offer an objective, noninvasive means of quantifying and monitoring facial nerve function during progression of or recovery from disease. In any case, the reflexes of interest are with the probe in the ear on the affected side, with contralateral probe reflex measurements serving as control values.

Case 6

Bell's palsy. The patient was a 33-yr-old male with a 1-month history of idiopathic right facial paralysis diagnosed as Bell's palsy. He reported no hearing complaints, no history of otologic disease, tinnitus, or balance disturbances, and was otherwise in good health. Medical therapy consisted of prednisone.

Audiometric findings are illustrated in Figure 7.9. Hearing sensitivity was well within normal limits bilaterally. Audiometric Weber (500 Hz) was referred to midline. There was no consistent difference between air- and bone-conducted pure tone thresholds on the right. Maximum word recognition scores were 100% in each ear, but there was asymmetric PI-PB rollover of 20% on the right. Immittance audiometry yielded normal (type A) tympanograms and static compliance values in the normal range bilaterally. Acoustic reflex thresholds for tonal stimuli were at expected hearing levels (80 to 95 dB) with probe in the left ear, but the crossed and uncrossed reflexes with probe right were relatively elevated (10 to 20 dB). There was no evidence of excessive reflex

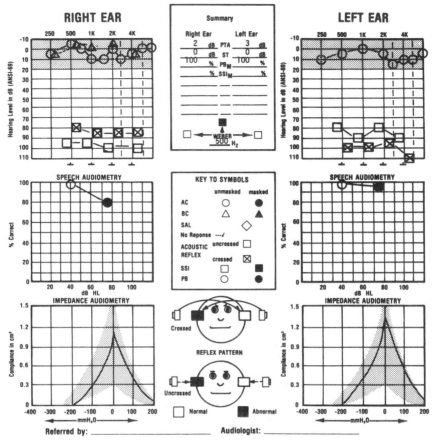

Figure 7.9. Audiometric findings for case 6, a 33-yr-old male with Bell's palsy. Note vertical pattern of acoustic reflex abnormalities (*right*) and ipsilateral evidence of rollover in word recognition performance.

decay. As depicted in the lower center portion of Figure 7.9, these reflex aberrations formed the vertical pattern (right side).

Abnormalities with a common probe (measurement) ear (vertical pattern; Jerger and Jerger, 1977, 1981) reflect disruption of the efferent portion of the acoustic reflex arc. Usually, they result from middle ear pathology, but they may be produced also by facial nerve dysfunction. In case 6, middle ear pathology was effectively ruled out by other immittance findings (symmetrically normal static compliance and tympanograms), by pure tone audiometry (no air-bone gap and midline Weber), and by normal otologic examination. The reflex threshold elevations with probe right were, therefore, secondary to facial nerve dysfunction proximal to the branching to the stapedius

muscle, and consistent with the diagnosis of Bell's palsy on the right. The unilateral evidence of decreased word recognition ipsilateral to this dysfunction is probably due to the reduced sound attenuation capacity of the right stapedial muscle having impaired facial nerve innervation. This finding is sometimes associated with facial nerve paresis (Borg and Zakrisson, 1973).

Age-related Central Auditory Dysfunction. As discussed earlier in this chapter, age is an important factor in acoustic reflex measurements. In many cases, age-related changes in middle ear or sensorineural function directly influence activity at the afferent or efferent portions of the reflex arc. There is some evidence, however, that integrity of the central reflex structures may also be involved in the age effect. For example,

Quaranta et al (1980) reported reflex abnormalities in 55% of a presbycusic population and attributed the finding to auditory brainstem aging processes. Supporting this contention was the tendency for abnormalities of crossed, rather than uncrossed, acoustic reflex thresholds. Comparable age effects are documented as well for other measures of central auditory functioning, including the auditory evoked responses (Fujikawa and Weber, 1977; Jerger and Hall, 1980) and complex speech perception tasks (Hall, 1983; Hayes and Jerger, 1979b; Jerger and Hayes, 1977).

Acoustic reflex amplitude-intensity functions are shown for two groups of elderly subjects in Figure 7.10. Subject characteristics are displayed in Table 7.2. Groups were comparable in age, hearing threshold levels, and maximum performance for word recognition. The centrally impaired group, however, demonstrated significant deficits for synthetic sentence identificaton (SSI) with a competing message, both in maximum percent correct score and degree of rollover. Ipsilateral and contralateral acoustic reflexes were simultaneously stimulated and then measured and computer-averaged with specially constructed dual probe apparatus, described in detail elsewhere (Hall, 1982a). Average magnitude of uncrossed

and crossed acoustic reflex activity was greater for the control group than the centrally impaired group. The difference is most apparent in the crossed reflex condition. These data suggest that age-related central nervous system changes (Hansen and Reske-Nielsen, 1965) may involve the brainstem auditory structures of the acoustic reflex arc, including, perhaps, the ventral cochlear nucleus region (Borg, 1973; Königsmark, 1969), as evidenced by the ipsilateral reflex magnitude deficit in the central group.

Cerebral Auditory Pathology. Whether or not suprabrainstem regions influence acoustic reflex activity is currently debated. On the one hand, there are case studies documenting normal acoustic reflex thresholds in patients with confirmed, bilateral damage to auditory temporal cortex (Jerger and Jerger, 1975b; Jerger, 1980). Gelfand and Silman (1982) also contend that cerebral damage does not affect reflex thresholds for tonal stimuli. Unfortunately, in this latter, retrospective study there were no control subjects. Furthermore, the site of CNS damage was not specified neuroradiologically, nor was there any documentation of associated neurologic deficits. These serious methodologic deficiencies cast doubt on the stated conclusions of the study. In contrast, Downs and Crum (1980) found abnormally

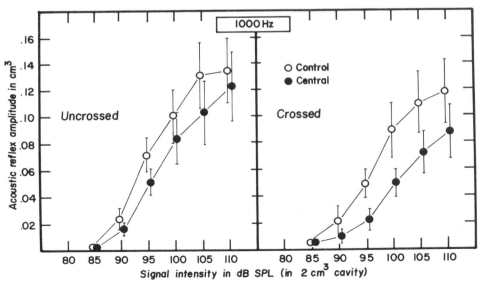

Figure 7.10.   Acoustic reflex amplitude intensity functions in elderly subjects with speech audiometry evidence of central auditory impairment and a control group. See Table 7.2 for description of subjects. Note depressed amplitude in centrally impaired group, expecially for crossed acoustic reflexes.

Table 7.2
Characteristics of Seventeen Subjects (Seven Male and Ten Female) with Evidence of Central Auditory Impairment by Speech Audiometry and Twenty-Three Subjects (Nine Male and Fourteen Female) with No Evidence of Central Auditory Impairment[a]

Group	Index Age (yr)	HTL[b] (dB) (1000 Hz)	Static compliance (cm³)	PBmax[c] (%)	SSImax[d] (%)	SSI-rollover[e] (%)
No central auditory impairment						
mean	69.2	15.5	0.76	93.0	91.1	2.4
SD	(5.0)	(11.2)	(0.36)	(15.0)	(17.5)	(7.6)
Central auditory impairment						
mean	72.5	15.4	0.64	90.9	65.9	25.0
SD	(5.1)	(9.8)	(0.23)	(9.7)	(20.9)	(22.8)
Difference in mean	3.3	0.2	0.12	2.1	25.2**	22.6**

[a] Audiologic data are averaged for both ears of each subject.
[b] Hearing threshold level (dB) at test signal frequencies of 1000 Hz or 500 to 1500 Hz (noise-band).
[c] Maximum score (%) for Phonetically Balanced (PB) word test.
[d] Maximum score (%) for Synthetic Sentence Identification (SSI) test.
[e] Decrease in SSI performance (%) between maximum score and score at highest speech intensity level.
[f] Difference in mean values between groups is significant at 0.01 level of confidence by t-test.

sensitive acoustic reflex threshold activity in four patients with neurophysiologic, neuroradiologic (e.g., computerized tomography), and/or neurologic evidence of cerebral lesions. Also, Peterson and Lidén (1972) described reduced reflex amplitude in a patient with a corpus callosum lesion. Experimental bilateral ablation of auditory cortex reduced middle ear muscle activity in cat (Baust and Berlucchi, 1964), and recent experimental investigations in monkey also provided preliminary evidence of a cortical modulation of suprathreshold acoustic reflex activity (B Stach, personal communication, 1983). The issue requires further experimental study and more carefully conducted clinical exploration to define the potential role of rostral brainstem, midbrain, thalamic, and/or cortical influences on the acoustic reflex.

Other Central Nervous System Dysfunctions

Scattered throughout the literature are reports of acoustic reflex findings in diverse confirmed and suspected central auditory nervous system dysfunctions. The suppressive acute influence of alcohol on acoustic reflex activity was noted previously in this chapter. In a recent study, Spitzer and Ventry (1980) found a significantly higher proportion of inexplicably absent acoustically measured reflexes in a group of *chronic al-coholics* than in an age-matched control group. Acoustic reflex threshold levels were equivalent for the two groups. The results of a diagnostic audiologic test battery, including these reflex findings, were consistent with brainstem auditory dysfunction.

Acoustic reflex measurements are clinically useful in patients with *speech-language and voice problems* of varied CNS etiologies, including autism, cerebral palsy, and mental retardation (Keith et al, 1977; Niswander and Ruth, 1977; Suria and Serra-Raventos, 1975). The main applications are in prediction of hearing loss and identification of middle ear pathology. There is no conclusive evidence of reflex abnormalities in these patient groups, assuming middle ear function is unequivocally normal (Keith et al, 1977). Hall and colleagues (Hall and Jerger, 1976, 1978; Hall, 1981) observed acoustic reflex aberrations in two speech-voice disorders of unknown etiology. A reflex latency measure (rise time) was longer in a group of six patients with *spastic dysphonia* than an age- and sex-matched control group (Hall and Jerger, 1976). In a subsequent study, uncrossed reflex amplitude was curiously larger in a group of 12 spastic dysphonics than in a control group, but crossed reflex amplitude showed no group differences. This deviant pattern (greater uncrossed reflex amplitude) had previously been associated with brainstem pathology (Bosatra and Russolo, 1976).

In addition, reflex amplitude aberrations were reported in *stuttering*, again with reference to control data (Hall and Jerger, 1978). Further investigation of reflex parameters in such patient populations may help to define the etiology and possible neurologic bases of these enigmatic communicative disorders.

In acutely and severely head-injured patients, acoustic reflexes are rarely observed, even in persons with normal middle ear function as determined by otologic examination and other acoustic immittance measures (Hall et al, 1982 a and b, 1983). Only 16% of a series of 25 patients showed evidence of any acoustic reflex activity within 3 days after a head injury defined as severe by the extent of coma. This high proportion of abnormal acoustic reflexes was probably related to their comatose state and neurosurgical management rather than to brainstem structural damage. That is, severe head injury impairing consciousness presumably affects the brainstem reticular activating system. Barbiturate-induced coma, as noted earlier in the chapter, is sometimes employed therapeutically in management of brain pathophysiology secondary to head injury and was used in six of the above patients with no reflex activity. Both findings lend further support to the role of the reticular formation in the central acoustic reflex arc in man.

PROMISING NEW DIRECTIONS FOR ACOUSTIC REFLEX MEASUREMENTS IN CNS PATHOLOGY

In the years since Griesen and Rasmussen (1970) first described reflex abnormalities in brainstem pathology, interest in neurodiagnostic applications has not abated but, rather, increased. This clinical popularity is not surprising. Acoustic reflexes offer a noninvasive, objective, simply administered, and cost-effective measure of eighth (acoustic) nerve, auditory brainstem and seventh (facial) nerve function, available in most audiology facilities (Jerger and Jerger, 1983).

The general diagnostic value of acoustic reflexes is now well-documented, yet the specific neuropathologic correlates of abnormal findings are not adequately defined. Also, pathophysiologic processes affecting acoustic reflex parameters are virtually un-

known. Particularly unclear is the influence of brainstem regions not traditionally considered part of the auditory system (e.g., reticular formation) and the suprabrainstem auditory anatomy. These basic and clinically important issues require further study.

The versatility of reflex measurements in central auditory dysfunction has expanded with the clinical application of latency, decay, and amplitude parameters, as well as threshold levels. In the literature, and in this chapter, are clinical cases illustrating the independence of these parameters. That is, the response parameters are characterized by differential sensitivity to brainstem lesions. Put another way, it is likely that different pathologic processes produce distinctive reflex aberrations, some affecting amplitude, others time course (decay), and still others temporal characteristics (rise time or latency). Defining these associations is a worthy objective for future clinical research. Among the response parameters, reflex amplitude especially has shown promise in identification of brainstem dysfunction (Borg, 1973; Brask, 1978). The clinical feasibility of amplitude measures, however, has been questioned on the basis of the troublesome variability of intersubject data, and, consequently, the difficulty in developing meaningful normative values. Recently developed amplitude indices that emphasize the intrasubject crossed vs uncrossed relationship appear to reduce the clinical problem posed by variability (Hall, 1982c; Hayes and Jerger, 1983).

Computer averaging of acoustic reflex activity for a series of stimuli is becoming clinically feasible and probably will contribute to the stability and reliability of measurements in patient populations. Often this is done by interfacing commercially available immittance audiometers with signal averaging evoked response systems. Multipurpose audiometric microprocessors offer another means of averaging acoustic reflexes. In addition to enhancing the sensitivity and reliability of acoustic reflex determinations, signal averaging over a brief time period (less than 500 msec) offers increased accuracy in temporal measurements, and data storage capacity with some microcomputers permits archiving and facilitates intersubject comparisons of reflex findings.

Finally, because it is noninvasive, cost-effective, and brief, acoustic reflex measurement is well-suited for serially monitoring auditory brainstem status, or eighth and seventh cranial nerve function, over time. This is likely to be a particularly important clinical application in dynamic neurologic pathologies, including multiple sclerosis, Bell's palsy, and even neuromuscular disorders, such as myasthenia gravis (Kramer et al, 1981; Neff et al, 1980). The extreme susceptibility of the acoustic reflex to the influence of many CNS depressants, such as barbiturates, suggests a potentially valuable application in anesthetic monitoring. In summary, the role of acoustic reflex measurements in neuroaudiology appears secure, and, indeed, will probably expand with further basic science and clinical investigation.

Acknowledgments. Grant Berry, Kristine Olsen, and Barbara Murray, audiologists at the Speech and Hearing Center of the Hospital of the University of Pennsylvania, provided invaluable assistance in collecting and analyzing audiometric data reported in this chapter.

I gratefully acknowledge the contributions of Stella Rodriguez in manuscript preparation.

References

Alberti PW: The diagnostic role of stapedius reflex estimations. *Otolaryngol Clin North Am* 11:251–261, 1978.

Alberti P, Fria T, Cummings F: The clinical utility of ipsilateral stapedius reflex tests. *J Otolaryngol* 6:466–472, 1977.

Alford BR, Jerger J, Coats A, Peterson C, Weber S: Neurophysiology of facial nerve testing. *Arch Otolaryngol* 97:214, 1973.

Anderson H, Barr B, Wedenberg E: Intraaural reflexes in retrocochlear lesions. In Hamburger C, Versall J (eds): *Nobel Symposium: Disorders of the Skull-Base Region.* Stockholm, Almquist and Wiskell, 1969, pp 49–55.

Anniko M, Wroblewski R: Ultrastructure and elemental composition of the stapedius muscle in guinea pig. *Arch Otorhinolaryngol* 230:109–112, 1981.

Baust W, Berlucchi G: Reflex response to clicks of cat's tensori tympani during sleep and wakefulness and the influence thereon of the auditory cortex. *Arch Ital Biol* 102:686–712, 1964.

Beedle RK, Harford ER: A comparison of acoustic reflex and loudness growth in normal and pathological ears. *J Speech Hear Res* 16:271–281, 1973.

Block MG, Wiley TL: Acoustic-reflex growth and loudness. *J Speech Hear Res* 22:295–315, 1979.

Borg E: Efferent inhibition of afferent acoustic activity in the unanesthetized rabbit. *Exp Neurol* 31:301–312, 1971.

Borg E: On the neuronal organization of the acoustic middle ear reflex. A physiological and anatomic study. *Brain Res* 49:101–123, 1973.

Borg E: Dynamic characteristics of the intra-aural muscle reflex. In Feldman AS, Wilber CA (eds): *Acoustic Impedance and Admittance—The Measurement of Middle Ear Function.* Baltimore, Williams & Wilkins, 1976, pp 236–299.

Borg E: The intra-aural muscle reflex in retrocochlear pathology: a model study in the rabbit. *Audiology* 16:316–330, 1977.

Borg E: Dynamic properties of the intra-aural reflex in lesions of the lower auditory pathways: an experimental study in rabbits. *Acta Otolaryngol (Stockh)* 93:19–29, 1982a.

Borg E: Time course of the human acoustic stapedius reflex. A comparison of eight different measures in normal-hearing subjects. *Scand Audiol* 11:237–242, 1982b.

Borg E, Counter SA, Rydquist B: Contraction properties and functional morphology of the avian stapedius muscle. *Acta Otolaryngol (Stockh)* 88:20–26, 1979.

Borg E, Møller A: Effect of ethylalcohol and pentobarbital sodium on the acoustic middle ear reflex in man. *Acta Otolaryngol (Stockh)* 64:415–426, 1967.

Borg E, Møller A: Effect of central depressants on the acoustic middle ear reflex in rabbits. *Acta Physiol Scand* 94:327–338, 1975.

Borg E, Ødman B: Decay and recovery of the acoustic stapedius reflex in humans. *Acta Otolaryngol (Stockh)* 87:421–428, 1979.

Borg E, Zakrisson J-E: Stapedius reflex and speech features. *J Acoust Soc Am* 54:525–527, 1973.

Bosatra A: Pathology of the nervous arc of the acoustic reflexes. *Audiology* 68:307–315, 1977.

Bosatra A, Russolo M: Oscilloscopic analysis of the stapedius muscle reflex in brain stem lesions. *Arch Otolaryngol* 102:284–290, 1976.

Bosatra A, Russolo M, Poli P: Modifications of the stapedius muscle reflex under spontaneous and experimental brain-stem impairment. *Acta Otolaryngol (Stockh)* 80:61–66, 1975.

Boudreau JC: Stimulus correlates of nerve activity in the superior-olivary complex of the cat. *J Acoust Soc Am* 37:779, 1965.

Brask T: Extratympanic manometry in man: clinical and experimental investigations of the acoustic stapedius and tensor tympani contractions in normal subjects and in patients. *Scand Audiol* 7(suppl):1–199, 1978.

Brodal A: *Neurological Anatomy in Relation to Clinical Medicine.* New York, Oxford Univ Press, 1981.

Bunch CC: Age variations in auditory acuity. *Arch Otolaryngol* 9:625–636, 1929.

Burgener J, Mayr R: Guinea pig stapedius muscle. A histochemical, light and electron microscopic study. *Anat Embryol* 161:65–81, 1980.

Citron D, Adour K: Acoustic reflex and loudness discomfort in acute facial paralysis. *Arch Otolaryngol* 104:303–306, 1978.

Clemis JD, Sarno CN: The acoustic reflex latency test: clinical application. *Laryngoscope* 90:601–611, 1980.

Cohill EM, Greenberg HJ: Effects of ethyl alcohol on the acoustic reflex threshold. *J Am Audiol Soc* 2:121–123, 1977.

Colletti V: Stapedius abnormalities in multiple sclerosis. *Audiology* 14:63–71, 1975.

Danaher EM, Pickett JM: Notes on an artifact in measurement of the acoustic reflex. *J Speech Hear Res* 17:505–510, 1974.

Djupesland G: The acoustic reflex. In Jerger J, Northern JL (eds): *Clinical Impedance Audiometry*, ed 2. Acton, MA, American Electromedics, 1980, pp 65–82.

Djupesland G, Sundby A, Flottorp G: Temporal summation in the acoustic stapedius reflex mechanism. *Acta Otolaryngol (Stockh)* 76:305–312, 1973.

Djupesland G, Zwislocki JJ: On the critical band in the acoustic stapedius reflex. *J Acoust Soc Am* 54:1157–1159, 1973.

Downs DW, Crum MA: The hyperactive acoustic reflex: four case studies. *Arch Otolaryngol* 106:401–404, 1980.

Draskovich E, Székely TH: Diagnostic value of the stapedius reflex examination by facial palsy (German). *HNO* 29:222–224, 1981.

Erulkar SD, Shelanski ML, Whitsel BL, Ogle P: Studies of the muscle fibers of the tensor tympani muscle of the cat. *Anat Res* 149:279–298, 1964.

Fernand VSV, Hess A: The occurrence, structure and innervation of slow and twitch muscle fibers in the tensor tympani and stapedius muscle of the cat. *J Physiol (Lond)* 200:547–554, 1969.

Flottorp G, Djupesland G, Winther FØ: The acoustic stapedius reflex in relation to critical bandwidth. *J Acoust Soc Am* 49:457–461, 1971.

Foley JO, Dubois FS: An experimental study of the facial nerve. *J Comp Neurol* 79:70–101, 1953.

Freyss G, Casteran J-M: Optimisation de l'utilisation du réflexe stapédien acoustique á la distinction des surdités endo- et rétro-cochléaires (French). *Rev Laryngol* 100:11–12, 1979.

Fujikawa SM, Weber BA: Effects of increased stimulus rate in brainstem electric response (BER) audiometry as a function of age. *J Am Audiol Soc* 3:147–150, 1977.

Gelfand SA, Silman S: Acoustic reflex thresholds in brain-damaged patients. *Ear Hearing* 3:93–95, 1982.

Gelfand SA, Silman S, Silverman CA: Temporal summation in acoustic reflex growth functions. *Acta Otolaryngol (Stockh)* 91:177–182, 1981.

Gersdorff C. Modifications du réflexe acoustico-facial chez l'homme en fonction de l'age, par etude impedance metrique. *Audiology* 17:260–270, 1978.

Giacomelli F, Mozzo W: An experimental and clinical study on the influence of the brainstem reticular formation on the stapedial reflex. *Int Audiol* 3:42–47, 1964.

Griesen O, Rasmussen P: Stapedius reflexes in otoneurological examination in brain stem tumors. *Acta Otolaryngol (Stockh)* 70:366–370, 1970.

Habener SA, Snyder MJ: Stapedius reflex amplitude and decay in normal hearing ears. *Arch Otolaryngol* 100:294–297, 1974.

Hall JW III: The effect of age and sex on static compliance. *Arch Otolaryngol* 105:153–156, 1979.

Hall JW III: Predicting hearing level from the acoustic reflex In Jerger J (ed): *Handbook of Clinical Impedance Audiometry*, ed 2. Acton, MA, American Electromedics, 1980, pp 141–163.

Hall JW III: Central auditory function in spastic dysphonia. *Am J Otolaryngol* 2:188–198, 1981.

Hall JW III: Acoustic reflex amplitude. I. Effect of age and sex. *Audiology* 21:294–309, 1982a.

Hall JW III: Acoustic reflex amplitude. II. Effect of age-related auditory dysfunction. *Audiology* 21:386–399, 1982b.

Hall JW III: Quantification of the relationship between crossed and uncrossed acoustic reflex amplitude. *Ear Hearing* 3:296–300, 1982c.

Hall JW III: Diagnostic applications of speech audiometry. *Semin Hear* 4(3):179–204, 1983.

Hall JW III, Huangfu M, Gennarelli TA: Auditory function in acute head injury. *Laryngoscope* 93:383–390, 1982b.

Hall JW III, Huangfu M, Gennarelli TA, Dolinskas CA, Olson K, Berry GA: Auditory evoked response, impedance measures and diagnostic speech audiometry in severe head injury. *Otolaryngol Head Neck Surg* 91:50–60, 1983.

Hall JW III, Jerger JF: Acoustic reflex characteristics in spastic dysphonia. *Arch Otolaryngol* 102:411–415, 1976.

Hall JW III, Jerger JF: Central auditory function in stuttering. *J Speech Hear Res* 21:324–337, 1978.

Hall JW III, Jerger JF: Impedance audiometry. In Lass NJ, Northern JL, Yoder DJ, McReynolds LV (eds): *Speech, Language and Hearing*. Philadelphia, WB Saunders, 1982, pp 968–981.

Hall JW III, Koval C: Accuracy of hearing prediction by the acoustic reflex. *Laryngoscope* 92:140–149, 1982.

Hall JW III, Spielman G, Gennarelli TA: Auditory evoked responses in acute severe head injuries. *J Neurosurg Nurs* 14:225–231, 1982a.

Hall JW III, Weaver T: Impedance audiometry in a young population: the effects of age, sex and minor tympanogram abnormality. *J Otolaryngol* 8:210–222, 1979.

Handler SS, Margolis RH: Prediction of hearing loss from stapedius reflex thresholds in patients with sensorineural impairment. *Trans Am Acad Ophthalmol Otolaryngol* 84:425–431, 1977.

Hannley M, Jerger JF, Rivera VM: Relationships among auditory brainstem responses, masking level differences and the acoustic reflex in multiple sclerosis. *Audiology* 22:20–33, 1983.

Hansen CC, Reske-Nielsen E: Pathological studies in presbycusis. *Arch Otolaryngol* 82:115–132, 1965.

Hayes D, Jerger J: Low-frequency hearing loss in presbycusis: a central interpretation. *Arch Otolaryngol* 105:9–12, 1979a.

Hayes D, Jerger J: Aging and hearing aid use. *Scand Audiol* 8:33–40, 1979b.

Hayes D, Jerger J: Signal averaging of the acoustic reflex: diagnostic application of amplitude characteristics. *Scand Audiol* Suppl. 17:31–36, 1983.

Hess K: Stapedius reflex in multiple sclerosis. *J Neurol Neurosurg Psychiatry* 42:331–337, 1979.

Hirayama M, Daly JF: Ultrastructure of middle ear muscle in the rabbit. I. Stapedius Muscle. *Acta Otolaryngol (Stockh)* 77:13–18, 1974.

Hirsch A, Anderson H: Audiologic test results in 96 patients with tumours affecting the eighth nerve. A clinical study, with emphasis on the early audiological diagnosis. *Acta Otolaryngol [Suppl] (Stockh)* 369:1–26, 1980a.

Hirsch A, Anderson H: Elevated stapedius reflex threshold and pathologic reflex decay. Clinical occurrence and significance. *Acta Otolaryngol [Suppl] (Stockh)* 368, 1980b.

Hung I, Dallos P: Study of the acoustic reflex in human beings. I. Dynamic characteristics. *J Acoust Soc Am* 52:1168–1180, 1972.

Jepsen O: The threshold of the reflexes of the tympanic

muscles in a normal material examined by means of the impedance method. *Acta Otolaryngol* 39:406–408, 1951.

Jerger JF: Clinical experience with impedance audiometry. *Arch Otolaryngol* 92:311–324, 1970.

Jerger J: Comment on the effect of aging on the stapedius reflex threshold (*J Acoust Soc Am* 66:735–738, 1979). *J Acoust Soc Am* 66:908, 1979.

Jerger J, Anthony L, Jerger S, Mauldin L: Studies in impedance audiometry. III. Middle ear disorders. *Arch Otolaryngol* 99:165–171, 1974a.

Jerger J, Burney P, Mauldin L, Crump B: Predicting hearing loss from the acoustic reflex. *J Speech Hear Disord* 39:11–22, 1974b.

Jerger J, Hall JW III: Effects of age and sex on auditory brainstem response. *Arch Otolaryngol* 106:387–391, 1980.

Jerger J, Harford E, Clemis J, Alford B: The acoustic reflex in eighth nerve disorders. *Arch Otolaryngol* 99:409–413, 1974c.

Jerger J, Hayes D: Diagnostic speech audiometry. *Arch Otolaryngol* 103:216–222, 1977.

Jerger J, Hayes D: Latency of the acoustic reflex in eighth-nerve tumor. *Arch Otolaryngol* 109:1–5, 1983.

Jerger J, Hayes D, Anthony L: Effect of age on prediction of sensorineural hearing level for the acoustic reflex. *Arch Otolaryngol* 104:393–394, 1978a.

Jerger J, Hayes D, Anthony L, Mauldin L: Factors influencing prediction of hearing level from acoustic reflex. *Monogr Contemp Audiol* 1:1–20, 1978b.

Jerger J, Jerger S: Audiological comparison of cochlear and eighth nerve disorders. *Ann Otol Rhinol Laryngol* 83:1–11, 1974a.

Jerger J, Jerger S: Auditory findings in brainstem disorders. *Arch Otolaryngol* 99:342–350, 1974b.

Jerger J, Jerger S: Clinical validity of central auditory tests. *Scand Audiol* 4:147–163, 1975.

Jerger J, Jerger S, Mauldin L: Studies in impedance audiometry: normal and sensori-neural ears. *Arch Otolaryngol* 96:513–523, 1972.

Jerger J, Mauldin L, Lewis N: Temporal summation of the acoustic reflex. *Audiology* 16:177–200, 1977.

Jerger J, Neeley JG, Jerger S: Speech, impedance and auditory brainstem response audiometry in brainstem tumors. Importance of a multiple test strategy. *Arch Otolaryngol* 106:218–223, 1980.

Jerger J, Northern J (eds): *Clinical Impedance Audiometry*, ed 2. Acton, MA, American Electromedics, 1980.

Jerger S: Diagnostic application of impedance audiometry in central auditory disorders. In Jerger J, Northern JL (eds): *Clinical Impedance Audiometry*, ed 2. Acton, MA, American Electromedics, 1980, pp 128–140.

Jerger S, Jerger J: Extra- and intra-axial brainstem auditory disorders. *Audiology* 14:93–117, 1975.

Jerger S, Jerger J: Diagnostic value of crossed versus uncrossed acoustic reflexes. Eighth nerve and brainstem disorders. *Arch Otolaryngol* 103:445–453, 1977.

Jerger S, Jerger J: *Auditory Disorders: A Manual for Clinical Evaluation*. Boston, Little, Brown, 1981.

Jerger S, Jerger J: Evaluation of diagnostic audiometric tests. *Audiology* 22:144–161, 1983.

Jerger S, Jerger J, Hall J: A new acoustic reflex pattern. *Arch Otolaryngol* 105:24–28, 1979.

Jerger S, Neely G, Jerger J: Recovery of crossed acoustic reflexes in brainstem auditory disorders. *Arch Otolaryngol* 101:329–332, 1975.

Johnson EW: Auditory test results in 500 cases of acoustic neuroma. *Arch Otolaryngol* 103:152–158, 1977.

Keith RW, Murphy KT, Martin F: Acoustic reflex measurement in children with cerebral palsy. *Folia Phoniatr (Basel)* 29:311–314, 1977.

Koike Y, Hojo K, Iwasaki E: Prognosis of facial palsy based on the stapedial reflex-test. In Fisch U (ed): *Facial Nerve Surgery*. Amstelveen, Netherlands, Kugler, Aesculapius, 1977, pp 159–164.

Königsmark BW: Neuronal population of the ventral cochlear nucleus in man. *Anat Res* 163:212–213, 1969.

Kramer LD, Ruth RA, Johns ME, Sanders DB: A comparison of stapedial reflex fatigue with jitter and single fiber EMG in the diagnosis of myasthenia gravis. *Ann Neurol* 9:531–536, 1981.

Kunoz H: The "eardrum artifact" in ipsilateral reflex measurements. *Scand Audiol* 6:163–166, 1977.

Laukli E, Mair IWS: Ipsilateral and contralateral acoustic reflex thresholds. *Audiology* 19:469–479, 1980.

Lehnhardt E: Audiometric localization of brainstem lesions. *Z Laryngol Rhinol Otol* 52:11–21, 1973.

Lehnhardt E, Schmidt W, Franke KE: Aspects in diagnostics of central neural hearing disorders. *Arch Otol Rhinol Laryngol* 234:73–95, 1982.

Leis BR, Lutman ME: Calibration of ipsilateral acoustic reflex stimuli. *Scand Audiol* 8:93–99, 1979.

Lidén G, Korsan-Bengtsen M: Audiometric manifestations of retrocochlear lesions. *Scand Audiol* 2:29–40, 1973.

Lilly DJ: Measurement of acoustic impedance at the tympanic membrane. In Jerger J (ed): *Modern Developments in Audiology*, ed 2. New York, Academic Press, 1973, pp 345–406.

Lilly DJ, Franzen R: Threshold of the acoustic reflex for pure-tones. *ASHA* 12:435, 1970.

Lorente de Nó R: The reflex contractions of the muscles of the middle ear as a hearing test in experimental animals. *Trans Am Laryngol Rhinol Otol Soc* 39:26–42, 1933a.

Lorente de Nó R: Anatomy of the eighth nerve. III. General plan of structure of the primary cochlear nuclei. *Laryngoscope* 43:327–350, 1933b.

Lorente de Nó R: The function of the central acoustic nuclei examined by means of the acoustic reflexes. *Laryngoscope* 45:573–595, 1935.

Lüscher E: Die funktion des musculus stapedius beim menschen. *Z Hal-Nasen-U Ohrenheilk* 23:105–132, 1929.

Lyon MJ: Localization of the efferent neurons of the tensor tympani muscle of the newborn kitten using horseradish peroxidase. *Exp Neurol* 49:439–455, 1975.

Lyon MJ: The central location of the motor neurons to stapedius muscle in cat. *Brain Res* 143:437–444, 1978.

Mangham CA Jr, Burnett PA, Lindeman RC: Standardization of acoustic reflex latency. A study in humans and nonhuman primates. *Ann Otol Rhinol Laryngol* 91:169–174, 1982.

Mangham CA, Lindeman RC, Dawson WR: Stapedius reflex quantification in acoustic tumor patients. *Laryngoscope* 90:242–250, 1980.

Mangham CA, Miller JM: A case for further quantification of the stapedius reflex. *Arch Otolaryngol* 105:593–596, 1979.

Margolis RH, Fox C: A comparison of three methods for predicting hearing loss from acoustic reflex thresholds. *J Speech Hear Res* 20:241–253, 1977.

Margolis RH, Popelka GR: Loudness and the acoustic reflex. *J Acoust Soc Am* 58:1330–1332, 1975.

Matzui H: The origin of diphasic impedance change in middle ear muscle reflex (Japanese). *Otolaryngol Jap* 53:1033–1037, 1981.

McCandless G, Harmer D: Abnormal intra-aural reflex in multiple sclerosis patients. *Impedance Newsletter* 4:16–22, 1975.

McPherson O, Thompson D: Quantification of the threshold and latency parameters of the acoustic reflex in human. *Acta Otolaryngol [Suppl] (Stockh)* 353:1–37, 1977.

Metz O: The acoustic impedance measured in normal and pathological ears. *Acta Otolaryngol [Suppl] (Stockh)* 63:1–249, 1946.

Metz O: Studies on the contraction of the tympanic muscles as indicated by changes in the impedance of the ear. *Acta Otolaryngol (Stockh)* 39:397–405, 1951.

Møller AR: Intra-aural muscle contraction in man examined by measuring acoustic impedance of the ear. *Laryngoscope* 68:48–62, 1958.

Møller A: Bilateral contraction of the tympanic muscles in man, examined by measuring impedance change. *Ann Otol Rhinol Laryngol* 70:735–752, 1961.

Møller AR: Acoustic reflex in man. *J Acoust Soc Am* 34:1524–1534, 1962.

Møller AR: The middle ear. In Tobias JV (ed): *Foundations of Modern Auditory Theory.* New York, Academic Press, 1972, pp 135–194.

Møller AR: *Auditory Physiology* New York, Academic Press, 1983.

Nagafuchi M: Delayed auditory feedback and acoustic reflex (Japanese). *Audiol Jpn* 25:1–6, 1982.

Neff PA, Morioka WT, Sample PA, Cantrell RW: Audiometry and tympanometric monitoring of a disease affecting muscle transmission. *Audiology* 19:293–309, 1980.

Niemeyer W, Sesterhenn G: Calculating the hearing threshold from the stapedius reflex threshold for different sound stimuli. *Audiology* 13:421–427, 1974.

Niswander PS, Ruth RA: Prediction of hearing sensitivity from acoustic reflexes in mentally retarded persons. *Am J Ment Defic* 81:474–481, 1977.

Niswander PS, Ruth RA: A discussion of some temporal characteristics of electroacoustic impedance bridges. *J Am Audiol Soc* 5:151–155, 1979.

Norris TW, Stelmachowicz PG, Bowling C, Taylor DJ: Latency measures of the acoustic reflex. Normal versus sensorineural. *Audiology* 13:464–469, 1974.

Olsen W, Noffsinger D, Kurdziel S: Acoustic reflex and reflex decay: occurrence in patients with cochlear and eighth nerve lesions. *Arch Otolaryngol* 101:622–625, 1975.

Olsen W, Stach B, Kurdziel S: Acoustic reflex decay in 10 seconds and 5 seconds for Ménière's disease and for 8th nerve tumor patients. *Ear Hearing* 2:180–181, 1981.

Papez JW: Subdivisions of the facial nucleus. *J Comp Neurol* 43:159–191, 1927.

Perlman HB, Case TJ: Latent period of the crossed stapedius reflex in man. *Ann Otol Rhinol Laryngol* 48:663–675, 1939.

Pestalozza G, Shore I: Clinical evaluation of presbycusis on the basis of different tests of auditory function. *Laryngoscope* 65:1136–1163, 1955.

Peterson J, Lidén G: Some static characteristics of the stapedius muscle reflex. *Audiology* 11:97–114, 1972.

Popelka G, Margolis R, Wiley T: Effect of activating signal bandwidth on acoustic-reflex threshold. *J Acoust Soc Am* 59:153–159, 1976.

Quaranta A, Cassano P, Amoroso C: Presbyacoustic et réflexométrie stapédienne. *Audiology* 19:310–315, 1980.

Rasmussen GL: The olivary peduncle and other fiber projections of the superior olivary complex. *J Comp Neurol* 84:141–219, 1946.

Reker U: Methodological problems in the determination of homolateral stapedius reflex thresholds. *Audiology* 16:487–498, 1977.

Reker U, Baumgarten D: Binaural summation of the ipsilateral and contralateral acoustic stapedius reflex (German). *HNO* 28:135–138, 1981.

Richards GB, Mitchell OC, Speights JL: Effects of phenobarbital on intra-aural muscle reflexes in retarded children. *Eye Ear Nose Throat Mon* 54:73–75, 1975.

Robinette MS, Brey RH: Influence of alcohol on the acoustic reflex and temporary threshold shift. *Arch Otolaryngol* 104:31–37, 1978.

Robinette MS, Rhoads DP, Marion MW: Effects of secobarbital on impedance audiometry. *Arch Otolaryngol* 100:351–354, 1974.

Russolo M, Poli P: Lateralization, impedance, auditory brainstem response and synthetic sentence audiometry in brainstem disorders. *Audiology* 22:50–62, 1983.

Ruth RA, Nilo ER, Mravec JJ: Acoustic reflex magnitude (ARM) in idiopathic facial paralysis. *Otolaryngology* 86:215–220, 1978.

Ruth R, Niswander P: Acoustic reflex latency as a function of frequency and intensity of eliciting stimulus. *J Am Aud Soc* 2:54–60, 1976.

Salomon G: Middle ear muscle activity. *Proc R Soc Med* 59:966–971, 1966.

Sanders JW, Josey AF, Glasscock ME III: Audiological evaluation in cochlear and eighth nerve disorders. *Arch Otolaryngol* 100:283–289, 1974.

Sheehy J, Inzer B: Acoustic reflex test in neurootologic diagnosis. *Arch Otolaryngol* 102:647–653, 1976.

Silman S: The effects of aging on the acoustic reflex thresholds. *J Acoust Soc Am* 66:735–738, 1979a.

Silman S: The acoustic reflex, aging and the distortion product: a reply to Jerger (*J Acoust Soc Am* 66:908, 1979*). J Acoust Soc Am* 66:909–910, 1979b.

Silman S, Gelfand SA: Effect of sensorineural hearing loss on the stapedial reflex growth function in the elderly. *J Acoust Soc Am* 69:1099–1106, 1981.

Silman S, Popelka GR, Gelfand SA: Effect of sensorineural hearing loss on acoustic stapedial reflex growth functions. *J Acoust Soc Am* 64:1406–1411, 1978.

Spitzer JB, Ventry IM: Central auditory dysfunction among chronic alcoholics. *Arch Otolaryngol* 106:224–229, 1980.

Sprague BH, Wiley TL, Block MG: Dynamics of acoustic reflex growth. *Audiology* 20:15–40, 1981.

Steinberger D, Lehnhardt E: Impedance changes in central hearing disturbances. *Z Laryngol Rhinol Otol*

51:693, 1972.

Stephens S, Thornton A: Subjective and electrophysiologic tests in brainstem lesions. *Arch Otolaryngol* 102:608–613, 1976.

Sterkers O, Barres F, Sterkers JM: The stapes reflex in acoustic tumors (French). *Ann Otolaryngol Chir Cervicofac* 97:597–607, 1980.

Strominger NL, Silver SM, Truscott TC, Goldstein JC: Horseradish peroxidase demonstration of motorneurons to the stapedius muscle in the rhesus monkey. *Soc Neurosci Abstr* 6:553, 1980.

Suria D, Serra-Raventos W: Acoustic impedance measurement and autistic children. *Folia Phoniatr* 27:387–388, 1975.

Thompson DJ, Sills JA, Recke KS, Bui DM: Acoustic reflex in the aging adult. *J Speech Hear Res* 23:393–404, 1980.

Thompson GC, Stach BA, Jerger JF: Effect of ketamine on the stapedius reflex in squirrel monkey. *Arch Otolaryngol* 110:22–24, 1984.

Thomsen J, Terkildsen K: Audiological findings in 125 cases of acoustic neuromas. *Acta Otolaryngol (Stockh)* 80:353–361, 1975.

Tieg E, Dahl HA: Actomysin ATPase activity of middle ear muscles in the cat. *Histochemie* 29:1–7, 1972.

Wersäll R: The tympanic muscles and their reflexes. *Acta Otolaryngol [Suppl] (Stockh)* 139:80–101, 1958.

Wilson RH: Factors influencing the acoustic-immittance characteristics of the acoustic reflex. *J Speech Hear Res* 22:480–499, 1979.

Wilson R, McBride L: Threshold and growth of the acoustic reflex. *J Acoust Soc Am* 63:147–154, 1978.

Wilson RH: The effects of aging on the magnitude of the acoustic reflex. *J Speech Hear Res* 24:406–414, 1981.

Woodford C, Henderson D, Hamernik R, Feldman A: Threshold-duration function of the acoustic reflex in man. *Audiology* 14:53–62, 1975.

Zwislocki JJ: Temporal summation of loudness: an analysis. *J Acoust Soc Am* 46:431–441, 1969.

CHAPTER 8

Overview of Disorders of the Central Nervous System

ALEXANDER G. REEVES, M.D.

This chapter is an overview of neurological disorders and, therefore, describes symptoms and lesions not necessarily seen in the central auditory system. However, the professional who does central auditory testing should be familiar enough with these disorders of the central nervous system so that he/she understands the neurologist's report of symptoms and his diagnosis.

INTRODUCTION

The pathways and way stations of the auditory system lie at all levels and in an almost ubiquitous fashion from the medulla through the auditory cortex of the cerebral hemispheres. Lesions of any portion of the brainstem and many regions of the cerebral hemispheres are capable of causing abnormalities that may be reflected symptomatically and assessed by various simple and sophisticated auditory system analyses. The descriptions of these techniques are extensively presented in this text. However, it is the more dramatic symptoms associated with involvement of the structures of the brainstem and hemispheres which are more frequently used by the neurologist to localize and identify the presence of pathology.

The purposes of this chapter are to discuss the general principles of pathological involvement of the nervous system and to review some aspects of clinical localization based on an understanding of functional neuroanatomy. This is an overview to familiarize the specialist in audiological disorders with neurological analysis. Further reading will hopefully be pursued.

GENERAL PRINCIPLES

It is extraordinary to find uniqueness in the effects of any one pathological process in the nervous system. Be it infarction, neoplasm, hemorrhage, infection, metabolic, or degenerative disease, the nervous system can only respond in a certain number of stereotyped ways, none of which is specific for that single disease entity. Even so, *patterns* of specific involvements can be diagnostic or at least lead to a statistical likelihood of certain pathologies, which can then be confirmed by appropriate laboratory studies.

There are four basic central and peripheral nervous system responses to pathologic processes.

1. *Ablative* or *deficiency phenomena* are associated with destructive (e.g., infarction, trauma, tumor) and depressing processes (e.g., anesthesia).

2. *Irritative manifestations* of various pathological processes are typified by epileptic seizures, the pins and needles or burning parasthesias of peripheral neuropathy, and the tinnitus of eighth nerve and cochlear disorders.

3. *Release phenomena* are exemplified by the hyperactive reflexes and spasticity of corticospinal involvement, the tremor of Parkinson's disease, sedative withdrawal hyperactive states, and the vertigo from unilateral peripheral vestibular system loss.

4. *Compensatory phenomena* are typified by the circumductive gait of a paretic leg, the high stepping gait to avoid tripping caused by a foot drop, and the visual-motor compensation for the nystagmus and vertigo of vestibular disease. There also may be

inappropriate compensatory phenomena such as tendon contractures.

As a rule these phenomena occur in combinations. For example, the individual who suffers a cerebral infarction is hemiparetic, develops spasticity, may develop seizures, and compensates for this hemiparesis with a circumducting gait. In the absence of physical therapy, flexion contracture develops in his paretic arm.

Momentum of disease is another phenomenon that should be considered. This refers essentially to the rate of involvement of the nervous system. An acute destructive lesion (e.g., infarction) causes an early maximal deficit, whereas a chronic, slowly progressive lesion (e.g., tumor) usually produces considerably less deficit because compensating mechanisms (e.g., mechanical adjustment, redundancy of function in other regions) parallel the destructive forces. We have seen a slow growing meningioma compressing the frontal lobes reach the size of a lemon over at least 25 yr and cause no clear-cut neurologic deficit; the patient was admitted to the hospital for onset of seizures. Malignant glial tumors (glioblastoma) frequently infiltrate neuronal tissue, and many neurons lying within the tumor continue to function; this is a reason for the surprisingly small deficit occasionally associated with very large tumors, which as a rule grow rapidly. It is not surprising, therefore, that removal of these tumors almost invariably leaves the patient with even greater neurologic deficits, because many functioning neurons are lost in the ablation.

Recuperation of function following the termination of a pathological process in the nervous system takes two basic forms: resolution and reorganization.

Resolution of the lesion (as seen by the clearing of edema, ischemia, hemorrhagic or tumor compression of tissue, and metabolic suppression of neurons, as for example, by drugs, uremia, hypoxia, etc.) is the main mechanism of recovery in adults and older children with major dysfunctions.

Reorganization derived from redundancy and/or multipotentiality of function in the remaining normal neurons is an important mode of recuperation following minor destructive lesions. In young children (5 yr or younger) this can be the major mode of recuperation following destructive lesions. In adults and older children, plasticity or multipotentiality of neuronal function is less, whereas in young children it can be very marked for certain major functions. An example is verbal language; left hemisphere lesions that leave an adult with permanent and severe aphasia can be compensated by development of speech in the right hemisphere in young children. Residual hemiparesis in children following large hemispheric lesions is less than that seen in adults. Redundancy assumes multifocal localization of function. Although it is not the major source of recuperation following large lesions, it is the reason for the lack of dysfunction in some capabilities. For example, memories of past events, well imprinted, are very resistant to hemispheric lesions because they are diffusely represented in the cortices of both cerebral hemispheres.

LOCALIZATION OF LESIONS

It is the segmental systems, i.e., the functional systems restricted to the various subdivisions of the brain and spinal cord, which are the key to localization of pathology. When the long tract motor and sensory systems which extend from the hemispheres through the spinal cord are involved alone, specific localization of the pathological process is more difficult.

Cerebral Hemispheres

Dysfunction associated with cerebral cortical destructive lesions (e.g., infarction, hemorrhage, tumor, trauma) can be divided into abnormalities of *complex* motor and sensory functions, which are segmental and may be specific for the hemisphere involved, and abnormalities of *elementary* motor and sensory functions. These latter are of less localizing value, because lesions at other levels of the descending motor systems (corticospinal tracts) and the ascending sensory systems (e.g., dorsal column, medial lemniscal-thalamic, and the spinal trigeminal-thalamic tracts) cause very similar deficits.

Bilateral diffuse cortical neuronal loss, as seen in degenerative processes such as Alzheimer's disease, is characterized by a general loss of cognitive function (dementia) in which learning processes are frequently affected early because of a preferential involvement of the hippocampal formations in the temporal lobes. The recrudescence of infantile reflexes such as sucking (pouting) in response to firm pressure on the lips by the examiner and forced grasping on stimulation of the palmar (flexor) surface of the hand are common symptoms. These reflexes are normally inhibited during development of cortical maturity only to reappear with loss of that inhibition as cortical neurons drop out.

A recent study with dichotic auditory stimulation showed deficits in patients with Alzheimer's disease. The abnormalities were shown only in the dichotic mode, while normal responses were obtained with unilateral stimulation (Grimes et al, 1983).

Unilateral cortical lesions cause abnormalities characteristic of the left or right brain.

Left-sided destructive lesions cause verbal language dysfunction in virtually all right-handers and approximately 70% of left-handers. Ninety percent of most populations are right-handed; the remaining 10% are left-handed. This means that 97% of individuals have verbal language function lateralized to the left hemisphere (Springer and Deutsch, 1982). Anterior (frontal lobe) lesions on the left cause difficulties executing speech, although comprehension remains almost intact (Broca's aphasia). Posterior lesions involving the temporal-occipital-parietal region cause problems with central verbal language function, i.e., thinking and comprehending words (Wernicke's aphasia). Lesions separating the posterior from anterior regions cause a defect characterized by difficulty repeating phrases on command (conduction aphasia). The typical middle cerebral artery distribution ischemic stroke is the most common destructive lesion of the language areas and involves both anterior and posterior language areas giving a mixed aphasia which may be predominantly Broca's or Wernicke's or a global aphasia.

Persons with large left cortical lesions also display disinhibited emotionality (easy to anger and cry), presumably secondary to release of the more emotional right hemisphere from left hemisphere inhibition (Benson, 1979).

Lesions of the right hemisphere, especially in the posterior regions in and around the temporal-occipital-parietal region, cause deficits in visuospatial capacities (e.g., problems with direction finding and constructing and deciphering three-dimensional figures), musicality (e.g., the ability to reproduce melodies), and emotionality. This latter dysfunction may include a striking indifference to loss of the contralateral elementary motor-sensory functions. The left hemiparesis and hemisensory defect may even be denied (anosognosia).

Lesions in and around the primary auditory cortex, extending onto the temporal operculum of the insula (see Chapter 2), are most often diagnosed by the symptoms from damage to the surrounding cortical areas as described above. However, there are several abnormalities which can be observed at the bedside. Bilateral simultaneous auditory stimulation using simple stimuli such as finger snapping or rubbing will result in **extinction** of the sound presented to the ear contralateral to the lesion, whereas unilaterally presented stimuli will be correctly perceived on either side. In Figures 8.1 and 8.2 results are shown from dichotic (see Chapter 12)

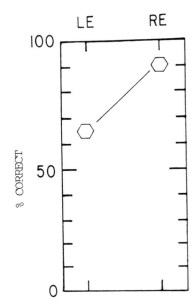

Figure 8.1. Scores on a dichotic speech test (digits) from a 39-yr-old male with infarction in the right middle cerebral artery. Note the typical left ear deficit contralateral to the hemisphere with the vascular disorder.

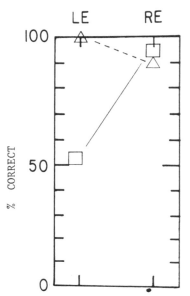

Figure 8.2. Results from a teenage girl with a right temporal lobe lesion on a dichotic sentence test (□———□) and on a monaural word recognition test (△-----△).

sentence testing and a monaural word recognition test. Note that the dichotic tests in which sentences or digits are presented to each ear simultaneously show a deficit in the ear contralateral to the lesion. However, the test which requires identification of words presented only to one ear at a time shows no deficit for either side (Fig. 8.2). Auditory extinction is not, however, unique to auditory cortex lesions. As with other stimuli (i.e., visual, tactile), extinction to double simultaneous stimulation will occur contralateral to parietal lesions on either side and also on occasion contralateral to frontal cortex lesions and in both instances in the absence of any direct involvement of primary sensory cortex or pathways. This extinction appears to be the result of an orienting or attentional deficit (Weinstein and Friedland, 1977).

Stimulus mislocalization is another striking abnormality of auditory integration which results from lesions of either hemisphere involving the auditory cortex, or, if the lesions are large, the parietal frontal cortex (Sanchez-Longo and Forster, 1958). Simple sounds presented within the cone of space subtended by the pinna opposite the cortical lesion are no longer well localized by the patient whose eyes are closed. In their classical study, Sanchez-Longo and Forster (1958) demonstrated impairment of sound localization ability in the auditory field contralateral to the temporal lobe lesion in five brain-damaged subjects. Sound lateralization tasks, such as the interaural intensity difference (IID) as discussed in Chapter 10, also appear sensitive to detecting lesions of the auditory cortex and surrounding neural tissue.

Bilateral involvement of the auditory cortex is rare, usually the result of tandem ischemic lesions, and is associated with cortical deafness (Graham et al, 1980). In the absence of involvement of the contiguous posterior verbal language zone on the left or the comparable visuospatial predominant zone on the right, this deafness cannot be differentiated at the bedside from peripheral deafness. This dilemma is easily remedied today by the availability of means to test the acoustic (stapedius) reflex and auditory brainstem response (ABR), both of which would reflect normal function (see Chapters 4 and 7). The midlatency evoked potentials (MLR), which appear to be dependent on the integrity of the auditory cortex, would be absent (see Chapter 6). These findings are well described in the article by Graham and associates (Graham et al, 1980).

Basal Ganglia

Destructive or degenerative loss of neurons in various parts of the basal ganglia give rise to relatively specific segmental signs. As a rule, aberrations of motor function are most pronounced. Parkinsonism and chorea are the two major disorder complexes associated with diseases of the basal ganglia.

Parkinsonism is a conglomeration of *rigidity* (a full range **plasticky** resistance to passive manipulation of the limbs which may be broken into a rhythmic stop and start (cogwheel) resistance by the presence of tremor), **bradykinesia** (more a slowness of initiation of movement than slowness of movement once begun), *postural abnormality* (a difficulty maintaining appropriate antigravity compensatory postures as exemplified by the stooped or flexed parkinsonism stance which counters an inappropriate retropulsive force), *tremor* (a three to eight per second rhythmic oscillation present during wakeful rest or posturing of the limbs and head), and varying degrees of *dementia.* The pathophysiological substrate for the first three dysfunctions is a deficiency in the dopamine transmitter system caused by loss of the source in substantia nigra neurons which degenerate in idiopathic and postencephaletic parkinsonism. The tremor may take origin from disruption of ascending cerebellar pathways which course through the substantia nigra in transit to the thalamus and motor cortex. The dementia, which is usually mild, is considered to be the result of loss of cortical neurons. When the dementia is severe, Alzheimer's disease with secondary basal ganglia involvement should be suspect.

Chorea is an involuntary movement disorder characterized by irregular and fleeting movements of the limbs and/or axial musculature including also the muscles of the face, jaw, and tongue. The intensity of movement varies from the very minimal buccolingual chorea characteristic of long-term neuroleptic use (tardive dyskinesia) to the wild and exhausting unilateral limb-flailing chorea called hemiballism. Excessive sensitivity to dopamine in the striatal complex (caudate nucleus and putamen) is the substrate for neuroleptic induced chorea, while small cell degeneration in the striated complex is the substrate for Huntington's chorea, a well publicized, although rare, autosomal dominant degenerative disorder also associated with progressive dementia from parallel cortical degeneration (Vinken and Bruyn, 1968).

A relative or absolute deficiency in the cholinergic transmission system or a relative or absolute excess in the dopamine transmission system is likely the major biochemical abnormality in chorea. The reverse, a relative or absolute deficiency in the dopamine system or a relative or absolute excess in the cholinergic system, is the substrate for the bradykinesia and rigidity of parkinsonism (Reeves, 1981b).

Although motor aberrations dominate the basal ganglia syndromes, it has become evident that destructive lesions, particularly when isolated to the striatum, are also associated with abnormalities of perception and language function. Left caudate-putamen lesions have been associated with expressive aphasia of the Broca's type, while right striatal lesions have been associated with extinc-

tion of contralateral auditory, visual, and tactile stimuli and also denial of dysfunction in the left limbs. We have observed a patient with left hemichorea from an ischemic right striatal lesion who denied the presence of the chorea which was so violent that it resulted in coronary insufficiency (Goldblatt et al, 1974).

It has been assumed that these syndromes reflect a loss of striatal influence on the respective left and right hemispheres with which the striatum has major interconnections.

Brainstem and Cranial Nerves

The major segmental markers of brainstem disorder are the cranial nerves (CN), in particular, cranial nerves III through XII which lie from the midbrain through the medulla (Reeves, 1981a).

The olfactory nerve (CNI) and optic nerve (CNII) and their respective systems are also useful segmental markers, but at a higher level. The olfactory system does not have a way station in contiguity with the brainstem. Olfactory input courses directly through the olfactory tracts from each olfactory bulb to the mesial cortex of the anterior temporal lobes. Beyond the arrival of the olfactory tracts at the posterior border of the orbitofrontal cortex, the system is entirely bilateral, and, therefore, lesions need to be bilateral to cause olfactory loss beyond this point. However, unilateral irritation as by an epileptiform discharge may produce olfactory hallucinations. The Foster Kennedy syndrome is an excellent example of the use of segmental localization. A unilateral loss of the sense of smell is associated with papilledema on the opposite side and optic atrophy on the same side. The lesion which usually causes this complex of signs is a neoplasm (meningioma or glioma) involving the orbitofrontal cortex on one side, compressing the ipsilateral olfactory tract and optic nerve while causing raised intracranial pressure from the intracranial mass effect, which can be reflected only in the contralateral noncompressed optic nerve head.

The optic system only touches base with the brainstem in the lateral geniculate relay which lies on the inferior posterolateral border of the thalamus. An elaborate description of the multiple characteristic and segmentally localizing visual field defects caused by lesions anywhere from the retina to the occipital cortex is beyond the scope of this presentation. In general, monocular field defects are caused by lesions anterior to the optic chiasm (the retina or optic nerve), while lesions at or posterior to the chiasm cause binocular field defects. An exception to this axiom is the contralateral monocular superior temporal crescentic defect caused by anterior temporal lobe lesions which destroy the rostral portion of Meyer's temporal loop of the visual radiations. This monocular system arises from the most peripheral nasal retina of each eye which has no comparable binocular representation in the opposite eye's temporal retina. Unless one is aware of this system, anterior temporal lobe lesions, most often caused by neoplasms, will be missed by field testing at bedside. Office perimetry is the only means to determine these very peripheral defects.

As a rule of thumb, visual field defects lie opposite the visual anatomy involved, and this holds from the retina to the occipital cortex. For example, destruction of the lower bank of the right occipital visual cortex or the right temporal visual radiations are associated with a left superior **homonymous** (binocular field) quadrant field loss while right upper bank or right parietal lesions will give a left inferior homonymous quadrantanopsia.

The oculomotor system is represented by cranial nerves III, IV, and VI. CNIII (the oculomotor nerve) and CNIV (the trochlear nerve) lie in the dorsum of the midbrain just below the aqueduct of Sylvius, while CNVI (the abducens nerve) lies in the dorsum of the caudal pons just deep to the floor of the fourth ventricle. Knowledge of the courses of each of these nerves from their nuclei through the brainstem and then from the brainstem to the superior orbital fissure of the orbit give the clinician a tool for accurately localizing lesions in and around the brainstem and posterior fossa of the cranium. Typically, persons with involvement of one or more of these three nerves complain of diplopia and display on examination extraocular motion deficiencies specific for the nerve or nerves involved. If the parasympa-

thetic segment of III is involved, the light and accommodation constrictor reflexes of the pupil will be depressed and the pupil will be dilated.

Involvement of the central oculomotor or **conjugate gaze** systems in the pons (the horizontal gaze system) or midbrain (the vertical gaze system) cause specific and easily recognized defects. Lesions, usually vascular, less often tumor compression, in the most rostral midbrain cause loss of vertical upwards and downwards gaze (also convergence), while lesions of the mid to lower pons cause defects in horizontal gaze towards the side of the lesion. If a lesion involves the medial longitudinal fasciculus (MLF), where it courses in the medial dorsal portion of the pons between CNVI and CNIII, the medial rectus portion of horizontal gaze will be unyoked from lateral rectus function. For example, if one MLF is involved (most often by multiple sclerosis in persons under 50 and ischemic lesions in persons over 50), on horizontal gaze to the opposite side the medial rectus will not function, while the lateral rectus (which is still connected to the paramedian lying horizontal gaze zone, situated in and around the sixth nerve nucleus) will function adequately. Because neither CNVI or III are directly involved, this is appropriately called an internuclear ophthalmoplegia.

The trigeminal nerve (CNV) subserves facial sensation and jaw movement. Its input to the midpons from the face is via three divisions: (1) the ophthalmic division which innervates the face from the eye to the vertex; (2) the maxillary division which innervates the face from the lower lid to the upper lip (also the maxillary gingiva and teeth and the hard palate); and (3) the mandibular division which innervates the lower lip, the skin covering the mandible, the mandibular gingiva and teeth, and the lower oral cavity and tongue. The motor supply to the jaw travels via the mandibular division. The fibers of the three divisions of CNV have their cell bodies in the single trigeminal or semilunar ganglion which lies on the medial rim of the middle cranial fossa, from whence it sends its single root into the lateral aspect of the midportion of the pons. Generally, lesions of the peripheral trigeminal branches cause loss of sensation in a divisional pattern, while lesions of the central connections in the lateral wall of the pons or medulla give defects which involve all three divisions in an overlapping fashion.

The auditory pathways which course through the brainstem are well described in Chapter 2. This pathway and its function can be affected by many of the pathologies mentioned earlier. There are two main categories of tumors of the brainstem, intra- and extraaxial. Intraaxial tumors arise from within the brainstem, whereas the more common extraaxial tumors arise from outside but immediate to the brainstem. The glioma is probably the most common intraaxial tumor of the brainstem, while the acoustic schwannoma has the highest incidence in regard to extraaxial lesions (Huertas and Haymaker, 1969).

Degenerative diseases such as multiple sclerosis can affect the auditory brainstem pathway (see Chapters 4 and 7). This disease is characterized by the loss of myelin with preservation of the axon. It is confined to the white matter and does not extend beyond the root entry zone (Wechsler, 1963). Auditory involvement is as common as optic dysfunction in this disease. If the myelinated segment of the auditory nerve becomes involved, hearing symptoms can become rather severe. As related by Noffsinger et al (1972) there is much disagreement in the literature as to the degree, type, and incidence of hearing loss associated with multiple sclerosis. Since most lesions in multiple sclerosis are in the brainstem, sophisticated tests of higher auditory function can be employed to assess the integrity of the system (Noffsinger et al, 1972).

There are other brainstem degenerative diseases which may affect the auditory pathway. Olivopontocerebellar degeneration has been shown to commonly affect the auditory brainstem response (ABR) (Lynn et al, 1983). Also, a recent report has shown Charcot-Marie-Tooth disease to initially manifest itself as a severe hearing disability (Musiek et al, 1982).

From an auditory assessment perspective, such tests as the ABR (see Fig. 8.3) and various competing speech tests can be of value in detecting lesions of the brainstem (see Chapters 4, 11, and 12).

Acoustic schwannomas usually arise from

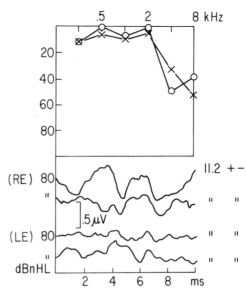

Figure 8.3. The pure tone audiogram and selected ABR tracings from a middle-aged patient with a known, long standing brainstem tumor affecting both sides, but with greater involvement on the left. Absolute wave V latencies were bilaterally abnormal (near 7 msec), and wave form morphology was poor for both ears. The left ear shows generally less amplitude and greater latency of wave V than the right ear (presentation rate of an alternating polarity click is shown on the right side of the figure). (From Musiek FE: ABR in eighth nerve and brainstem disorders. *J Otol* 3:243–248, 1982.)

the vestibular division of the eighth nerve in or very near to the internal auditory meatus and comprise between 5 to 10% of all intracranial tumors. The best technique for determining the presence of these masses is use of the auditory brainstem response (ABR), which is abnormal in over 90% of patients (see Chapter 4). Unilaterally depressed hearing usually brings the patient to the clinician. The finding of a combination of involvement of the vestibular and trigeminal systems, less often the facial nerve, is almost diagnostic. Depression of response to bedside external auditory canal caloric irrigation ipsilateral to the tumor in parallel with a depression of the corneal response is characteristic. The corneal reflex involves input from the cornea via the ophthalmic division of V and output via the seventh nerve to the

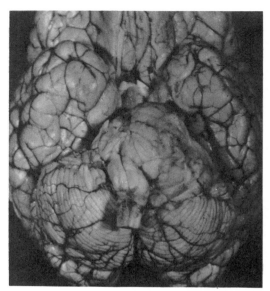

Figure 8.4. An example of a brainstem tumor primarily infiltrating and expanding the pons into the cerebellopontine recess. (From Dublin WB: *Fundamentals of Sensorineural Auditory Pathology, 1976.* Courtesy of Charles C Thomas, Publisher, Springfield, Illinois.)

orbicularis muscle of the eye. It is affected early by eighth nerve tumors which have grown into the angle between the cerebellum and the pons, not because the first division of V is compressed (the first division is much too far rostral and the third and second divisions would, therefore, have been affected earlier), but because the tumor compresses the lateral wall of the pontomedullary junction wherein lies the descending spinal tract of V, the most superficial fibers of which come from the ophthalmic division. Some decrease in the corneal reflex may be attributed to seventh nerve dysfunction. However, it is extraordinary how stretched and compressed the facial nerve can become by these very slowly growing tumors (may take 10 to 30 or more years to reach significant size) without affecting facial movement.

An important concept to grasp is that the seventh (facial) nerve has easily distinguishable **supranuclear** and nuclear or nerve dysfunction. The facial nuclei which lie in the lower pons are bilaterally innervated from the motor system originating in cerebral cortex. Therefore, unilateral supranuclear lesions cause contralateral weakness of the face and not paralysis. Further, the frontalis muscles which elevate the brow are evenly innervated (50/50) from each hemisphere, and unilateral lesions cause no weakness of this movement. As a general rule, 50% supranuclear innervation is adequate for normal function of any movement. However, the lower facial movements have a variably but persistently predominant (60 to 80%) contralateral supranuclear innervation, and, therefore, the lower face contralateral to the supranuclear lesion will be weak. Facial nucleus or nerve lesions typically cause equal weakness of both the upper and lower face on the side of the lesion(s).

Lesions of the facial nerve in its course through the temporal bone are most often idiopathic, commonly called Bell's palsy. Typically various functional systems of VII are involved in addition to the motor portion. Thus, taste may be depressed from chorda tympani or geniculate ganglion involvement, and there may be pain in the auditory canal and mastoid region from irritation of the somatosensory portion of VII. The seventh nerve courses circuitously from the facial nucleus in the lateral aspect of the lower pons, up and over the sixth nerve nucleus as the genu of the seventh nerve, before turning laterally and ventrally to exit from the lateral pons. It joins the eighth nerve at the internal auditory meatus. The sensory portion of VII separates from the nerve at the border of the brainstem to travel to various way stations in the brainstem (e.g., taste to the nucleus solitarious and tactile sensation to the trigeminal complex). As a rule, therefore, weakness from lesions of the intrapontine portion of the seventh nerve is not associated with loss of taste or with pain in and around the ear. Acoustic reflex testing (see Chapter 7) can be valuable in assessing the level of the seventh nerve lesion. This tests the contraction of the stapedius muscle on presentation of auditory stimulation and, therefore, reflects an eighth nerve through brainstem to seventh nerve reflex.

Because most of this text concerns evaluations of the auditory system, we will discuss only the vestibular portion of the eighth nerve in this section.

At the bedside the vestibular nerve is traditionally evaluated predominantly through observation and testing of the vestibulooculomotor systems. Tests of equilibrium are supplementary. An understanding of the substrates of vestibular-driven horizontal reflex conjugate eye movements (tonic, slow, or reflex component) and the counteracting cerebral hemispheric driven horizontal eye movements (phasic, fast, or checking component), which together comprise nystagmus, allows one to evaluate most acute and chronic disorders of the vestibular apparatus. It is unusual to find isolated involvement of the vertically driven vestibulooculomotor systems in the absence of horizontal system involvement; for the substrates of both overlap at most levels of the brainstem. The exception to this rule is the presence of vertical up or down nystagmus (termed for the direction of the fast component), which isolates pathology to the brainstem, possibly also to the cerebellum. Involvement of the vestibular nerve or peripheral apparatus (semicircular canals, sacculus, and utriculus), unless bilateral and symmetrical, will cause only horizontal or rotary beating nystagmus. This is because isolated involvement of the vertical (anterior and posterior) semicircular canals must be rare, and if, indeed, it does occur in absence of horizontal canal involvement, it would have to be bilateral and symmetrical. This is due to the fact that each anterior and posterior canal innervates rotary vertical movements in one eye and purely vertical movements in the opposite eye. Bilateral simultaneous caloric irrigation of each external auditory canal gives this symmetry and is a way of eliciting vertical nystagmus at the bedside, although it adds little information which cannot be garnered by unilateral caloric irrigations which predominantly test the horizontal systems. The anterior and posterior canal sections of the side irrigated essentially cancel each other out as is so with unilateral disease of the vestibular apparatus.

Brainstem involvement can result in vertical, horizontal, or rotary beating nystagmus. An additional point contrasting central and peripheral vestibular apparatus involvement is the presence of relatively little sensation of motion of self or environment (vertigo) with central disease in spite of all degrees of nystagmus, while peripherally associated vertigo is, as a rule, as severe as the nystagmus (Weinstein and Friedland, 1980).

Analysis of the vestibular apparatus at the bedside is particularly useful in evaluating pathological depression of consciousness (stupor and coma) (Plum and Posner, 1980). The reticular activating system responsible for cerebral alerting spans between the midpons and diencephalon (thalamus and hypothalamus) before dispersing to the cerebral hemispheres. Bilateral involvement of this primitive network of neurons causes varying degrees of depression of consciousness. Strokes, ischemic or hemorrhagic, neoplasms, and traumatic damage are the major causes of direct mechanical involvement of the reticular formation. However, the most common cause of depression of consciousness is either endogenous metabolic suppression (e.g., hypoxia, hypoglycemia, acidosis, uremia, liver failure, etc.) or exogenous metabolic suppression (e.g., sedative or other drug excess) of the reticular formation which is preferentially susceptible to these abnormalities. The central vestibular oculomotor systems span the pons and midbrain and lie within the reticular formation, making analysis of vestibular driven eye movement the key to localizing primary destructive processes causing coma. In contrast, metabolic processes suppressing the reticular formation do not suppress the vestibular oculomotor reflex system until very late. Typically, the vestibular oculomotor reflex, elicited by caloric irrigation or rotation of the head (oculocephalic or doll's eyes maneuver), remains full, while the fast or checking component is lost early for it is dependent upon cerebral hemisphere-reticular formation relays.

Cranial nerves IX (glossopharyngeal) and X (vagus) are frequently considered together by the clinician because of a considerable overlap in their functions and nuclear substrates. Along with cranial nerve XI (spinal accessory), these nerves exit the lateral border of the medulla along the upper surface of the inferior medulla and then course together through the jugular foramen to appear in the pharyngeal-cervical region. IX and X supply the pharyngeal-palatal musculature and receive afferents from the same region. The symmetry of palatal elevation in making the sound "aaah" (weakness of one side causes elevation and deviation to the strong side—the "curtain sign") tests predominantly IX. The gag reflex, tested on each side of the posterior pharyngeal wall, evaluates a combination of IX–X input from and IX–X output to the pharyngeal wall.

Hoarseness, a sign of vocal cord dysfunction, should be considered extraordinary beyond 3 weeks' duration, the maximal allowable length for an upper respiratory infection with laryngitis. A direct or indirect examination of the vocal cords should be undertaken at that time to determine the presence or absence of vocal cord paralysis, tumor, or other chronic process. If paralysis is found, then a search should be made for involvement of the recurrent laryngeal nerves of the vagus in their respective circuitous routes. This should encompass the neck for the right branch and the neck and mediastinum of the chest for the left branch.

The most common brainstem pathology involving IX and X is infarction in the distribution of the posterior inferior cerebellar artery (PICA), which arises from the vertebral artery on each side to supply the dorsolateral portion of the medulla and the posterior inferior cerebellum. For some unknown reason this is the most common brainstem stroke and usually is the result of thrombotic occlusion of a short portion of the vertebral artery trapping the opening of the PICA. The combination of signs gives a precise clinical localization. They are: (1) ipsilateral loss of the gag reflex and palatal elevation (IX and X-nucleus ambiguous): (2) ipsilateral pupillary narrowing (miosis), ptosis, and decreased sweating (*Horner's syndrome* from involvement of the descending sympathetic fibers in the brainstem); (3) ipsilateral loss of facial sensation (spinal tract and nucleus of V) and contralateral depression of pain and temperature sensation over the whole body if the spinothalamic system is involved; (4) varying degrees of nystagmus and vertigo, depending upon how much of the dorsolaterally lying vestibular nuclear complex is involved; and (5) ipsilateral ataxia and intention tremor from involvement of the cerebellum. An interesting exception in this lateral medullary syndrome is the absence of involvement of the acoustic portion of VIII, i.e., the cochlear nuclei and superior olivary complexes which lie just rostral to the maximal limits of the usual zone of PICA ischemia.

Dysfunction of the eleventh (spinal accessory) cranial nerve can occur with lesions, usually compressive, from the cervical cord, from which the nerve arises, up through the foramen magnum to where it joins the ninth and tenth nerves to exit via the jugular foramen. It innervates the sternomastoid and trapezius muscles, which, respectively, turn the head to the opposite side and shrug the shoulders. These muscles obey the rule of bilateral supranuclear innervation of axial movements. Therefore, unilateral cerebral hemisphere lesions cause only weakness of a mild degree. Peripheral lesions, as a rule, cause more severe weakness and also atrophy. Also, the sternomastoid movement innervation obeys the rule that each hemisphere *moves* the body into and the limbs within the opposite world. It just happens that the sternomastoid used to *move* the head towards the opposite side is ipsilateral to the hemisphere initiating the movement, that is, the right cerebral hemisphere turns the head to the left using the right sternomastoid, an ipsilateral muscle. It is, therefore, *movements* that are orchestrated by the hemispheres; the muscles needed for these movements may be ipsilateral, contralateral, or bilateral.

Disorders of the twelfth (hypoglossal) nerve are obvious before specific examination. Slurring of speech caused by weakness of the tongue is the giveaway. On examination unilateral weakness is indicated by deviation towards the weak side when the tongue is protruded. Lesions involving the hypoglossal nucleus or nerve cause atrophy and weakness, while contralateral supranuclear lesions cause mild weakness (axial movement rule) and no atrophy. Overwhelmingly the most common cause of tongue weakness is involvement of the cerebral hemispheres by ischemic stroke. The tongue weakness is, therefore, only part of the contralateral and poorly localizing hemiparesis of the body, while the hemispheric signs (cortical or less often of the basal ganglia) are the segmental localizers. Lesions of the hypoglossal nucleus or intramedullary portion of the twelfth nerve, where it lies in the dorsal midline of the medulla, are minutely localizing but unusual, frequently ischemic also, and associated with a contralateral hemiparesis. This crossed weakness occurs because the medullary pyramid is usually also involved before it decussates in the lower medulla.

Cerebellum

Tremor, ataxia, and hypotonia of the axial and limb systems are characteristic of cerebellar systems dysfunction. These dysfunctions arise from involvement of the major functional cerebellar unit, the neocerebellum, which comprises the overwhelming majority of the cerebellum. It has developed in parallel with the neocortex of the cerebral hemispheres and is comprised of the massive lateral lobes which overlap in the midline to form the vermis which contains the remnants of the more primitive paleo- and archicerebellar systems.

The cerebellum disobeys the general rule of contralaterality in the nervous system. Each cerebellar hemisphere modulates motor activity, predominantly through inhibition, of the ipsilateral limbs. Therefore, a destructive lesion, such as a neoplasm or stroke of one side of the cerebellum or its projections, causes ipsilateral limb tremor and hypotonia. Trunk and other axial movements (e.g., oculomotor, articulation, respiration) are represented in the vermis and, therefore, affected by lesions of the midline of the cerebellum and its projections.

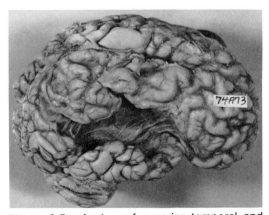

Figure 8.5. A view of superior temporal and inferior parietal lobe destruction as a result of an infarction of the right middle cerebral artery. (From Dublin WB: *Fundamentals of Sensorineural Auditory Pathology*, 1976. Courtesy of Charles C Thomas, Publisher, Springfield, Illinois.)

The tremor of cerebellar disease occurs during intention, as opposed to that of parkinsonism which occurs during wakeful rest or posturing (and disappears during intention), as tested by such maneuvers as alternating finger to nose pointing. The cerebellar intention tremor is an oscillatory over- and undershooting (**dysmetria**) of the target, which becomes characteristically worse as the hand or foot or, for that matter, the eyes approach the target.

The ataxia or staggering gait may be caused by lateral hemisphere involvement and, therefore, ipsilateral limb dysmetria with an associated tendency to stagger to the involved side, or it may be the result of dysmetria of the trunk from midline involvement. One of the most common causes of relatively pure trunk ataxia in our society is the cerebellar degeneration which occurs in chronic alcoholics and involves the anterior cerebellar vermis, which somatotopically represents the trunk. In this condition the lateral portions of the neocerebellum and, therefore, the limbs are involved later. Anterior midline neoplasms or strokes may give a similar picture.

Hypotonia is considered a classic finding associated with neocerebellar disease. Nevertheless, it is an unusual finding in patients with cerebellar involvement. This may well be because many pathologic processes involving the cerebellum in isolation (i.e., without concomitant involvement of the brainstem and its descending cerebral and basal ganglia motor systems) are chronic in nature (e.g., tumors and degenerative processes), allowing compensatory processes to keep up with the ablative effects. When it is present, more often with acute lesions such as ischemia or hemorrhage, the hypotonia is best seen as the to and fro unchecked (pendular) swinging of the leg when the knee jerk reflex is elicited. In contrast, in the normal state, when the quadriceps muscle contracts on patellar tendon tapping, the antagonist hamstring muscles are stretched and almost immediately contract and damp the leg movement.

A less common cerebellar syndrome is seen with a childhood midline tumor, the medulloblastoma, which arises from cells in the posterior midline archicerebellum. The archicerebellum, so named because it is the most primitive part of the cerebellum, has major reciprocal connections with the vestibular nuclear complex of the underlying brainstem. Ipsilateral vestibular complex inhibition is the predominant function of the archicerebellum, so it is not surprising to see early on in these children nystagmus and vestibular dysequilibrium. These appear before enlargement of the neoplasm involves neocerebellar structures and underlying brainstem, thereby causing a much broader syndrome with added neocerebellar, other cranial nerve, and long tract motor and sensory difficulties.

An overview of neurological evaluation using various disorders as models has been presented.

References

Benson FD: *Aphasia, Alexia, and Agraphia.* New York, Churchill Livingston, 1979.

Dublin WB: *Fundamentals of Sensorineural Auditory Pathology.* Springfield, IL, Charles C Thomas, 1976.

Goldblatt D, Markesberry WR, Reeves AG: Recurrent hemichorea following striatal lesions. *Arch Neurol* 31:51–54, 1974.

Graham J, Greenwood R, Lecky B: Cortical deafness: a case report and review of the literature. *J Neurol Sci* 48:35–49, 1980.

Grimes A, Grady A, Foster N, Sunderland T: Performance on the SSW in Alzheimer's Disease. Presented at the annual meeting of the American Speech-Language and Hearing Association, Cincinnati, Nov 20, 1983.

Huertas J, Haymaker W: Localization of lesions involving the statoacoustic nerve. In Haymaker W (ed): *Bing's Localization in Neurological Disease,* ed 15. St. Louis, CV Mosby, 1969.

Lynn G, Cullis P, Gilroy J: Olivoponto cerebellar degeneration: effects on auditory brainstem responses. *Semin Hearing* 4:375–384, 1983

Musiek FE, Weider DJ, Mueller R: Audiological findings in Charcot-Marie-Tooth syndrome. *Arch Otolaryngol* 108:595–599, 1982.

Noffsinger D, Olsen W, Carhart R, Hart C, Sahgal V: Auditory and vestibular aberrations in multiple sclerosis. *Acta Otolaryngol,* Suppl 303, 1972.

Plum F, Posner JB: *The Diagnosis of Stupor and Coma,* ed 3. Philadelphia, FA Davis, 1980.

Reeves AG: Cranial nerve evaluation. In *Disorders of the Nervous System.* Chicago, Year Book Medical Publishers, 1981a, pp 26–70.

Reeves AG: Disorders of basal ganglia function. In: *Disorders of the Nervous System.* Chicago, Year Book Medical Publishers, 1981b, pp 147–155.

Sanchez-Longo L, Forster F: Clinical significance of impairments in sound localizations. *Neurology (Minneap)* 8:119–125, 1958.

Springer SP, Deutsch G: *Left Brain, Right Brain.* San Francisco, WH Freeman, 1982.

Vinken PJ, Bruyn GW: Diseases of the Basal Ganglia. Amsterdam, North Holland Publishing Company, 1968, vol 6, pp 298–409.

Wechsler IS: *Clinical Neurology,* ed 9. Philadelphia, WB Saunders, 1963, pp 514–520.

Weinstein EA, Friedland RP: *Advances in Neurology.* New York, Raven Press, 1977, vol 18.

CHAPTER 9

The Central Auditory System and Issues Related to Hemispheric Specialization

ROBERT EFRON, M.D.

Dr. Efron's chapter cautions the professional who does central auditory testing to beware of facile interpretation of dichotic data. He points out a possible role for a cortical efferent pathway and describes results of auditory experiments on patients with anterior temporal lobe lesions.

INTRODUCTION

"Central Auditory Processing," a phrase of postcomputer vintage, refers to the functional role of those parts of the auditory system which lie within the brain itself as distinct from the cochlea and its neural output through the eighth cranial nerve. In terms of the volume or weight of neural substrate, the central auditory system (as is true also of the central visual system) is enormously larger than its peripheral sensory end organ. Though small unilateral lesions in the central visual system often produce clinically dramatic contralateral perceptual deficits which can be studied at the bedside, even large unilateral lesions in the central auditory system appear to give rise to only subtle functional contralateral deficits which have been identified finally in the second half of the present century and then only by using highly sophisticated laboratory techniques.

The reason for this difference between the central visual and auditory systems is usually attributed to the extensive redundancy of the auditory system in that each ear is strongly—almost equally—represented in each hemisphere. Thus, it can be argued that the occurrence of a clinically significant auditory deficit would be surprising following a unilateral cerebral lesion. Implicit in this argument is its corollary, that further study of central auditory processing disorders following unilateral lesions may prove to be clinically futile and of limited scientific value.

Such a negative view can be maintained, however, only by excluding from our anatomical and physiological definition of the central auditory system those areas of the brain which have come to be identified as language or speech "centers," since unilateral damage to any of these structures (particularly on the left side) results in clinically dramatic and personally devastating functional deficits. By tautologically defining these regions as "speech centers" and by ignoring the anatomical and physiological evidence that the same areas critically important for speech processing are *coextensive* with auditory association cortex, the "central auditory system" necessarily shrinks in size and, of course, in clinical significance. As a consequence of this historical evolution of our concepts, the study of the effects of damage to this part of the central auditory system has been coopted by the fields of aphasiology and the speech sciences, the conceptual relationship between language processing and audition has been virtually severed, and the role of the hearing scientist is generally perceived as being concerned with the study of cochlear mechanisms with permissible forays into the lower brainstem. Given this historical context, it is not surprising that very little research has been performed on the *auditory* consequences of lesions of cerebral cortex, that almost all of the limited auditory research which has been conducted has employed speech stimuli, and that, as a consequence, some significant distortions in interpretation of the meaning of results have occurred.

CONTRALATERAL AUDITORY DEFICITS AFTER UNILATERAL CEREBRAL LESIONS

Although considerable anatomical, electrophysiological, and clinical evidence attests to the fact that the neural pathways from each ear reach both auditory cortices, the critically important work of Tunturi (1946) in dogs and Rosenzweig (1951) in cats was the first to reveal that each ear has a somewhat more extensive physiological (and presumably a functionally more potent) connection to the contralateral than to the ipsilateral primary auditory cortex. The implications of this fact for human hearing were first reported by Bocca et al (1955) who found that speech recognition was impaired in the ear contralateral to a temporal lobe tumor, *regardless of the side of the lesion*, if the speech signal to that ear was degraded by low-pass filtering. Sinha (1959) subsequently reported that the addition of white noise, rather than low-pass filtering, had a similar contralateral effect on monaural speech recognition in patients with atrophic temporal lobe lesions. These findings were then extended by Kimura (1961a), who used dichotic presentation of spoken digits to patients with unilateral anterior temporal lobe resections (most of whom had no aphasic symptoms). She found that these patients made more errors in identifying speech sounds presented to the ear contralateral to the lobectomy, while control patients with frontal lobe resections did not exhibit this contralateral deficit. In the same studies, Kimura showed that patients who had larger resections of the anterior temporal lobe, extending more posteriorly and possibly encroaching on the primary auditory cortex, had an even larger asymmetry in error rate than those with smaller anterior resections.

Although Kimura's studies have received wide attention and have led to a virtual orgy of experimental work using dichotic speech signals, it is curious that no one has wondered (at least in print) why an *anterior* resection of the temporal lobe—a lesion which does not encroach on *any* of the previously identified speech areas, and to the best of our present understanding, even spares the primary auditory cortex and auditory association cortex—should result in any auditory disturbance, let alone a disturbance of speech processing. Since electrophysiological studies of this anterior region of the temporal lobe fail to show evoked potentials following auditory stimuli (Celesia and Puletti, 1969), it is presumed that the anterior temporal lobe has no afferent input from the medial geniculate. The results of Bocca et al, Sinha, and Kimura prompt yet another question. Is the contralateral deficit of speech processing which these investigators described an *auditory* deficit (one which happened to be revealed by the incidental use of speech signals) or an aphasic-like deficit (one which uniquely affects only speech processing)? If the former is the case, then we would expect essentially similar findings to be obtained with nonspeech signals, and we would need to explore the auditory functions of the anterior temporal lobe in some detail. If the latter is the case, we would be forced to conclude that a mild, contralateral, aphasic-like syndrome can be restricted to speech signals presented to only one ear—a conclusion which would significantly undermine our present view of aphasia as a high-level, supramodality, cognitive disorder involving speech, reading, and writing. The data to be reviewed below strongly support the conclusion that the deficit described by Bocca, Sinha, and Kimura is a consequence of unilateral damage to *auditory* pathways, possibly efferent pathways, which lie within the superior temporal gyrus on both sides of the brain, and that this deficit is not restricted to the processing of speech sounds.

Although the studies discussed previously employed speech or speech-like stimuli to demonstrate a contralateral auditory deficit following temporal lobe lesions, a number of contralateral auditory deficits have also been reported with nonspeech signals. These include impairments of temporal summation (Gersuni et al, 1971; Baru, 1971), temporal resolution (Lackner and Teuber, 1973; Chedru et al, 1978), threshold detection of brief stimuli (Allard and Zeffiro, 1983) and sound localization (Whitfield, 1977; Whitfield et al, 1972; Sanchez-Longo et al, 1957; Sanchez-Longo and Forster, 1958; Klingon and Bontecou, 1966). It should be noted that in these studies extensive damage to Heschl's gyrus and other hemispheric structures was present. However, in more precisely defined surgical resections of the anterior temporal lobe (similar to those described by Kimura), Sherwin and Efron (1980) reported an elevation of temporal order threshold for two consecutive pure tones of different frequencies presented monaurally in the ear contralateral to the lobectomy, and Efron et al (1985) have recently described a degradation in the ability to detect a gap (a brief silent interval) in a wide-band noise stimulus in the contralateral ear.

In sum, the data presently available indicate that the contralateral auditory deficit reported by Bocca et al, Sinha, and Kimura using speech sounds is not the only contralateral auditory deficit following unilateral lesions. The processing of other attributes of acoustic stimuli is similarly compromised. Although the relationship of these other deficits to the deficit in speech processing remains to be determined by future work, there appears to be good reason for caution in continuing to believe that speech sounds represent a "special" type of stimulus, or that their use will necessarily provide any unique insight into the underlying contralateral *auditory* mechanisms—except that, from a physical standpoint, they happen to be unusually complex in their temporal and spectral characteristics. However, this conclusion makes it more imperative that we explore still further the auditory functions of an area of the brain (the anterior temporal lobe) which heretofore has not been thought to have any role in audition. (The historical trend of anatomical and functional "shrinkage" of the central auditory pathways potentially might be reversed!)

Several recent studies from the author's laboratory, using nonspeech stimuli, justify some description, as they suggest a possible role of this most anterior part of the auditory system. For some years we have been studying the perceptual experiences which result when two pure tones of different frequencies are presented dichotically. In this experimental paradigm the subject is not required to recognize, name, or identify any familiar sound pattern (as is usually the case in dichotic listening experiments which test memory as well as "real-time" perceptual processing) but is asked to report only if one of these dichotic tone pairs has a higher or lower pitch than a second tone pair, presented only 300 msec later with a reversed ear-frequency relationship. For almost all normal hearing subjects the pitch of the tone presented to one ear (either right or left depending on the subject, see also "Right-Left Auditory Asymmetries in Normal Subjects") is perceptually more salient in the pitch mixture than the tone simultaneously presented to the other ear. We have called this right-left asymmetry in the binaural integration of dichotically presented pure tones an "ear-dominance for pitch." (See Gregory et al (1983) for a summary of this extensive body of work, its primary characteristics, and references to the original reports.)

In our initial attempt to determine if cerebral mechanisms play a role in this asymmetry, ear dominance for pitch was studied in a number of subjects who had had a complete hemispherectomy in infancy (Efron et al, 1977). These subjects revealed an unusually strong ear dominance: the dominant ear was always ipsilateral to the side of the hemispherectomy. In contrast, commissurotomized subjects (Efron et al, 1977) appeared to be unaffected. The finding of a contralateral effect on binaural pitch integration resulting from a unilateral lesion led us to measure the strength and direction of ear dominance before and after anterior temporal lobe (ATL) resections (Efron and Crandall, 1983). Every subject tested exhibited a postoperative decrease in the contribution of the contralateral ear pitch information to the dichotic pitch mixture compared to performance prior to the resection. In brief, the effect of ATL resection was to decrease the perceptibility of the tone presented to the contralateral ear. This result suggests: (a) that the contralateral auditory deficits in "identification" or "recognition" of speech signals following ATL resection reported by others actually reflect a diminished perceptibility of the contralateral ear stimulus, and (b) that the *intact* ATL might be dynamically involved in *enhancing* the perceptibility of a sound source located contralaterally (see Efron and Crandall, 1983, for the details of methods and reasoning). Such a mechanism would enable us more efficiently to perceive a biologically (or socially) relevant sound source when more than one concurrent stimulus was present in our auditory field. We have also suggested that this perceptual enhancement of the acoustic signal of interest might be performed most efficiently if the ATL was a component of an *efferent* auditory system. This argument is supported by the recent discovery (in rhesus) (in Seltzer and Pandya, 1978) of an efferent multisynaptic auditory pathway which courses anteriorly within the superior temporal gyrus and appears to extend even to the temporal pole before descending to as yet unidentified regions. The location of this pathway (if it is present also in man) is such that it would be severely damaged by an ATL resection. Briefly, our hypothesis is that the contralateral auditory deficits following ATL resections are not due to the slight functional preponderance of the contralateral *afferent* pathway (as first suggested by Kimura) but may result from damage to a contralaterally organized *efferent* pathway which is located within each temporal lobe. Activation of this efferent pathway may significantly enhance our ability to perceive a stimulus on the contralateral side of auditory space.

If this hypothesis is valid, then a patient with a unilateral ATL resection would be expected to have more difficulty perceiving and then identifying a sound source on the side of space contralateral to the lesion at a cocktail party (where multiple different sound sources fill his entire auditory field) because he could not selectively enhance the set of spectral components at each (contralateral) spatial locus. Further, this problem also should be apparent with nonspeech signals. This prediction was tested and confirmed in a recent experiment (Efron et al, 1983a) which warrants a brief description. Thirty common environmental sounds (of

which only two were speech) of 10 sec duration were used in a simulated "cocktail party" task. When these highly overlearned sounds were presented one at a time (via earphones) monaurally or binaurally, they were recognized with virtually no errors by all subjects. The subjects thus were familiar with all 30 sounds prior to the main experiment. From this set of 30 sounds various subsets of five simultaneous sounds were presented under two conditions. In the first the sounds were presented *binaurally* in such a fashion that each of the five sounds was heard in a different (intracranial) locus determined by the interaural intensity differences employed for that particular sound. In the second condition the five simultaneous sounds were presented *monaurally.* For both conditions the subject's task was to name the five sounds presented on that trial. While normal subjects exhibited no difference in the accuracy of identifying *spatially distributed* sounds in the right or left auditory field, the ATL subjects had a 60% higher error rate for the sounds spatially located contralateral to their lesions compared to their error rate in the ipsilateral auditory field. Since their error rate for sounds in the auditory field ipsilateral to their lesion was the same as that obtained by normal subjects, the contralateral deficit in the ATL population could not be dismissed merely as a *nonspecific* performance degradation following a cerebral lesion. When the five sounds were presented monaurally, and thus had the same spatial localization, the normal subjects, as expected, exhibited a significantly ($p < 0.00001$) higher error rate than with spatially separated sounds. Quite clearly, the additional information provided by spatial separation of the sound images in a cocktail party improves our ability to "tune in" to conversation in the babble of sounds usual at such social functions. Although the error rate for normal subjects was increased in the monaural condition, the accuracy for the left and right sides remained the same. The ATL subjects differed from the controls in two ways in their response to monaural stimuli. Firstly, their error rates in *both* ears were more than 70% higher than the normal subjects, and, secondly, their error rates in the ear contralateral to their lesion did *not* increase compared to their performance with spatially distributed stimuli in the same auditory field. That is to say, the effect of anterior temporal lobectomy was to completely eliminate the subject's ability to utilize the information provided by spatial separation of the sounds in the contralateral field to improve his performance—his ability to eavesdrop at a cocktail party would be significantly impaired on one side of space.

This conclusion was supplemented in a separate experiment (Efron et al, 1983a), in which the subjects were informed prior to hearing a subset of five spatially distributed simultaneous sounds that one particular sound, e.g., a violin, would be present. They were required to report whether this "target" sound was lateralized to the left or right of the midline. The ATL subjects exhibited a *normal* localization accuracy for target sounds ipsilateral to the lesion but more than three times the normal error rate for targets which were located contralateral to their lobectomy. It is of interest to note that some patients spontaneously reported (when the "target" was located contralateral to their ATL resection) that they "heard" the sound, but that it was so poorly localized (subjectively) or that it was "so close to the midline" that they were unsure of its location. Thus, the evidence from these experiments indicates that these patients have a deficit in the ability to utilize information pertaining to the localization of sounds in the auditory field contralateral to their lesions of the *anterior* temporal lobe. [Contralateral deficits in sound localization in human subjects having more posterior temporal lobe lesions involving Heschl's gyrus have been reported (Sanchez-Longo et al, 1957; Sanchez-Longo and Forster, 1958) but disputed on methodological grounds (Klingon and Bontecou, 1966) (see also Chapter 10). (But see also Altman et al, 1979; Bisiach et al, 1984.) More recent studies in cats (Jenkins and Masterton, 1982), however, have demonstrated clearly that unilateral lesions of primary auditory cortex result in contralateral deficits of sound localization (see also Chapter 5). The result of our own experiment is of particular interest as it is the first to reveal contralateral deficits in sound localization (at least when multiple simultaneous stimuli are employed) in temporal lobe lesions which *spare* primary auditory cortex.]

The other deficit observed in the ATL subjects, the elevation of error rates in both ears for monaurally presented stimuli, is quite puzzling. Since their performances with spatially separated sounds in the auditory field ipsilateral to the lesion were not abnormal, we cannot easily account for these elevated monaural error rates as a nonspecific effect of brain injury. Thus, we are forced to conclude that a bilateral deficit in auditory processing can result from a unilateral lesion. It should be emphasized that this deficit was observed when the subject was required to process an acoustic signal of approximately the same temporal and spectral complexity as that of speech. Such bilateral auditory deficits following a unilateral lesion have been observed heretofore for auditory temporal patterns (Chapter 13) and for the processing of speech signals in aphasic subjects. It is worth noting, however, that aphasic patients frequently complain that they have their greatest difficulty understanding speech in noisy environments, a complaint which suggests that at least one aspect of their bilateral problem with speech may be related closely to a bilateral problem observed even with nonspeech signal processing.

In conclusion, the findings of a number of recent studies revealed that unilateral cerebral lesions result in deficits in both contralateral and bilateral auditory processing and suggest that these auditory deficits may underlie significant aspects of speech analysis.

RIGHT-LEFT AUDITORY ASYMMETRIES IN NORMAL SUBJECTS

The previous section was primarily concerned with the effects of unilateral lesions on central auditory processing but avoided dealing directly with one of the most striking aspects of central auditory processing, namely, the right-left asymmetry of performance observed in numerous studies of speech as well as nonspeech signals in normal subjects. These findings of an asymmetrical performance of normal subjects in auditory experiments have significantly altered (indeed, they have come to dominate) contemporary investigations of central auditory processing. Such asymmetries are usually explained in terms of hemispheric specialization in the processing of different classes of acoustic stimuli, an explanation inferred principally from the results of dichotic listening experiments—an experimental paradigm which also requires other, often dubious assumptions to be made in interpreting the results. Dichotic stimuli,[1] however, have great value as they permit the study of physiological and/or psychological interactions between two concurrent acoustic stimuli under experimental conditions in which the interaction could not take place in the peripheral mechanisms of the ear itself but must occur somewhere central to the point of entry of each eighth nerve into the medulla.

While the experimental power of this research tool is indisputable, the interpretation of results of dichotic experiments has relied on a number of additional, apparently plausible, assumptions which have had the unfortunate effect of confounding the concept of "central auditory processing" with an ill-defined concept of "hemispheric specialization" of function. In this section we will refer to some of these widely accepted assumptions as "myths" in the hope that this provocative terminology will serve to alert the reader to a number of key logical and methodological problems in this area of research. These problems all too frequently have not been appreciated.

The Myth of "Symmetrical" Hearing

Although various populations of different age, sex, handedness, and brain damage have been studied, the universal (and not unreasonable) procedure among experimenters is to exclude from their experiments subjects who do not have normal hearing. However, "normal hearing" is operationally defined by most researchers in this field as normal *detection* thresholds in both ears, with right-left threshold differences of less than 10 dB at any frequency. A review of the dichotic

listening literature reveals that rarely is any other study of monaural function performed. It is not generally recognized, except by most psychoacousticians and audiologists, that symmetry of thresholds does not necessarily reflect a symmetry in other monaural functions measured at suprathreshold levels *where dichotic listening experiments are always performed.* Thus, measurements of right-left asymmetries in loudness recruitment, frequency discrimination, speech discrimination, gap detection thresholds, binaural diplacusis, masking levels, "psychophysical tuning" functions, and more recently, sound localization (all functions measured at suprathreshold levels) are seldom performed by those who report results of various dichotic listening experiments. From this nearly universal practice of defining symmetrical hearing *only* in terms of detection thresholds for pure tones, it can be inferred that any asymmetries which exist at suprathreshold levels are not believed to be relevant or significant to the analysis of the asymmetrical results of dichotic listening experiments. While this implicit assumption might conceivably be valid in some cases, it is surely premature to attribute *all* right-left performance asymmetries to hemispheric specialization without at least providing some evidence that the functional asymmetry in question could not be accounted for by suprathreshold peripheral, brainstem, or thalamic asymmetries in the processing of auditory information.

The Myth of "Earphone Reversal"

The accepted practice among experimenters using dichotic listening paradigms is to reverse earphones between blocks of trials to ensure that any avoidable *transducer* asymmetries are properly counterbalanced in the experimental design. This procedure does indeed achieve this limited goal.

Unfortunately, earphone reversal does not counterbalance (a) any right-left asymmetry of acoustic coupling between the earphones and the ear, (b) any asymmetries which exist in the resonance characteristics of the two external auditory canals (Shaw, 1966), or (c) any asymmetries in pitch mechanisms—most notably binaural diplacusis (van Den Brink, 1970). In sum, even these well-known right-left asymmetries, found in individuals

---

[1] The term "dichotic stimuli" generally refers to an experimental arrangement in which the two ears simultaneously receive "different" acoustic inputs. Experiments employing differences in interaural intensity, phase, and fine timing, while literally fitting the above definition, are not usually referred to as "dichotic." Such stimuli have been employed in the analysis of the mechanisms of sound localization and have historically been referred to as "binaural" stimuli.

with normal and symmetrical thresholds, are apparently thought by many investigators to be either counterbalanced by earphone reversal or to be irrelevant to their interpretation of the performance asymmetries they have observed in dichotic experiments. The point here is not that earphones should *not* be reversed, but that investigators should not continue to believe that earphone reversal alone magically ensures a completely counterbalanced experiment.

The Myth of Pooling Data

The third myth has its origins in the valid observation that no two subjects are identical and, thus, cannot be expected to produce identical results in any experiment. One acceptable method of dealing with this problem is to perform the same experiment on many subjects and to rely on a statistical analysis of the pooled data to reveal the important findings. This powerful technique often enables the investigator to extract a valid broad conclusion from intrinsically "noisy" data and protects him from the danger of forming an erroneous conclusion on the basis of a few idiosyncratic subjects.

Two underlying (implicit) assumptions are made in pooling the data of many subjects. The first is that the observed differences between individuals are likely to be of lesser biological significance than the generalizations based on the group performance; the second is that the results have a normal (gaussian) distribution. While these assumptions may be true in many cases, it is a myth to believe that averaging the results of many subjects is always the preferred mode of data analysis. It is a particularly risky scientific procedure in those instances where *marked* individual differences are found—as is the case for *every* dichotic listening experiment so far reported. Although it may at times be scientifically justifiable to ignore the results obtained in a few idiosyncratic subjects, the results of most dichotic listening experiments reveal that performances of 20 to 30% (or more) of the subjects do not, in fact, correspond to the conclusion based on the pooled data. Despite this unacceptably high incidence of "aberrant" data, surprisingly little effort has been made to discover why such individual variability exists [particularly notable exceptions being Lauter (1982);

and Speaks et al (1982)]. If 20 to 30% of some species of animals failed to develop clinical signs of tuberculosis when injected with tubercle bacilli, it is unlikely that the importance of individual differences in host response would be so ignored. That equivalent variations in individual responses have been largely ignored in the field of dichotic listening experiments derives, we believe, from the widespread conviction that myth 4, to be discussed below, so adequately "explains" the experimental results that the aberrant responses can be disregarded.

The Myth of Inferring "Hemispheric Specialization" from "Ear Advantages"

The fourth, and by far most conceptually damaging belief, is the view that a performance asymmetry found in a dichotic listening experiment provides *direct* and *sufficient* evidence of right-left differences in hemispheric specialization for that type of stimulus. This belief can be traced to the reports by Kimura (Kimura, 1961a and b, 1964) that a right ear advantage (REA) is observed with dichotically presented speech sounds, while a left ear advantage is obtained with dichotically presented melodies. Despite the fact that Gordon (1970) failed to confirm the latter finding, he has nevertheless offered one of the most concise formulations of myth 4; "It is accepted that the contralateral ear-to-cortex pathways are the stronger and, as a result, ipsilateral pathways tend to be more blocked out during dichotic stimulation. Consequently, superior performance by one ear reflects superior performance by the contralateral hemisphere" (Gordon, 1974). Subsequent investigations using many other types of dichotic stimuli,[2] however, have provided data which require that myth 4 be revised radically or abandoned.

---

[2] The following list, containing only the most often cited studies, gives some indication of the variety of dichotic stimuli which have been employed: pure tones, pure tones with added harmonics, broadband tonal stimuli with temporal asymmetries and with frequency transitions, pulse trains, orchestral melodies, alto and soprano recorded melodies, musical chords, tonal patterns, musical instruments, Morse codes, harmonics with missing fundamentals, natural speech sounds (digits or words), synthetic speech sounds (consonant vowel tokens, consonant-vowel-consonant tokens, vowels), speech played backward.

Six major problems with this interpretation of dichotic experiments are now apparent.

1. For the cerebral function in which the evidence of hemispheric specialization is indisputable, speech analysis in the left hemisphere, the right ear advantage (REA) for dichotically presented speech sounds is a weak effect, exhibiting a large intrasubject variability from test to test and only a mean right ear advantage of 6.6% (Speaks et al, 1982). Although it might be argued that only a small effect could be expected, since there is only a slight preponderance of the contralateral vs the ipsilateral projections from ear to cortex, the same study (which employed the highest number of trials of any reported experiment) found that only 62.5% of normal subjects exhibited a significant ($p <$ 0.025) right *or* left ear advantage, and less than 80% of these subjects displayed a right ear advantage, i.e., about 50% of the population. In another recent study (Wexler et al, 1981), only 45% of listeners had a right ear advantage. Even if we accept the *highest* reported incidence of a REA for dichotically presented speech sounds (80%), it is still difficult to understand why less than 95% of right-handed subjects reveal a REA when more than 95% would be presumed, on the basis of the incidence of aphasia, to have their speech centers in the left hemisphere. Given the clinical evidence that speech is the most *strongly* lateralized cerebral function in man, these results do not generate any confidence that hemispheric specializations for *less* strongly lateralized functions can be directly inferred from performance in a dichotic listening experiment.

2. Although such weak ear advantages and poor correlations with a *known* hemispheric specialization have been widely noted, no attempts have been made to account for the problems of myth 4 in terms of suprathreshold peripheral auditory asymmetries despite reports (Sherwin and Efron, 1980; Efron et al, 1984; Bakker, 1968; Murphy and Venables, 1970; Catlin et al, 1976; Morais and Darwin, 1974; Young and Ellis, 1980; Vroon et al, 1977; Divenyi et al, 1977a; Haydon and Spellacy, 1973) that significant ear advantages have been observed in *monaural* experiments—even in baboons (Pohl, 1983). Such findings significantly undermine one of the major ad hoc assumptions underlying myth 4—that the various ear advantages observed with dichotic stimulation derive from a "competition" between the two channels of information. While ear advantages may be potentiated by "competition," they have been readily observed even under monaural presentations where such competition does not exist.

3. The contribution to the subject's performance asymmetries from any right-left asymmetries in the anatomy or functional capacity of the cochleas, brainstem, and thalamic auditory nuclei, and even from the primary auditory cortex itself, has been neglected. Appreciable evidence now exists that at least some subcortical auditory functions are not always symmetrical. Brainstem evoked responses (BSER) performed on subjects with symmetrical absolute thresholds using suprathreshold monaural stimuli exhibited substantial right-left differences in wave form amplitude and morphology (Chiappa et al, 1979) in 42% of the subjects tested. Further, an unexplained difference has been described between the binaural computer summation of the averaged evoked potentials produced by "identical" right and left monaural stimuli and the actual average evoked potential obtained when these same two stimuli are presented simultaneously (Dobie and Berlin, 1979; Decker and Howe, 1981; Berlin et al, 1981). Anatomical evidence (von Economo and Horn, 1930; Campain and Minckler, 1976; Chi et al, 1977) also indicates that the primary auditory cortex may be smaller on the left side, perhaps inversely related to the very large planum temporale (auditory association cortex) on the left (Galaburda et al, 1978; Geschwind and Levitsky, 1968; Witelson and Pollie, 1973). Although these asymmetries in BSERs and primary auditory cortices have not been correlated yet with any specific asymmetry in cognitive performance, their very existence should at least restrain investigators from making an unwarranted conceptual leap from the mere discovery of an ear advantage (using a particular type of dichotic stimulus) to the conclusion that the contralateral hemisphere is specialized for the processing of that type of stimulus. This last point is further emphasized by other studies (Efron et al, 1979) which have provided evidence that at least

some of the right-left asymmetries observed when pure tones of different frequencies are presented dichotically can be attributed to differences between the acoustic-to-neural transduction mechanism in the two cochleas.

4. Even if it should be the case that peripheral, brainstem, and cortical asymmetries in any individual or groups of individuals are minor and/or average out across subjects, it leaves unresolved the critical question of what particular function each hemisphere is presumably specialized to perform. Excluding the magnitude of the effect, there are only two possible results from any dichotic listening experiment—a right or a left ear advantage. (The failure to find any asymmetry can always be accounted for by an inadequate number of trials). Since there are more than two types of dichotic stimuli which have been used in such experiments, several different types of stimuli must necessarily produce the *same* ear advantage. Only two (equally unpalatable) interpretations of this result are consistent with myth 4. On the one hand, it may be argued that the same ear advantage was obtained because the two types of stimuli were not, in fact, fundamentally different with respect to the specific (as yet unidentified) function the "superior" hemisphere is specialized to perform. For example, the right ear advantages observed with speech sounds and with speech sounds played backward (Kimura and Folb, 1968) have been considered to arise from the left hemispheric specialization for speech, despite the fact that the latter stimulus has no linguistic meaning. Thus, one might argue that it is not speech per se which gives rise to a REA, but merely the use of dichotic stimuli which are highly complex in the spectral and temporal domain. However, a right ear advantage also occurs for pure tones (Deutsch, 1974), tonal stimuli having a relatively broad spectrum (Halperin et al, 1973), and for Morse code (Papcun et al, 1974). If these five types of stimuli, which all give rise (in pooled data) to a REA, are not fundamentally different, then what is their common feature which the left hemisphere is specialized to process? No satisfactory answer to this question has been provided. Alternatively, it may be argued that the left hemisphere has multiple, different specializations—one for each of the five types of stimuli used in this example. However, if we adopt this second argument, we must be prepared to accept an apparently endless number of differential hemispheric specializations, as imaginative investigators use still further types of dichotic stimuli yielding the same ear advantage. It is apparent, therefore, that the continued acceptance of myth 4 requires an ever increasing number of ad hoc assumptions.

5. For each type of dichotic stimulus, a different methodology is usually required. Is the ear advantage which results in a given experiment due to the specific acoustic stimulus which is employed, or is it due to the particular method selected to study that type of dichotic stimulus? For example, in some experiments subjects are required to name the stimulus in each ear; in others they must select the two stimuli from a subsequently presented set of alternatives; in still others they must identify the temporal pattern of the stimulus in each ear. Since the nature of the stimuli employed necessarily dictates the use of different methods, and each method in turn makes different cognitive demands on the subject, the advocate of myth 4 is logically required to (but rarely does) determine whether the observed ear advantage derives from the type of acoustic stimulus used or the cognitive task associated with the method employed. A further complication stems from the fact that for some types of dichotic stimuli, e.g., natural speech sounds, melodies, Morse code, etc., the presentation to the two ears cannot be strictly simultaneous (dichotic). At any moment one ear may be receiving an input, while the other ear may or may not have an input. Such types of stimuli might permit subjects to use a different cognitive strategy than the strategy used when the acoustic stimuli are fully simultaneous.

6. Evidence exists that relatively minor changes in the parameters of a dichotic stimulus may produce changes in the strength of an ear advantage and also in the direction of an ear advantage in some subjects even when the *same* method is used.

Five different experiments illustrating the difficulty encountered in an attempt to infer hemispheric specialization from ear advantages (using dichotic stimuli) warrant particular attention, since within each of the five there was no change of method as the parameters were varied.

1. Sidtis (1980; 1981) used two pure tones of low frequency and required his right-handed subjects to report whether a subsequent test tone was or was not one of the dichotic tones. Under these conditions he found no ear advantage. When he added higher harmonics of the fundamental frequency to each of the dichotic tones, a left ear advantage was observed. Sidtis, apparently accepting myth 4, concluded from this second study that the right hemisphere was specialized "for the analysis of steady state harmonic information." However, in a third study, in which the frequency difference between the fundamentals of the two dichotic stimuli was progressively increased, the left ear advantage steadily decreased and virtually disappeared. Then it increased once again when the fundamental frequencies had an octave relationship. If the right hemisphere is specialized for steady-state harmonic analysis, as Sidtis claimed, why did the left ear advantage decrease when the difference between the fundamentals increased? The same number of harmonics was still present presumably requiring analysis. (It should be noted that as Sidtis presented only pooled data, it is likely that in the third experiment some of his subjects displayed a right ear advantage at frequency differences for which the left ear dominance of the group was very weak.)

2. In right-handed subjects Divenyi et al (1977) also studied the ear advantage (they used the term "ear dominance") for two pure tones of different frequencies using a variety of center frequencies. Although about 75% of "normal hearing" subjects exhibited a *left* ear dominance at a center frequency of 1700 Hz (Gregory, 1982), Divenyi et al observed that a subject might be left ear dominant at one center frequency but right ear dominant at another, or the reverse. If one concluded from a study at a single center frequency that one hemisphere was specialized for some particular function, then one would be obliged by the same reasoning to conclude that the other hemisphere was specialized for the same function at a slightly different center frequency—an implausible state of affairs.

3. Deutsch (1974), using a different paradigm with dichotic tones of 400 and 800 Hz (i.e., a frequency difference (Δf) of 400 Hz at a center frequency (f_c) of 600 Hz), reported that most of her right-handed subjects ex-

hibited a *right* ear dominance. However, Efron et al (1983b), using an identical paradigm but with a smaller ratio of $\Delta f / f_c$, observed a shift towards left ear dominance at center frequencies of 600 as well as 1700 Hz. Once again, a change of the parameters of a dichotic stimulus, even in pure tone stimuli, demonstrably altered the ear dominance.

4. In the study by Efron et al (1983b), employing dichotically presented pure tones around a center frequency of 1700 Hz, 71.4% of 63 right-handed subjects exhibited a left ear dominance when the Δf was 100 Hz. However, increasing the Δf to 400 caused a statistically significant (at the 0.001 level) rightward shift of ear dominance, and a number of subjects actually reversed their ear dominance between the two conditions.

5. In another study, using the paradigm described above and employing only subjects who were strongly left ear-dominant for pure tones, Divenyi and Efron (1979) showed that the progressive addition of temporal and spatial information (ultimately using speech tokens) caused a rightward shift of ear dominance.

These five experiments provide data demonstrating that relatively minor changes in the parameters of a dichotic stimulus pair can result in a shift of ear advantage in a group of subjects or in an individual, even when the *same* method is used. If myth 4 is accepted, then one must conclude that these minor parametric changes have somehow created a new category or class of dichotic stimuli for which the opposite hemisphere is mysteriously specialized—a conclusion which strains credulity! Myth 4 thus appears to have the essential characteristics of a self-perpetuating and irrefutable belief system. The results of any new experiment or the failure to replicate a previous study can always be accounted for by postulating still one more (albeit previously unsuspected) right-left asymmetry in hemispheric specialization. The logical status of this belief system is curiously reminiscent of the last phases of Ptolemaic theory, when it became necessary to postulate yet another and another planetary epicycle in a futile attempt to salvage a disintegrating theory.

In conclusion, the acceptance of these four "myths" has made the concepts of central auditory processing and hemispheric specialization of function almost indistinguishable. To the extent that hemispheric specialization plays a role in the processing of certain (as yet unspecified) aspects of auditory analysis, some overlap between these concepts may be necessary. However, to assume prematurely that all performance asymmetries observed in the presence of symmetrical thresholds derive from *hemispheric* specializations can only retard our understanding of those central auditory processing mechanisms which are fundamentally unrelated to the phenomenon of hemispheric specialization and may be due instead to asymmetrical processes which occur in the many subcortical structures subserving audition.

CONCLUSION

It is the author's hope that this limited review of some recent advances in our understanding of central auditory processing mechanisms and the effects of cerebral lesions on auditory function has emphasized that unilateral lesions produce distinctive auditory deficits which can be contralateral as well as bilateral; that these deficits can be readily observed even when explored with nonspeech stimuli; that some of these deficits may involve damage to efferent (feedback) pathways from cortex to subcortical auditory structures rather than degradation of the afferent input to the auditory cortex; and finally, that appreciably more caution is required than is presently exhibited in the interpretation of the possible role of hemispheric specialization(s) on central auditory processing.

Acknowledgment. This study was supported by the Medical Research Service of the Veterans Administration.

References

Allard T, Zeffiro TA: Contralateral Deficits in Human Auditory Perception after Unilateral Cerebral Lesions. Society for Neuroscience, Boston, 1983.

Altman, JA, Balonov LJ, Deglin VL: Effects of unilateral disorder of the brain hemisphere function in man on directional hearing. *Neuropsychologia* 17:295–301, 1979.

Bakker D: Ear asymmetry with monaural stimulation. *Psychonom Sci* 12:62, 1968.

Baru AV: Absolute thresholds and frequency difference limens as a function of sound duration. In Gersuni GV, Rose J (eds): *Sensory Processes at the Neuronal and Behavioral Levels.* New York, Academic Press, 1971, pp 265–285.

Berlin C, Allen P, Parrish K: Asymmetries in the binaural interaction of the auditory brainstem response. *J Acoust Soc Am* 70(suppl):S-71, 1981.

Bisiach E, Cornacchia L, Sterzi R, Vallar G: Disorders of perceived auditory lateralization after lesions of the right hemisphere. *Brain* 107:37–52, 1984.

Bocca E, Calearo C, Cassinari V, Migliavacca F: Testing "cortical" hearing in temporal lobe tumors. *Acta Otolaryngol (Stockh)* 45:289–304, 1955.

Campain R, Minckler J: A note on the gross configurations of the human auditory cortex. *Brain Lang* 3:318–323, 1976.

Catlin J, Vanderveer NJ, Teicher RD: Monaural right-ear advantage in a target identification task. *Brain Lang* 3:470–481, 1976.

Celesia GG, Puletti F: Auditory cortical areas of man. *Neurology* 19:211–220, 1969.

Chedru F, Bastard V, Efron R: Auditory micropattern discrimination in brain damaged subjects. *Neuropsychologia* 16:141–149, 1978.

Chi JG, Dooling EC, Giles FH: Gyral development of the human brain. *Ann Neurol* 1:86–93, 1977.

Chiappa KH, Gladstone KJ, Young RR: Brainstem auditory evoked responses: studies of waveform variations in 50 normal human subjects. *Arch Neurol* 36:81–87, 1979.

Decker TN, Howe SW: Auditory tract asymmetry in brainstem electrical responses during binaural stimulation. *J Acoust Soc Am* 69:1084–1090, 1981.

Deutsch D: An auditory illusion. *Nature* 251:307–309, 1974.

Divenyi PL, Efron R: Spectral vs. temporal features in dichotic listening. *Brain Lang* 7:375–386, 1979.

Divenyi PL, Efron R, Yund EW: Ear dominance in dichotic chords and ear superiority in frequency discrimination. *J Acoust Soc Am* 62:624–632, 1977a.

Divenyi PL, Efron R, Yund EW: Ear dominance in dichotic chords and ear superiority in frequency discrimination. *J Acoust Soc Am* 62:624–632, 1977b.

Dobie RA, Berlin CE: Binaural interaction in brainstem-evoked responses. *Arch Otolaryngol* 105:391–398, 1979.

Efron R, Bogen JE, Yund EW: Perception of dichotic chords by normal and commissurotomized human subjects. *Cortex* 13:137–149, 1977.

Efron R, Crandall PH: Central auditory processing: effects of anterior temporal lobectomy. *Brain Lang* 19:237–253, 1983.

Efron R, Crandall PH, Koss B, Divenyi PL, Yund EW: Central auditory processing. III. The "Cocktail Party" effect and anterior temporal lobectomy. *Brain Language* 19:254–263, 1983a.

Efron R, Dennis M, Yund EW: The perception of dichotic chords by hemispherectomized subjects. *Brain Lang* 4:537–549, 1977.

Efron R, Koss B, Yund EW: Central auditory processing. IV. Ear dominance—spatial and temporal complexity. *Brain Lang* 19:264–282, 1983b.

Efron R, Yund EW, Divenyi PL: Individual differences in the perception of dichotic chords. *J Acoust Soc Am* 66:75–78, 1979

Efron R, Yund EW, Nichols D, Crandall PH: An ear asymmetry for gap detection following anterior temporal lobectomy. *Neuropsychologia* 23:43–50, 1985.

Galaburda AM, Sanides F, Geschwind N: Cytoarchitectonic left-right asymmetries in the temporal speech region. *Arch Neurol* 35:812–817, 1978.

Gersuni GV, Baru AV, Karaseva TA, Tonkonogii IM: Effects of temporal lobe lesions on perception of sounds of short duration. In Gersuni GV, Rose J (eds): *Sensory Processes at the Neuronal and Behavioral Levels.* New York, Academic Press, 1971, pp 287–300.

Geschwind N, Levitsky W: Human brain: left-right asymmetries in temporal speech region. *Science* 161:186–187, 1968.

Gordon HN: Hemispheric asymmetries in the perception of dichotic chords. *Cortex* 6:387–398, 1970.

Gordon HN: Auditory specialization of the right and left hemispheres. In Kinsbourne M, Smith WL (eds): *Hemispheric Disconnection and Cerebral Function.* Springfield, IL, Charles C Thomas, 1974.

Gregory AH: Ear dominance for pitch. *Neuropsychologia* 20:89–90, 1982.

Gregory AH, Efron R, Divenyi PL, Yund EW: Central auditory processing. I. Ear dominance—a perceptual or an attentional asymmetry. *Brain Lang* 19:225–236, 1983.

Halperin Y, Nachson I, Carmon A: Shift of ear superiority in dichotic listening to temporally patterned nonverbal stimuli. *J Acoust Soc Am* 53:46–50, 1973.

Haydon SP, Spellacy FJ: Monaural reaction time asymmetries for speech and non-speech sounds. *Cortex* 9:288–294, 1973.

Jenkins WM, Masterton B: Sound localization: effects of unilateral lesions in central auditory system. *J Neurophysiol* 47:987–1015, 1982.

Kimura D: Some effects of temporal-lobe damage on auditory perception. *Can J Psychol* 15:156–165, 1961a.

Kimura D: Cerebral dominance and the perception of verbal stimuli. *Can J Psychol* 15:166–171, 1961b.

Kimura D: Left-right differences in the perception of melodies. *Q J Exp Psychol* 14:355–358, 1964.

Kimura D, Folb S: Neural processing of backwards speech sounds. *Science* 161:395–396, 1968.

Klingon GH, Bontecou DC: Localization in auditory space. *Neurology* 16:879–886, 1966.

Lackner JR, Teuber H-L: Alterations in auditory fusion thresholds after cerebral injury in man. *Neuropsychologia* 11:409–415, 1973.

Lauter J: Dichotic identification of complex sounds: absolute and relative ear advantages. *J Acoust Soc Am* 71:701–707, 1982.

Morais J, Darwin CJ: Ear differences for same-different reaction time to monaurally presented speech. *Brain Language* 1:383–390, 1974.

Murphy EH, Venables PH: Ear asymmetry in the threshold of fusion of two clicks: a signal detection analysis. *Q J Exp Psychol* 22:288–300, 1970.

Papcun G, Krashen S, Terbeek D, Remington R, Harshman R: Is the left hemisphere specialized for speech, language and/or something else? *J Acoust Soc Am* 55:319–327, 1974.

Pohl P: Central auditory processing. V. Ear advantages for acoustic stimuli in baboons. *Brain Lang* 20:44–53, 1983.

Rosenzweig M: Representation of the two ears at the auditory cortex. *Am J Physiol* 167:147–158, 1951.

Sanchez-Longo LP, Forster FM: Clinical significance of impairment of sound localization. *Neurology* 8:119–125, 1958.

Sanchez-Longo LP, Forster FM, Auth TL: A clinical test for sound localization and its applications. *Neurology* 7:655–663, 1957.

Seltzer B, Pandya DN: Afferent cortical connections and architectonics of the superior temporal sulcus and surrounding cortex in the Rhesus monkey. *Brain Res* 149:1–24, 1978.

Shaw EAG: Ear canal pressure generated by circumaural and supraaural earphones. *J Acoust Soc Am* 39:471–479, 1966.

Sherwin I, Efron R: Temporal ordering deficits following anterior temporal lobectomy. *Brain Language* 11:195–203, 1980.

Sidtis JJ: On the nature of the cortical function underlying right hemisphere auditory perception. *Neuropsychologia* 18:321–330, 1980.

Sidtis JJ: The complex tone test: implications for the assessment of auditory laterality effects. *Neuropsychologia* 19:103–112, 1981.

Sinha SP: The Role of the Temporal Lobe in Hearing. Master's thesis, McGill University, Montreal, 1959.

Speaks C, Niccum N, Carney E: Statistical properties of responses to dichotic listening with CV nonsense syllables. *J Acoust Soc Am* 72:1185–1194, 1982.

Tunturi AR: A study on the pathway from the medial geniculate body to the acoustic cortex in the dog. *Am J Physiol* 147:311–319, 1946.

van Den Brink G: Experiments on binaural diplacusis and tone perception. In: Plomp R, Smoorenburg GF (eds): *Frequency Analysis and Periodicity Detection in Hearing.* AW Sijhoff, Leiden, Netherlands, 1970, pp 362–374.

von Economo C, Horn L: Uber windungsrelief, masse und rindenarchitektonik der supratemporalflache, ihre individuellen und ihre scitenunterschiede. *Z Gesamte Neurol Psychiatr* 130:678–757, 1930.

Vroon PA, Timmers H, Tempelaars S: On the hemispheric representation of time. In Dornic S (ed): *Attention and Performance VI.* New York, Wiley, 1977, pp 231–245.

Wexler E, Halwes T, Heninger GR: Use of a statistical significance criterion in drawing inferences about hemispheric dominance for language function from dichotic listening data. *Brain Lang* 13:13–18, 1981.

Whitfield IC: 'Auditory Space' and the role of the cortex in sound localization. In Evans EF, Wilson JP (eds): *Psychophysics and Physiology of Hearing.* London, Academic Press, 1977.

Whitfield IC, Cranford J, Ravizza R, Diamond IT: Effects of unilateral ablation of auditory cortex in cat on complex sound localization. *J Neurophysiol* 35:718–731, 1972.

Witelson SF, Pallie W: Left hemisphere specialization for language in the newborn: neuroanatomical evidence of asymmetry. *Brain Res* 96:641–646, 1973.

Young AW, Ellis HD: Ear asymmetry for the perception of monaurally presented words accompanied by binaural white noise. *Neuropsychologia* 18:107–110, 1980.

CHAPTER 10

Binaural Interaction Tasks

HENRY TOBIN, Ph.D.

This chapter by Henry Tobin describes binaural interaction tasks most frequently used clinically to evaluate the integrity of the central auditory system. These include binaural fusion, rapidly alternating speech, interaural intensity difference, and masking level difference. The author reviews the literature on normal and pathological subjects and points out the strengths and weaknesses of the tests.

Binaural interaction is the most efficient of the two possible conditions for binaural transfer of information, interaction or relative noninteraction (Durlach et al, 1981). This chapter will focus specifically on those tasks that will be referred to as noncongruent binaural interaction tasks. Operationally these tasks require the two ears to effect closure for dichotic signal information separated by time, frequency, or intensity factors. This chapter will not include congruent interaction tasks such as those using dichotically presented words. (Read Chapter 12 for congruent tests.) Examples of noncongruent central auditory tests include Binaural Fusion (BF), Rapidly Alternating Speech (RASP), the Interaural Intensity Difference for Intracranial Lateralization (IID), and Masking Level Difference (MLD).

Many central auditory tasks have been designed to exploit the two-sidedness of the system. When the two ears are stimulated simultaneously, the signals may be in a competing (congruent) mode or a complementary (noncongruent) mode. The congruency in competing signals may be in similar onset times, intensity levels, wave envelopes, and/ or linguistic structure, as in the Staggered Spondee Words test (Arnst and Katz, 1982). Noncompeting exploitation of two eared-

ness is noncongruent and complementary in nature.

When the binaural system behaves normally for noncongruent tasks, it is possible to transmit a message by providing a different portion of the information to each of the two ears. From a psychoacoustic point of view the derivation of the message can be inferred, if there has been improvement in threshold for signals in noise, full lateralization to one ear, or the ability to discriminate a resynthesized speech event. All of these tasks depend on successful binaural interaction, i.e., the ability of the brain—the total system—to take disparate information delivered to the two ears and unify it, making it into one perceptual event. For noncongruent events the listener is forced to utilize the information from both ears in order to complete the task successfully.

Terms that have been associated with binaural response phenomena include binaural advantage (MacKeith and Coles, 1971), binaural summation (Reynolds and Stevens, 1960), binaural unmasking (Licklider, 1948; Hirsh, 1948), binaural integration (Tobias and Zerlin, 1959), binaural fusion (Broadbent and Ladefoged, 1957; Cherry, 1961), dichotic listening (Kimura, 1967), binaural shadowing (Cherry, 1953), dichotic shadowing (Moray, 1959), localization (Mills, 1972), lateralization (Moushegian and Jeffress, 1959; Békésy, 1960), and binaural interaction. These terms fall into three categories: (1) those that infer something about the physiological process; (2) the perceptual effect; or (3) the psychophysical task. Binaural interaction, binaural summation, binaural integration, and binaural fusion are *physiologic* terms based on mathematical ways of viewing the system, i.e., the calculus, addition, and/or geometry of the nervous system. Terms such as binaural advantage, binaural unmasking, localization, and lateralization focus on the *perceptual* end product. Dichotic listening, dichotic shadowing, binaural shadowing, as well as binaural congruency imply something about the *psychophysical* task, i.e., they are an attempt to define the signal-response paradigm, the foremost responsibility of the psychophysicist. Ultimately, the attention to psychophysical detail, not the task label, determines the ability to address response parameters that may be related to central auditory functioning.

The operational examples of interaction phenomena that are focused on in this chapter follow.

1. The speech signal for *Binaural Fusion* (BF) is divided in such a way that neither spectral portion individually is sufficient to produce recognition. When each spectral portion is presented, one to each ear, there is the expectation of fusion or synthesis—a reunifying merger of the whole.

Example

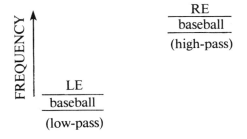

2. In *Rapidly Alternating Speech* (RASP) the signal is not divided by spectral parameters, but rather by time. A speech event, such as a short sentence, is chopped up into equal time segments. The time segments are alternated between the two ears, i.e., the first segment to the right ear, the second segment to the left ear, the third segment to the right ear, and so on to the completion of the speech event.

Example

The fire engine raced down the street.
```
LE: Th   re   ine   ced   wn   e st   t
RE:   e fi   eng   ra   do   th   ree
```
If the listener hears only the odd segments

or only the even segments, it should not be enough to produce the integration of the signal, i.e., the formation of a whole perceptual event by the combination of the parts.

3. For the *Interaural Intensity Difference* for intracranial lateralization (IID) a perceptually equal amount of noise (20 dB sensation level) is delivered to the two ears so that the sound cannot be referred to either ear. It is heard in the middle of the head. By successively adding increments of sound to one ear in 1 dB steps, the intensity of loudness sensation is moved toward that side, and localization (or more specifically lateralization, since the signals are presented under earphones and thus heard inside the head) is said to have occurred when the sound is perceived to be located at the ear. Lateralization can be thought of as a form of summation in which a cumulative effect is produced.

4. There is a reciprocal action/influence between a masking event and a signal of interest that depends upon the respective time of arrival of these events at the two ears, i.e., their phase relationship. It is this phase relationship between the two ears which produces the end result of binaural advantage, binaural unmasking, or release from masking, i.e., the *Masking Level Difference* (MLD). The relative phase relationship between the two ears offers the opportunity to produce a phenomenological separation of the signal and the noise.

A CLINICAL MODEL FOR BINAURAL INTERACTION

The interaction effect, when viewed as a behavioral response to binaural signaling, is a response by the complete auditory system. Interaction through the synaptic stations of the central auditory system can only be inferred. The inferences made are based on knowledge of the anatomic and neurophysiologic structure of the system and its decussating nature, bioacoustic studies of animals, and clinical studies of humans including autopsy information (Matzker, 1959; Deatherage, 1966; Baru and Karaseva, 1972). (See also Chapters 2 and 5.)

For clinical purposes it is convenient to have a model which can represent the neurophysiology of the auditory system and binaural interaction. Although Colburn and

Durlach (1978) pointed out that there is no satisfactory model of binaural interaction, clinicians have need of some kind of working model. Such a model has been available since the development of speech spectrography in the early 1940s. Speech spectrography, as Joos (1948) pointed out:

... is superior in that it presents only what the ear can hear, and presents it in a form closely analogous to the manner of hearing ... In the hair cells and nerve fibers, in the lowest levels of the hearing center in the brain, and from these levels onward for some distance toward the speech center, we find that harmonic analysis has taken place and the neural equivalents of the component frequencies are present IN DIFFERENT PLACES, just as their graphical equivalents—in a spectrogram. (From Joos M: Acoustic phonetics. *Language (Monograph no. 23),* 24(suppl):66–67, 1948).

The Visible Speech Translator can serve as a clinical model, as it provides real-time analysis and probably is instrumentally most analogous to the behavior of the auditory system. In this instrument the spectrographic analysis enters the display window in right-left fashion simultaneously with the acoustic signal (Potter, 1946; Steinberg and French, 1946; Koenig et al, 1946; Riesz and Schott, 1946; Dudley and Gruenz, 1946; Kopp and Green, 1946; Potter et al, 1947). It sweeps across the face of the oscilloscope, leaving behind an afterimage in the form of phosphor persistence. The subsequent acoustic signals enter in a similar manner and overlie the previous afterimages initially without completely obliterating them, finally leaving their own phosphor trace to be overlapped by the signals which follow. It is likely that something akin to this is going on in those portions of the auditory system where there is tonotopic organization and stacking of neural cells (Imig and Adrián, 1977; Middlebrooks et al, 1980). The phosphor persistence is suggestive of a holding mechanism that would permit fusion, integration, summation, and interaction (Neff and Diamond, 1958). It permits the formation of a geometric analog which represents weighting, as in lateralization, and embedding, as with phase relationships associated with binaural unmasking. With some elaboration it can provide for autocorrelation and cross-correlation comparisons which are so critical for binaural interactive events (Sayers and Cherry, 1957; Licklider, 1959). Thus, a neurophysiologic Visible Speech Translator with binaural representation seems capable of accepting the five categories of models of binaural interaction reviewed by Colburn and Durlach (1978), i.e., count-comparison models, interaural difference detector models, noise suppression models, cross-correlation models, and auditory nerve-based models.

The auditory system, as information servant of the brain, and the brain itself appear to have great flexibility in signal processing (Feldmann, 1965). Psychoacoustic and perceptual challenges of differing complexity presented monaurally or binaurally are met by a system that can modify its mode of operation in its search for appropriate solutions. It is anything but a parsimonious system. As Bocca and Calearo (1963) pointed out, there is a wealth of redundancy: extrinsic redundancy of the message as well as intrinsic redundancy of the neural centers and pathways. The decussating nature of the brainstem pathways and the interconnections within the brain make it difficult to demonstrate when and where pathology may exist. The clinician, by reducing the natural redundancy of the message, tries to "trick" the system into revealing its flaw. In order to do so, he must be a good psychoacoustician and carefully define the signal that is presented.

REVIEW OF LITERATURE

Psychoacoustic Parameters

Pinheiro (1969) found research on sound localization going back as far as 1796 by Venturi and 1798 by Jurine. Boring (1942) and Woodworth (1938) reported studies of binaural interaction tasks dating to the early 1900s. There is now a considerable fund of modern literature in this area (Durlach and Colburn, 1978). The portion that will be reviewed here will be highly selective and pertain only to the noncongruent binaural interaction tasks previously noted.

Fusion

Probably the earliest demonstration of binaural fusion (sometime during the 1920s) was conducted by Fletcher (1953) at the Bell Telephone Laboratories. The frequency components below 1000 Hz were delivered to the left ear, while the components above 1000 Hz were delivered to the right ear. When speech signals in both channels were played together, the fusion provided good sound quality. If either channel were turned off, the speech was severely degraded and difficult to understand. Subsequent application of speech resynthesis as a test of central auditory functioning involved dividing the speech signal into two filtered portions separated by a gap. Matzker (1959) accomplished this by using a low-frequency band between 500 and 800 Hz for one channel and a high-frequency band between 1815 and 2500 Hz for the other channel. The reader may wish to examine the relative contribution of these low- and high-pass bands to speech intelligibility by reviewing French and Steinberg's (1947) discussion on the articulation index. It should be kept in mind that the redundancy of the message is affected by the type of speech signal chosen as the testing vehicle (Kryter, 1962). The greater the signal's natural redundancy, the more readily closure and fusion will occur despite the limiting pass bands.

Integration

Alternation of a signal train between ears offers an opportunity to tax the central auditory system (Cherry, 1953; Cherry and Taylor, 1954). Cherry found the central switching time for normal listeners to be between 100 and 500 msec. The integration of alternating segments of short sentences turned out to be a relatively easy task because of the natural redundancy of meaningful sentences. Scrambled messages or synthesized nonmeaningful short sentences of the type used by Speaks and Jerger (1965) might limit response to the integration phenomenon by limiting language involvement. In the 1950s Bocca and Calearo (1963) adapted the Cherry procedure clinically for assessment of central auditory function.

Lateralization

One of the most fascinating studies of interaction did not involve the auditory system. This is the study by Békésy (1967) on lateral inhibition on the surface of the skin. It is summarized here because it is illustrative of the interaction process. Békésy found that one vibrator, separated from a second vibrator by 2 cm, had to have a differential of 10 dB greater intensity for complete lateralization to its site on the skin surface. Curiously, when the vibrators were 10 cm apart, an intensity difference of only 3 dB produced full lateralization. In addition, desensitizing the skin surface by warming it when the vibrators were only 2 cm apart gave results that were similar to the 10 cm separation, i.e., a small energy difference produced lateralization. It seemed as if there were some kind of short circuit, with the vibratory sensation jumping from one site to the other. Békésy hypothesized a decrease in neural activity in the region of the warmed skin that produced the 3 dB lateralization. Since the findings were similar, it is supposed that reduced neural activity also must have been present when the separation was 10 cm. The actual processing of these neural messages probably occurred at some central region remote from the source of the input information. Békésy offered an hypothesis of neural funneling produced by lateral inhibition (1967) as a partial explanation of this lateralization phenomenon (or phenomena).

Sensory systems can be thought of as difference detectors. The theory of signal detection (Green and Swets, 1966) has as its central theme the differentiation between the noise only condition and the signal with noise condition. In the latter condition the greater the noise the greater the signal must be to be perceived in the background of noise. The noise can take the form of intrinsic physiologic noise produced by neural activity. The greater the neural activity (the 2 cm unwarmed condition), the greater the intrinsic noise, and the higher the threshold of the signal. The less the neural activity (the 10 cm or warmed 2 cm condition), the less the intrinsic noise, and the lower the resulting threshold for the signal.

From an information theory point of view (Shannon and Weaver, 1949) fewer neural connections vs greater numbers of neural connections imply a time difference. The processing of more information requires a longer time. When a message is clear, there is little information transmitted, and the reaction time appears to be faster. The un-warmed 2 cm condition probably required more information processing, i.e., a 10 dB intensity difference, because there was greater uncertainty. The dynamic neural display was clearer for the 10 cm and warmed 2 cm conditions, thus requiring less information, i.e., only a 3 dB intensity difference.

Whatever the actual form neural processing takes, the study on skin lateralization has contributed greatly to the understanding of auditory lateralization. Békésy (1959) was also able to show that lateralization for the intact hearing system similarly required 10 dB of information. The Pinheiro and Tobin study (1969) provided the auditory correlation for Békésy's observations on reduced neuronal interaction.

Unmasking

Another way of looking at binaural interaction is to manipulate the phase relationship between signals and masking foils. The companion studies by Licklider (1948) and Hirsh (1948) established the way to examine this for speech signals and tones. Licklider used speech while Hirsh employed tones, and both used white noise as foils.

Licklider tested speech intelligibility at three noise levels with six interaural phase conditions (as well as a monaural condition which will be discussed later). He categorized the phase conditions as: homophasic, if the speech and noise were both either in-phase or out-of-phase; antiphasic, if either the speech or noise signal was out-of-phase, while the other signal was held in-phase and if the speech or noise signal was either in- or out-of-phase and the other signal was permitted to vary in a random phase manner. For the in-phase interaural condition the two eardrums are made to move in unison, while for the out-of-phase condition the membranes are directly opposite in position, i.e., 180° out-of-phase in relation to each other. As it turned out, the phase relationship of the earphones and the similarly imposed relationship of the eardrums were a major factor in speech intelligibility only under the severest of the signal to noise ratio (S/N) conditions, although speech intelligiblity was better in either of the two antiphasic conditions. In general, when a signal is presented in phase to the two ears, the listener reports that the signal seems to be located in the center of the head. When the signal is out-of-phase, the listener typically reports that the signal is located at the ears. The introspective reports of the listeners in this study were as interesting as the testing data and revealed the listeners natural awareness of the relative congruency of the binaural signals. Licklider (p 154) reported three impressions relating to observations of phenomenologic space and positions:

1. The speech "moves over" a little, as though to get out of the noise, when the speech and noise are presented together.
2. The noise obscures primarily that part of the speech that occupies the same position as the noise in phenomenal space.
3. The speech and noise overlap less when the interaural phase relations are antiphasic than they do when the interaural phase relations are homophasic.

It is interesting to note that even in the homophasic condition the speech signal can slightly disengage itself from the effects of the masker. A conclusion that might be drawn is that speech is a species-specific event, and inhibition is operating. Speech and the masker used in Licklider's study have different spectral and dynamic characteristics and, therefore, would occupy slightly different areas of phenomenologic space, even in the homophasic condition. If a masker that faithfully followed the wave envelope of the speech event had been used, this separation might not have occurred. The use of speech-modulated white noise as a masker might have provided a constant S/N ratio and avoided the vocalic transitions and consonantal spectra cues that probably contributed to the impression of separation (Horii et al, 1971). This type of masker might also be expected to have had some effect on intelligibility scores in the antiphasic condition. Its use might have limited the contributions of the spectral and dynamic differences between the signal and noise and provided results more completely based on phase angle.

In 1948 Hirsh also found the greatest release from masking for binaural threshold to be that antiphasic condition in which the tone was out-of-phase and the noise in-phase.

Similar to Licklider's finding, the highest intensity noise condition produced the greatest relative separation. Throughout all conditions it was the lower frequency tones which could be affected the most by phase, i.e., timing differences, which showed release from masking. Licklider, reflecting on Hirsh's findings, surmised that speech was not totally masked by the white noise because the white noise was least effective as a masker in the low-frequency region.

The monaural findings of both Licklider and Hirsh are of some interest. A binaural in-phase signal, whether speech or a low frequency tone, masked by a binaural in phase noise was not as efficient in the transmission of information as a monaural signal with a binaural in-phase masking foil. (The antiphasic results mentioned earlier were still superior to those provided by the monaural conditions.) When the signal was in competition with noise in the out-of-phase condition, binaural presentation, even when homophasic, was better than monaural presentation. These findings provided a clear indication that central processing was taking place, the only conclusion that could be drawn when the phase angle of noise in the opposite ear affected monaural signal processing.

A comprehensive clinical study of this central auditory unmasking phenomenon, the MLD, was done in the mid-1970s by Olsen et al (1976). They examined masking level differences in several populations exhibiting auditory anomalies and other clinical conditions.

Binaural Clinical Tasks

Binaural Fusion (BF)

At the writing of his 1959 report Matzker had used a test of BF with over 1700 patients. Autopsy information on some of these patients implicated the lower brainstem as site of lesion. Matzker felt that the "binaural test," as he called it, would be reliable for determining lower brainstem involvement. However, the very large number of patients assessed with the "binaural test" did not help to clarify its use as an indicator of lower brainstem involvement. An assumption of retrograde degeneration or intracranial pressure on the brainstem had to

be made for most of the patients showing positive response to this test. Of the five categories of central involvement, i.e., brain tumors, brain atrophy, hypertension, multiple sclerosis, and skull trauma, none is uniquely associated with the lower brainstem. In addition to the uncertainty of location of the lesion and its effects, the test itself was not clearly delineated. The test contained 41 two-syllable words that were phonetically balanced. Vowel recognition rather than word recognition was used as the criterion for correctness. The test was given three times. The first and third presentations were the filtered bands, while second presentation was diotic in nature. The diotic presentation, of course, did not require fusion. The few examples given suggested that learning was also a factor.

Lindén (1964) attempted an adaptation of the Matzker test for resynthesis. The low-pass band, 560 to 715 Hz, was essentially the same as the one Matzker chose, while high-pass filter was actually more restrictive. Lindén created nine Swedish spondaic word lists of 15 items each. Simple recognition was chosen as the response criterion rather than the less certain method Matzker had chosen. Although presentation level through the high-pass filter did not show great variation for normal listeners, the Sensation Level (SL) established with the low-pass filter significantly affected intelligibility of the spondees. Lindén felt SLs above 40 dB for the lower filter band would contribute too much to intelligibility. By using a 40 dB or lower SL the low- and high-pass bands, when played independently, produced equally poor recognition scores. For normal hearing subjects the average recognition score for resynthesized speech improved with increases in SL, i.e., 35% at 25 dB SL, 62% at 30 dB SL, 81% at 35 dB SL, and 89% at 40 dB SL. Lindén also presented the combined bands to a single ear, calling this monaural listening task a "distorted speech test." Interestingly, the scores were almost identical to those obtained with the binaural resynthesis test at each of the SLs cited above.

Lindén then tested 18 patients with known intracranial expanding lesions. Lindén took the position that binaural resynthesis scores would be lower than the monaural scores for distorted speech if BF did *not* occur. Spondaic function curves were derived for both monaural distorted speech and binaural speech resynthesis at several SLs to obtain the optimal recognition level for both tests. As a result of negative findings for the resynthesis test, Lindén completely rejected its use for assessing central auditory function.

Just as Matzker had been too sanguine about his findings, Lindén was too pessimistic. Negative findings can be just as helpful as positive findings, if the test or measure truly assesses the activity or behavior it is supposed to evaluate. Lindén's psychoacoustic methodology appeared superior to that employed by Matzker. He probably was testing BF at the lower brainstem level, and his patients may not have been as severely involved as some of Matzker's patients who were found to have ganglionic cell involvement at autopsy. Reinterpretation of Lindén's findings suggests that 4 of the 18 patients reported were beginning to show BF problems. For example, one of the patients had an 80% score on the ipsilateral ear for the distorted speech test and only 33% on the ear contralateral to the lesion. When the bilateral resynthesis test (BF) was given, the score was 47%. Based on the type of testing materials used, i.e., the spondiac words, it is possible that even the patient showing 93% for the ipsilateral ear, 60% for the contralateral ear, and 80% for BF was showing an early stage of lower brainstem involvement (possibly due to edema or intracranial pressure). A variation of Lindén's protocol is used today as the test for BF (Palva, 1965; Hayashi et al, 1966; Ohta et al, 1967; Ivey, 1969; Smith and Resnick, 1972; Lynn and Gilroy, 1975; Willeford, 1977).

Smith and Resnick (1972) chose to use phonetically balanced monosyllabic words for their study of BF. They believed that lower redundnacy of the signal (compared to spondees) would tax the auditory system further, but this fact would limit application of the BF test to those individuals with at least fair speech recognition ability. By using three presentation modes they overcame the limitations imposed by end organ involvement to a great extent. Two resynthesis tasks and a diotic task were developed. For one of the resynthesis tasks the low-pass portion of the signal was presented to the right ear. For the other task it was presented to the left ear, counterbalancing the tasks. The recog-

nition scores obtained with these fusion tasks were then compared to those obtained in the diotic task which required no fusion (since both the low- and high-pass bands were fed to both ears simultaneously). If all three scores were similar, there was no problem with BF. If the diotic score was "substantially better" than either of the resynthesis scores, the finding was considered positive for pathology. Four brainstem cases were examined, and all were found to be positive on BF. One of the cases showed a differential response based on sidedness: 74% (diotic), 62% (low-pass to right), and 40% (low-pass to left). To control for test bias, listener bias, fatigue, and other vagaries of monsyllabic test administration, the three listening conditions were continuously switched, i.e., first word, low-pass to the right ear; second word, diotic presentation; third word, low-pass to the left ear; and so on in this order. Although there is merit in the protocol used by Smith and Resnick, it has not been adopted by others, probably because of the use of monosyllabic words. The Modified Rhyme Test (House et al, 1965; Kryter and Whitman, 1965; Kreul et al, 1968) with its closed response format might serve as an interesting measurement vehicle for this type of procedure. The closed response feature might offset the use of low redundancy monosyllabic words.

The version of the BF test most commonly used now is the one developed by Willeford and Ivey (Ivey, 1969). The low-pass band for the spondaic words is 500 to 700 Hz and the high-pass band is 1900 to 2100 Hz. Lynn and Gilroy (1975) reported on the use of this test with individuals with various brain anomalies. The BF was abnormal for a patient with a left posterior temporal lobe tumor that was producing pressure on the brainstem. Both Willeford (1976, 1977), Pinheiro (1977, 1978), and Roush and Tait (1984) have applied this test to children with learning disabilities. Willeford reported on several children with poor BF scores, implicating brainstem integrity. Of six subjects illustrated by Pinheiro only two 6 to 7 yr of age showed abnormal results for one ear on BF. When BF scores were somewhat poorer than normal on both ears in children of this age, it was believed to be immaturity of the central nervous system (see Chapter 15). Nineteen dyslexic children

7 to 14 yr old generally had scores within the low normal range (Pinheiro, 1978). However, several individuals had abnormal scores for one ear. In 1977 Willeford published his normative data for his BF test, and he discusses further cases in this book in Chapter 14.

Willeford's 1976 report included the case of a 13-yr-old boy who scored 65% for his right ear and only 15% for his left ear.

Also of interest were his results for a 31-year-old woman who had had a learning disability as a child. Her scores were 45% for the right ear and 0% for the left ear. When the test was repeated at a 10 dB greater intensity level, scores shifted slightly, but there was no improvement. If such findings could be obtained in a statistically significant number of patients (see Chapter 9), it might imply that no improvement in fusion occurs in individuals over time. For example, though Pinheiro's 1978 study showed an improvement in overall scores for the learning-disabled children in the older age group when compared to the scores of the younger group of learning-disabled children, the *difference* between normal subjects and the learning-disabled of the same ages remained the *same*. Unfortunately, little is known about possible brain involvement in learning disabilities. Roush and Tait (1984) in comparing normal and language learning-disabled children demonstrated that binaural fusion performance was significantly depressed for the learning-disabled group.

There have also been some findings of poor BF scores for adults with brain lesions. The study of a 19-yr-old male who survived a gunshot wound to the brainstem in the area of the right pons resulted in a chance level score for the left ear on Willeford's BF test (Pinheiro et al, 1982). As for consideration of BF as a task limited to brainstem auditory function occasional patients with cortical lesions also achieve poor BF scores. Two such case examples evaluated by Pinheiro include a 16-yr-old with a glioma invading the left thalamus and extending into the anterior temporal lobe of the left hemisphere (Fig. 10.1) and a 27-yr-old with an uncontrollable psychomotor seizure disorder with a focus in the right hippocampus and amygdaloid area who underwent a right

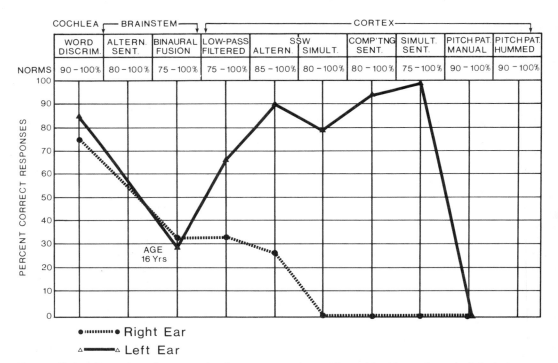

Figure 10.1. Central auditory graph of test results for a 16-yr-old with a glioma in left thalamus, invading left hemisphere at left anterior temporal lobe.

anterior temporal lobectomy (Fig. 10.2). Of course, both of these patients could also have had compromised brainstem function. Both had anterior temporal lobe involvement. However, it should be remembered that the speech redundancy is considerably reduced in this task, and a patient with a left hemisphere lesion might do poorly on the language processing of the verbal response to the words. Note the right ear results of the other central auditory tests on these two patients.

BF tapes can be obtained commercially for either the spondaic words or the NU-6 monosyllabic words. (Alternatively, the same task can be accomplished with a speech audiometer feeding high quality electronic filters.) There are differences in the pass bands used by the creators of different tapes. Not only must normative data be derived for each clinical setting, but it is suggested that each subject serve as his own control by combining high- and low-pass bands for each ear to obtain a recognition score at an overall 40 to 50 dB Sensation Level (SL).

Unfortunately, few of the clinical researchers have used the same methods for the BF task. Probably the best mode for presenting it would be to deliver the low-pass band to each ear in turn. (The ear receiving the low-pass band is considered the test ear.) The test should be presented at no higher intensity level than 40 to 50 dB SL referenced to the speech detection threshold (SDT) for the combined bands for each ear. This method would result in six scores: two scores for the low-pass segment, one for each ear; two scores for the high-pass segment, one for each ear; and two scores for the combined segments, one for each ear. The SDT will vary, depending on whether spondees or monosyllabic words are used. A normal BF score (for the low-pass ear) should be similar to the score for the same ear on the combined low-pass, high-pass presentation. If there is brainstem (or, possibly, brain) dysfunction sensitive to spectral fusion, the BF scores for the low-pass bands will be poorer than the scores for the combined bands in the same ear.

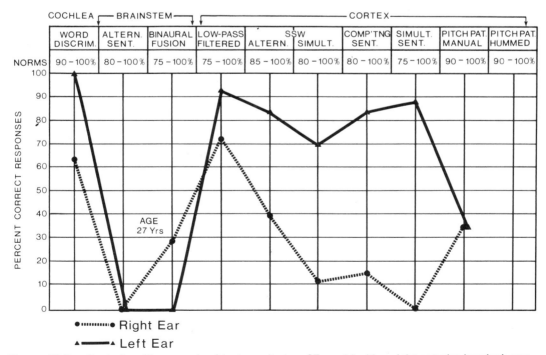

Figure 10.2. Central auditory graph of test results in a 27-yr-old with a right anterior hemispherectomy for an uncontrollable psychomotor seizure disorder. Note poor binaural fusion scores, worse for the left ear. All other test scores were poor for the right ear. This patient could not perform the RASP task at all.

Rapidly Alternating Speech Perception (RASP)

It seems that the number of alterations per second on the RASP test does not make a difference for normal listeners (Hennebert, 1955; Bocca and Calearo, 1963; Lynn and Gilroy, 1977). Bocca and Calearo employed alternating segments of running speech ranging from about 20 to 500 msec in duration without any disruption in intelligibility. Lynn and Gilroy selected 300 msec for their work with RASP, but this rate was based on experienced listeners. It is not known what alteration rate would reveal minimal degrees of brainstem involvement. There is some question as to whether the RASP test is sensitive to other than grossly abnormal brainstem function. Six of the 47 patients (who had medically evident brainstem involvement) tested by Lynn and Gilroy (1977) showed clearly positive (abnormal) results.

BF and RASP are not necessarily testing the same binaural interactive function. BF is a spectral function, while RASP requires the integration of segments over time. RASP may tax the "holding system" on at least one side of the brain, if there is a reduced number of neurons or nonfunctioning neurons in the brainstem nuclei or pathways. BF would not be affected in the same way because it requires fusion of spectral information and depends far less on temporal integration. The message in the RASP may be transmitted in an all or none fashion. If it reaches the "holding system" and there is sufficient holding capability, the alteration rate does not seem to be important. However, the integrity of each side of the system transmitting the message is vital for adequate message reception.

The familiarity of the RASP sentences in their present form may affect the results. An SL of 40 dB in each channel relative to the Speech Reception Threshold (SRT) is recommended. Willeford's testing protocol requires two trials with the sentence material; the ear which receives the first 300 msec of each sentence determines the so-called "Lead Channel." The "Lead Channel" is assigned to one ear, and ten sentences are presented. Then the "Lead Channel" is switched to the opposite ear. Testing experience indicates that this procedure may be unnecessary. A binaural score may be a more accurate representation in that there is interaction between ears.

Interaural Intensity Difference (IID)

Pinheiro and Tobin (1969) used two sources for presentation of noise signals in a dichotic manner for the IID. (A single source for diotic presentation could have been used in order to have minimized trivial signal differences, although it is unlikely that the results would have changed appreciably.) The IID for white noise bursts and low-pass-filtered noise bursts for normal subjects was about 10 dB, similar to what Békésy (1959) found was required for lateralization of a 100 Hz signal on the skin. Two signal durations were used, 76 and 506 msec. The results for all three test groups (17 normal subjects, 17 with high-frequency sensorineural hearing loss, and 17 with predominantly unilateral cerebral disease or trauma) showed no appreciable effect due to the type of noise used or to the duration of the signal. The IID for the sensorineural group (which included subgroups of nine subjects showing complete recruitment, four with partial recruitment, and four with no recruitment) was essentially the same as that shown by normal subjects, i.e., 10 dB. No difference was noted for better ear or poorer ear in subjects with hearing losses. For those with central lesions the ear ipsilateral to the site of the lesion required a greater IID than that shown for normal subjects or sensorineural subjects. The ear contralateral to the site of lesion for those with central involvement required an IID of only about 4 dB for lateralization. This finding coincides with that obtained by Békésy (1967) for his skin warming experiment. It should be noted that intrasubject variability across trials was less than 1 dB, indicative of a highly reliable procedure.

To obtain the IID, a threshold for the noise bursts in each ear was established. A 20 dB SL was used for the respective ears, and subjective midline or centering was established. This sometimes required a slight change in intensity at one ear or the other to achieve equal loudness in order to produce the centering phenomenon. For some patients within the central group full lateralization occurred at equal SLs. From the subjective center point the signal was increased in 1 dB steps in one ear until lateralization occurred. Midline was then reestablished, and the other ear tested.

In their 1971 report Pinheiro and Tobin reported the testing of 40 neurologically involved patients using the IID procedure. Patients who exhibited abnormal IIDs showed neurologic signs of temporal and/or parietal lobe involvement. Patients with frontal lobe and occipital lobe lesions had normal IID scores. The critical processing for the IID probably does not take place at the cortical level. It is more likely that it is a brainstem response. However, the perception of the location of the sound is a cortical function (see Chapter 5).

Goldberg and Brown (1969) found that excitatory-inhibitory neural units in the dog's superior olivary complex were responsive to interaural intensity differences. Other studies have found this same responsiveness at the level of the inferior colliculus, medial geniculate, and dorsal nucleus of the lateral lemniscus (Møller, 1983). (See also Chapters 3 and 5.) Mediation for the IID probably takes place at either the superior olivary level or at the inferior colliculus level (Hall, 1965; Moushegian et al, 1975; Masterton et al, 1975; Kuwada et al, 1979). However, it may be the nature of the IID that interference at any level within the system produces abnormal lateralization.

While Pinheiro and Tobin (1969) studied lateralization effects, there have been many studies employing sound field localization. A comprehensive review of research on localization and lateralization is presented by Durlach et al (1981). In general, the localization procedure is cumbersome, requiring an array of speakers placed in sound field. For clinical purposes lateralization under earphones is more convenient and easily administered. For localization the sound source is subjectively located at some point outside the head (extracranial), while lateralization usually, although not always, is experienced inside the head (intracranial).

Among the earliest studies to show a contralateral effect for a localization task was the one by Sanchez-Longo and Forster (1958). The test was proposed as a clinical procedure for localizing lesions of the temporal cortex. In 19 of 21 cases of reported temporal lobe involvement localization was found to be impaired in the contralateral field. Interestingly, in three cases that received radiation therapy for temporal lobe tumors two patients reverted to normal localization and one showed marked improvement.

Masking Level Difference

There are many variations in the method of binaural presentation for the MLD. The most typical methods applied to the clinical population have been the homophasic and antiphasic modes described by Licklider (1948) and Hirsh (1948). Today these are usually designated by the symbols SoNo for the homophasic condition (in which both signal and noise are in-phase at both ears) and $S\pi No$ or $SoN\pi$ for the two antiphasic conditions (in which either the signal is 180° out-of-phase at the two ears and the noise in-phase at both ears, or, as in the latter symbol, the signal is held in-phase, and the noise is 180° out-of-phase at the two ears).

Since the Licklider and Hirsh studies in 1948, there have been many laboratory experiments and a number of clinical experiments on the MLD (see Durlach et al, 1981). However, there remain unanswered questions concerning its application to a clinical population.

Typically, spondaic words or a low frequency tone (usually 500 Hz) have been chosen as the testing vehicle (Stubblefield and Goldstein, 1977). Most often the speech reception threshold (SRT) is used to demonstrate unmasking. Lynn et al (1981) reported on the MLD as a diagnostic tool for neurologic disorders. In this study the MLD was obtained using recorded consonant-vowel syllables, and a speech detection threshold (SDT) was used for the response task rather than the SRT. The SDT is probably more comparable to the tonal response without some of its inherent limitations.

Quaranta et al (1978) recommended that the tonal MLD be used only with patients exhibiting thresholds within normal limits because of the potential for peripheral auditory problems affecting release from masking and confounding the central signs. Degree of sensorineural impairment and asymmetry of loss can be compensated for to some extent when using the MLD. However, in general, if an MLD can be obtained at all, it will be smaller than that obtained with normal listeners (Schoeny and Carhart, 1971; Quaranta and Cervellera, 1974; Olsen and Noffsinger, 1976; Pengelly et al, 1982).

Establishing levels at the two ears when there is hearing loss is not a trivial problem. Clinically it may be desirable to preevaluate some of these patients for binaural interaction integrity. Quaranta and Cervellera (1974) required a centering ability for their clinical subjects before proceeding with the MLD. If an individual could not place an image in the center of the head after intensities at the two ears were adjusted to permit such a balance, the subject was rejected for testing with the MLD. Centering ability demonstrates at least minimal interaural correlation and cross-correlation. It is rudimentary evidence of binaural interaction. If the two sides of the auditory system cannot communicate with each other at the most elementary level, it is highly questionable whether the results of an MLD should be interpreted with any clinical weight. As Langford and Jeffress (1964, p 1458) pointed out:

Interaural correlation for the noise masker is an important factor in determining the masking-level difference obtained under antiphasic conditions. Reducing the correlation produces a reduction in the MLD regardless of whether the reduction is obtained by adding random noise or by adding a time delay in one noise channel.

Another important variable in the administration of the MLD is in the selection of the suprathreshold level (Hirsh and Pollack, 1948; Feldmann, 1965). Townsend and Goldstein (1972), using 250 Hz and 500 Hz sinusoids, found that the antiphasic release from masking phenomenon of the MLD decreased in size as the SL for presentation of the signals was increased. The degree of binaural unmasking reported in the literature varies considerably (Durlach and Colburn, 1978). Townsend and Goldstein surmised that the presentation levels of the signals could account for much of this variability. The size of the MLD is affected by both the masking level chosen as well as the frequency of the tone. The 500 Hz signal appeared less variable than the 250 Hz signal, but its binaural advantage was very limited at 20 dB SL. The largest MLD, approximately 15 dB, was found at 250 Hz at 0 dB SL with a masker with a 55 dB spectrum level. Using a masker with a 40 dB spectrum level, 250 Hz produced an MLD of about 12 dB at 0 dB SL and 8 dB at 5 dB SL. Comparable findings existed for 500 Hz: 11 dB at 0 dB SL and 8 dB at 5 dB SL.

It is not known whether SDT or SRT are similarly affected by presentation level, but it is likely that the SDT is more stable across SLs than either the 250 or 500 Hz sinusoids. However, as a general rule until these factors can be further studied, MLD administration using SDT should be as close to 0 dB SL as possible, i.e., 5 dB SL for 250 Hz or 500 Hz, and probably no more than 10 dB SL for the SDT. It is not clear what SL should be used when the SRT is selected as the testing vehicle.

A review of the MLD literature gives the impression that there is something special about the low frequency signal for release from masking (Flanagan and Watson, 1966; Durlach and Colburn, 1978). As Mosko and House (1971) found, maximum release from masking does occur for 250 and 500 Hz when these signals are presented as discrete frequencies. However, for vocalic signals unmasking may not be a function of the fundamental frequency but rather may be related to the spectral component that has the highest amplitude. For uniformity of signal for SDT and SRT tests, it may prove desirable to select syllables or spondaic words in which the fundamental frequency represents the highest amplitude component.

Consideration also needs to be given to the type of masker used as the foil for the MLD signals. Pengelly et al (1982) found no difference for a broadband or narrow band masker for normal subjects, but for a high frequency hearing-impaired group narrow band noise produced significantly larger MLDs for the 500 Hz signal. For further discussion of narrow band masking, see Metz et al (1968) and Durlach and Colburn (1978). This same effect might be found with the SDT, if speech-modulated white noise were used as the masker.

The size of the MLD also seems to be dependent on the duration of the masker (Green, 1966; McFadden, 1966). A continuous masker tends to produce a greater MLD. Maskers that are gated to follow the duty cycle of the signal produce smaller

MLDs. The size of the MLD is not really the issue, as long as the MLD is not so small as to make the test insensitive to phase changes. The real issue is how much one wants to tax the neurologically impaired system and what signal masker configuration would be most sensitive for the target population. When the target population for the MLD is neurologically impaired, even apparent minor psychophysical factors may lead to equivocal results.

A further question that needs to be explored is whether the SRT or any other material requiring speech intelligibility function should be used. As Carhart (1967) pointed out, a large change in a speech intelligibility score is not necessarily indicative of a large change in central masking. Olsen and Noffsinger (1976), however, concluded that the MLD using speech, i.e., SRT, is more sensitive to central auditory problems than 500 Hz signals. The SDT may be the better compromise. If the MLD is the result of binaural interaction at the level of the superior olivary complex (Cranford et al, 1978), the additional redundancy of meaningful material might obscure a problem of lower brainstem processing.

According to Stubblefield and Goldstein (1977), the MLD procedure employing the SRT for spondaic words and/or the 500 Hz tone is a highly reliable test. This is probably true for sentence material as well as the SDT, consonant rhyme test, vowel rhyme test, and other types of materials (Goldstein and Stephens, 1975; Bocca and Antonelli, 1976; Henning and Gaskell, 1981).

Almost all clinical applications of the MLD have used SoNo as reference, with $S\pi$No and/or SoNπ as indicative of release from masking. The Pengelly et al (1982) study found that $S\pi$No provided greater release from masking than the SoNπ condition. Olsen et al (1976) confirmed this relationship for 50 normal subjects and eight groups of variously impaired patients for both spondees and the 500 Hz signal.

The Lynn et al (1981) study is the only well-documented analysis currently available that reports the MLD responses for individuals with brainstem involvement. MLD was determined with the SDT by the $S\pi$No and SoNπ procedures. All subjects showed normal audiograms and less than 15 dB interaural differences. Ten subjects were

normal; 12 had cerebral lesions; 5 had upper pontine, midbrain or thalamic lesions; and 9 had pontomedullary lesions. Pathologies were confirmed by some combination of neurologic, roentgenographic, and/or surgical examination and by brainstem evoked response audiometry. The nine patients with lower brainstem involvement showed no release from masking or very limited release from masking for both $S\pi$No and SoNπ conditions (Fig. 10.3). The findings for the other patients were not unlike those exhibited by the control group. Although their scores were within normal limits, some subjects in the upper pontine, midbrain, and thalamic group showed a tendency toward limited release from masking. The 80 dB SPL white noise level seemed unnecessarily high, even though it did not seem to affect MLD responses.

In another recent study Noffsinger and colleagues (1982) demonstrated an interesting relationship between MLD and ABR in patients with brainstem lesions. It appeared that subjects with ABR abnormalities in waves I, II, or III yielded small or no MLDs. Conversely, patients with ABR abnormali-

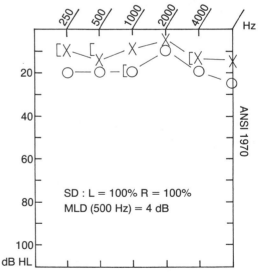

Figure 10.3. A 40-yr-old female with multiple sclerosis and essentially normal hearing bilaterally and excellent speech discrimination ability yielded an abnormal 500 Hz MLD (4 dB). This masking level difference indicates probable low brainstem dysfunction consistent with the diagnosis of multiple sclerosis. This MLD was achieved in comparing the SoNo and $S\pi$No listening conditions.

ties which commenced with waves IV or V yielded normal MLDs.

DISCUSSION

Special Cases

In a recent study in which BF and RASP were given to patients with brainstem lesions, the overall results led to the conclusion that the procedures lacked sensitivity (Musiek and Geurkink, 1982). However, in some individual cases RASP or BF tests were strikingly abnormal. For example, one woman who suffered a left pontine contusion yielded a score of only 5% on the RASP (Table 10.1). There may be another way of looking at these tasks in relation to brainstem lesions. It may be that brainstem pathology will not reveal abnormal results for every signal-processing mode. The MLD seems to be exploring cross-correlational intensity timing effects, whereas the IID explores cross-correlational intensity effects.

Table 10.1.
Normal and Abnormal Results on RASP and Binaural Fusion (BF) Tests in Patients with Brainstem Lesions[a]

Subject	Diagnosis	RASP	BF	Side of lesion
1	Brainstem contusion	X	—	?
2	Right brainstem tumor (extraaxial)	—	X	R
3	Left brainstem tumor (extraaxial)	X	X	L
4	Demyelinating disease	X	—	?
5	Right brainstem tumor (extraaxial)	—	—	R
6	Left upper pons mini-stroke	X	X	L
7	Demyelinating disease	—	—	?
8	Left brainstem contusion	X	—	L
9	Demyelinating disease	—	—	?
10	Demyelinating disease	—	—	?

[a] X, abnormal results; —, normal results. Results of the RASP and BF tests for ten subjects with brainstem lesions. The tests (Willeford, 1977) were administered at 50 dB SL (re:SRT). All lesions were neurologically or neurosurgically diagnosed. Abnormal results were based upon the normative data published by Musiek and Guerkink, 1981. (Modifed from Musiek FE: the evaluation of brainstem disorders using ABR and central auditory tests. *Monogr Contemp Audiol*, vol 4, no 2, 1983.)

BF is tapping spectral fusion ability, while the RASP relies on the integration over time of a signal message. It should not be expected that a brainstem lesion will lead to a decrement in all modes of operation except in the most severe of cases.

Recently it has become apparent that some of these central auditory tests may be sensitive to physiologic changes over time. The author has had four patients with facial paresthesia. One was a woman in her early 60s, two were women in their early 20s and one was a boy of 15. Chief complaint was a feeling of tingling from the top of the head down along the side of the face. In the older woman's case the sensation lasted a few months, while for the other three, it disappeared in less than 2 months. In the case of the boy it was related to a diving accident in which he hit the top of his head. A precipitating cause could not be established for the other three. Neurologic examination was unremarkable. The IID was administered at various intervals several times to each of these individuals. In all cases the initial IID was abnormally small. Over time the IID increased, and by the time the tingling sensation stopped the IID had returned to normal limits. These findings are not unlike those reported by Sanchez-Longo and Forster (1958).

James McDonald, of the Hearing and Speech Clinic of Johns Hopkins University, reported an interesting case in which the IID was helpful in localizing a lesion (JM McDonald, personal communication, 1983). This was the case of a 41-yr-old white female with a 3-yr onset of right facial paresthesia. A battery of special audiometric tests was performed. Tone decay, PI/PB function, MLD, BF, RASP, low-pass filtered speech, and SSW were all negative. Brainstem-evoked response was absent only at low intensity level. Pitch pattern recognition was very poor on both ears. IID was positive on the right (4 dB) and negative on the left (10 dB). The CAT scan revealed a right inferior colliculus intraaxial lesion. The diagnosis was multiple sclerosis.

Procedural Essentials

In order to be clinically useful central auditory evaluation procedures need to be easily administered, require little time, and make use of available equipment with very little expense for additional devices. Minimally a two-channel audiometer is necessary for administration of the noncongruent brainstem tasks. Most of the more complete diagnostic audiometers are capable of simultaneous presentation of both channels. The IID requires nothing more than this type of audiometer. BF and RASP require specially prepared tapes and a two channel recorder whose presentation levels can be controlled through the audiometer. In using BF tapes it is very important to check the intensity level of each channel. Some available tapes do not have good acoustic control of the intensity of the stimuli in each channel (Plakke et al, 1981). The MLD requires a special phase-controlling device. Some newer audiometers have this capability built in. If not, an easily installed add-on device is available.

The clinician is advised to obtain his own normative data for all tests that have not been standardized or have shown variability from laboratory to laboratory. This is particularly true for such recorded materials as the BF and RASP. The quality of the tape recording, the functioning of the recorder including head alignment, and the relative speed of the recording compared to the speed of the playback unit will contribute to variations in performance from one test facility to another. The maintenance of the equipment and the deterioration of the tape over time also can affect performance so that there must be periodic recalibration and reestablishment of norms.

At this stage in the development of tests to determine brainstem integrity, the clinician should be encouraged toward applications suggested by the experimental literature. However, the ultimate configurations for these tests should be determined by clinical trial. Each of the four tests discussed contributes information toward an understanding of brainstem function, but none is so far developed and refined that it does not warrant further investigation and possible modification.

It is not merely the manipulation of signal difficulty that will determine the usefulness of a procedure for assessment of central auditory function. There are two types of sensitivity, i.e, one to the test and the other related to the type of lesion. There is a need to study systematically signal-processing capabilities and their relationship to site of lesion with these tests or better tests. The growing neurophysiological literature is providing insights into the types of signal processing that take place at the various levels of the brainstem (See Chapter 3). Psychophysical test design and the clinical manner of test delivery must be improved. A test battery should be based on well-defined psychoacoustic parameters as well as on knowledge of expected psychophysical performance at the various levels of the brainstem.

References

Arnst D, Katz J (eds): *Central Auditory Assessment: The SSW Test, Development and Clinical Use.* San Diego, College Hill Press 1982.

Baru AV, Karaseva TA: *The Brain and Hearing: Hearing Disturbances Associated with Local Brain Lesions.* New York, Consultants Bureau, 1972.

Békésy von G: Neural funneling along the skin and between the inner and outer hair cells of the cochlea. *J Acoust Soc Am* 31:1236–1249, 1959.

Békésy von G: *Experiments in Hearing.* New York, McGraw-Hill, 1960.

Békésy von G: *Sensory Inhibition.* Princeton, NJ, Princeton Univ Press, 1967, pp 35–90.

Bocca E, Antonelli AR: Masking level difference: another tool for the evaluation of peripheral and cortical defects. *Audiology* 15:480–487, 1976.

Bocca E, Calearo C: Central hearing processes. In Jerger J (eds): *Modern Developments in Audiology.* New York, Academic Press, 1963, ch 4, pp 337–370.

Boring EG: *Sensation and Perception in the History of Experimental Psychology.* New York, Appleton-Century-Crofts, 1942, pp 381–398.

Broadbent DE, Ladefoged P: On the fusion of sounds reaching different sense organs. *J Acoust Soc Am* 29:708–710, 1957.

Carhart R: Binaural reception of meaningful material. In Graham B (ed): *Sensorineural Hearing Processes and Disorders.* Boston, Little, Brown, 1967, pp 153–175.

Cherry EC: Some experiments on the recognition of speech with one and with two ears. *J Acoust Soc Am* 25:975–979, 1953.

Cherry EC: Two ears—but one world. In Rosenblith WA (ed): *Sensory Communication.* Cambridge, MA, MIT Press, 1961, pp 99–117.

Cherry EC, Taylor WK: Some further experiments upon the recognition of speech, with one and with two ears. *J Acoust Soc Am* 26:554–559, 1954.

Colburn HS, Durlach NI: Models of binaural interaction. In Carterette EC, Friedman MP (eds): *Handbook of Perception.* New York, Academic Press, 1978, vol IV, ch 11, pp 467–518.

Cranford JL, Stramler J, Igarashi M: Role of neocortex in binaural hearing in the cat. III. Binaural masking-level differences. *Brain Res* 151:381–385, 1978.

Deatherage BH: Examination of binaural interaction. *J Acoust Soc Am* 39:232–249, 1966.

Dudley HW, Gruenz OO Jr: Visible speech translators

with external phosphors. *J Acoust Soc Am* 17:62–73, 1946.

Durlach NI, Colburn HS: Binaural phenomena. In Carterette EC, Friedman MP (eds): *Handbook of Perception.* New York, Academic Press, 1978, vol IV, ch 10, pp 365–466.

Durlach NI, Thompson CL, Colburn HS: Binaural interaction in impaired listeners: a review of past research. *Audiology* 20:181–211, 1981.

Feldmann H: Experiments on binaural hearing in noise: the central nervous processing of acoustic information. *Trans. Beltone Inst. Hear Res* 18:1–42, 1965.

Flanagan JL, Watson BJ: Binaural unmasking of complex signals. *J Acoust Soc Am* 40:456–468, 1966.

Fletcher H: *Speech and Hearing in Communication.* New York, D. Van Nostrand Company, 1953, p 216.

French NR, Steinberg JC: Factors governing the intelligibility of speech sounds. *J Acoust Soc Am* 19:90–119, 1947.

Goldberg JM, Brown PB: Responses of binaural neurons of dog superior olivary complex to dichotic tonal stimuli: some physiological mechanisms of sound localization. *J Neurophysiol* 32:613–636, 1969.

Goldstein DP, Stephens SDG: Masking level difference: a measure of auditory processing capability. *Audiology* 14:354–367, 1975.

Green DM: Interaural phase effects in the masking of signals of different durations. *J Acoust Soc Am* 39:720–724, 1966.

Green DM, Swets JA: *Signal Detection Theory and Psychophysics.* New York, Wiley, 1966.

Hall JL II: Binaural interaction in the accessory superior-olivary nucleus of the cat. *J Acoust Soc Am* 37:814–823, 1965.

Hayashi R, Ohta F, Morimoto M: Binaural fusion test: a diagnostic approach to central auditory disorders. *Int Audiol* 5:133–135, 1966.

Hennebert D: L'integration de la perception auditive et l'audition alternante. *Acta Otorhinolaryngol Belg* 9:344–346, 1955.

Henning GB, Gaskell H: Binaural masking level differences with a variety of waveforms. *Hearing Res* 4:175–184, 1981.

Hirsh IJ: The influence of interaural phase on interaural summation and inhibition. *J Acoust Soc Am* 20:536–544, 1948.

Hirsh IJ, Pollack I: The role of interaural phase in loudness. *J Acoust Soc Am* 20:761–766, 1948.

Horii Y, House AS, Hughes GW: A masking noise with speech-envelope characteristics for studying intelligibility. *J Acoust Soc Am* 49:1849–1856, 1971.

House AS, Williams CE, Hecker MHL, Kryter KD: Articulation testing methods: consonantal differentiation with a closed-response set. *J Acoust Soc Am* 37:158–166, 1965.

Imig TJ, Adrián HO: Binaural columns in the primary field (AI) of cat auditory cortex. *Brain Res* 138:241–257, 1977.

Ivey RG: Tests of CNS Auditory Function. Masters thesis, Colorado State University, Fort Collins, CO, 1969.

Joos M: Acoustic phonetics. *Language (Monograph no. 23),* 24(suppl):66–67, 1948.

Jurine L: Extrait des experiences de jurine sur les chauves-souris qu'on a prive de la vue. *J Physiol* 46:145–148, 1798.

Kimura D: Functional asymmetry of the brain in dichotic listening. *Cortex* 3:163–178, 1967.

Koenig W, Dunn HK, Lacy LY: The sound spectrograph. *J Acoust Soc Am* 17:19–49, 1946.

Kopp GA, Green HC: Basic phonetic principles of visible speech. *J Acoust Soc Am* 17:74–89, 1946.

Kreul EJ, Nixon JC, Kryter KD, Bell DW, Lang JS, Schubert ED: A proposed clinical test of speech discrimination. *J Speech Hear Res* 11:536–552, 1968.

Kryter KD: Validation of the articulation index. *J Acoust Soc Am* 34:1698–1702, 1962.

Kryter KD, Whitman EC: Some comparisons between rhyme and PB-word intelligibility tests. *J Acoust Soc Am* 37:1146, 1965.

Kuwada S, Yin TCT, Wickesberg RE: Response of cat inferior colliculus neurons to binaural beat stimuli: possible mechanisms for sound localization. *Science* 206:586–588, 1979.

Langford TL, Jeffress LA: Effect of noise correlation on binaural signal detection. *J Acoust Soc Am* 36:1455–1458, 1964.

Licklider JCR: The influence of interaural phase relations upon the masking of speech by white noise. *J Acoust Soc Am* 20:150–159, 1948.

Licklider JCR: Three auditory theories. In Koch S (ed): *Psychology: The Study of a Science.* New York, McGraw-Hill, 1959, vol 1, pp 41–144.

Lindén A: Distorted speech and binaural speech resynthesis tests. *Acta Otolaryngol (Stockh)* 58:32–48, 1964.

Lynn GE, Gilroy J: Effects of brain lesions on the perception of monotic and dichotic speech stimuli. In Sullivan MD (ed): *Central Auditory Processing Disorders.* Proceedings of a Conference at the University of Nebraska Medical Center, Omaha, 1975, pp 47–83.

Lynn GE, Gilroy J: Evaluation of central auditory dysfunction in patients with neurological disorders. In Keith RW (ed): *Central Auditory Dysfunction.* New York, Grune & Stratton, 1977, pp 177–221.

Lynn GE, Gilroy J, Taylor PC, Leiser RP: Binaural masking-level differences in neurological disorders. *Arch Otolaryngol* 107:357–362, 1981.

MacKeith NW, Coles RRA: Binaural advantages in hearing of speech. *J Laryngol Otol* 85:213–232, 1971.

Masterton B, Thompson GC, Bechtold JK, Robards MJ: Neuroanatomical basis of binaural phase-difference analysis for sound localization: a comparative study. *J Comp Physiol Psychol* 89:379–386, 1975.

Matzker J: Two methods for the assessment of central auditory functions in cases of brain disease. *Ann Otol Rhinol Laryngol* 68:1155–1197, 1959.

McFadden D: Masking-level differences with continuous and with burst masking noise. *J Acoust Soc Am* 40:1414–1419, 1966.

Metz PJ, von Bismark G, Durlach NI: Further results on binaural unmasking and the EC model. II. Noise bandwidth and interaural phase. *J Acoust Soc Am* 43:1085–1091, 1968.

Middlebrooks JC, Dykes RW, Merzenich MM: Binaural response-specific bands in primary auditory cortex (AI) of the cat: topographical organization orthogonal to isofrequency contours. *Brain Res* 181:31–48, 1980.

Mills AW: Auditory localization. In Tobias JV (ed): *Foundations of Modern Auditory Theory.* New York,

Academic Press, 1972, vol 2, ch 8, pp 303–348.

Møller AR: *Auditory Physiology.* New York, Academic Press, 1983, pp 251–299.

Moray N: Attention in dichotic listening: affective cues and the influence of instructions. *Q J Exp Psychol* 11:56–60, 1959.

Mosko JD, House AS: Binaural unmasking of vocalic signals. *J Acoust Soc Am* 49:1203–1212, 1971.

Moushegian G, Jeffress LA: Role of interaural time and intensity differences in the lateralization of low-frequency tones. *J Acoust Soc Am* 31:1441–1445, 1959.

Moushegian G, Rupert AL, Gidda JS: Functional characteristics of superior olivary neurons to binaural stimuli. *J Neurophysiol* 38:1037–1048, 1975.

Musiek FE: The evaluation of brainstem disorders using ABR and central auditory tests. *Monogr Contemp Audiol,* vol 4, no 2, 1983.

Musiek FE, Geurkink NA: Auditory brain stem response and central auditory test findings for patients with brain stem lesions: a preliminary report. *Laryngoscope* 92:891–900, 1982.

Neff WD, Diamond IT: The neural basis of auditory discrimination. In Harlow HF, Woolsey CN (eds): *Biological and Biochemical Bases of Behavior.* Madison, WI, University of Wisconsin Press, 1958, pp 101–126.

Noffsinger D, Martinez C, Schaefer A: Auditory brainstem responses and masking level differences from person with brainstem lesion. *Scand Audiol,* suppl 15, 1982.

Ohta F, Hayashi R, Morimoto M: Differential diagnosis of retrocochlear deafness: binaural fusion test and binaural separation test. *Int Audiol* 6:58–62, 1967.

Olsen WO, Noffsinger D: Masking level differences for cochlear and brain stem lesions. *Ann Otol* 85:820–825, 1976.

Olsen WO, Noffsinger D, Carhart R: Masking level differences encountered in clinical populations. *Audiology* 15:287–301, 1976.

Palva A: Filtered speech audiometry: basic studies with Finnish speech towards the creation of a method for the diagnosis of central hearing disorders. *Acta Otolaryngol [Suppl] (Stockh)* 210, 1965.

Pengelly M, Mueller HG, Hill B: Masking Level Difference: Effects of High Frequency Hearing Loss and Masking Stimuli. Presentation at the Convention of the American Speech-Language-Hearing Association, Toronto, Canada, 1982.

Pinheiro ML: The Interaural Intensity Difference for Intracranial Lateralization of White Noise Bursts. Ph.D. dissertation, Case Western Reserve Univ, Cleveland, 1969.

Pinheiro ML: Tests of central auditory function in children with learning disabilities. In Keith RW (ed): *Central Auditory Dysfunction.* New York, Grune & Stratton, 1977, pp 223–256.

Pinheiro ML: A central auditory test profile of learning-disabled children with dyslexia. *Communicative Disorders: An Audio Journal for Continuing Education.* New York, Grune & Stratton, 1978.

Pinheiro ML, Tobin H: Interaural intensity difference for intracranial lateralization. *J Acoust Soc Am* 46:1482–1487, 1969.

Pinheiro ML, Tobin H: The interaural intensity difference as a diagnostic indicator. *Acta Otolaryngol (Stockh)* 71:326–328, 1971.

Pinheiro ML, Jacobson GP, Boller F: Auditory dysfunction following a gunshot wound of the pons. *J Speech Hear Disord* 47:296–300, 1982.

Plakke B, Orchik D, Beasley D: Children's performance on a binaural fusion task. *J Speech Hear Res* 24:520–525, 1981.

Potter RK: Introduction to technical discussions of sound portrayal. *J Acoust Soc Am* 17:1–3, 1946.

Potter RK, Kopp GA, Green HC: *Visible Speech.* New York, D. Van Nostrand, 1947.

Quaranta A, Cassano P, Cervellera G: Clinical value of the tonal masking level difference. *Audiology* 17:232–238, 1978.

Quaranta A, Cervellera G: Masking level difference in normal and pathological ears. *Audiology* 13:428–431, 1974.

Reynolds GS, Stevens SS: Binaural summation of loudness. *J Acoust Soc Am* 32:1337–1344, 1960.

Riesz RR, Schott L: Visible speech cathode-ray translator. *J Acoust Soc Am* 17:50–61, 1946.

Roush J, Tait CA: Binaural fusion, masking level differences, and auditory brain stem responses in children with language-learning disabilities. *Ear Hear* 5:37–41, 1984.

Sanchez-Longo L, Forster FM: Clinical significance of impairment of sound localization. *Neurology* 8:119–125, 1958.

Sayers B McA, Cherry EC: Mechanism of binaural fusion in the hearing of speech. *J Acoust Soc Am* 29:973–987, 1957.

Schoeny ZG, Carhart R: Effects of unilateral Ménière's disease on masking-level differences. *J Acoust Soc Am* 50:1143–1150, 1971.

Shannon CE, Weaver W: *The Mathematical Theory of Communication.* Urbana, IL, Univ of Illinois Press, 1949, p 15.

Smith BB, Resnick DM: An auditory test for assessing brain stem integrity: preliminary report. *Laryngoscope* 82:414–424, 1972.

Speaks C, Jerger J: Method for measurement of speech identification. *J Speech Hearing Res* 8:185–194, 1965.

Steinberg JC, French NR: The portrayal of visible speech. *J Acoust Soc Am* 17:4–18, 1946.

Stubblefield JH, Goldstein DP: A test-retest reliability study on clinical measurement of masking level differences. *Audiology* 16:419–431, 1977.

Tobias JV, Zerlin S: Lateralization threshold as a function of stimulus duration. *J Acoust Soc Am* 31:1591–1594, 1959.

Townsend TH, Goldstein DP: Supra-threshold binaural unmasking. *J Acoust Soc Am* 51:621–624, 1972.

Venturi JB: Considerations sur la connaissance de l'etendue que nous donne le sens de l'ouie. *Ma Encycl J Lett Arts* (later title, *Ann Encycl*), 3:29–37, 1796.

Willeford JA: Central auditory function in children with learning disabilities. *Audiol Hearing Educ* 2:12–20, 1976.

Willeford JA: Assessing central auditory behavior in children: a test battery approach. In Keith RW (ed): *Central Auditory Dysfunction.* New York, Grune & Stratton, 1977, pp 43–72.

Woodworth RS: *Experimental Psychology.* New York, Henry Holt and Company, 1938, pp 501–538.

CHAPTER 11

Monaural Speech Tests in the Detection of Central Auditory Disorders

WILLIAM F. RINTELMANN, PH.D.

Dr. Rintelmann's chapter presents thorough explanations of monaural undistorted and low redundancy degraded speech tests and competing message tasks. Applications of these tests to central auditory patients, especially when peripheral hearing disorders and aging factors are involved, is discussed. He illustrates his chapter with case examples.

INTRODUCTION

Assessment of both the locus and extent of pathology within the middle ear and cochlea has been a relatively straightforward and routine procedure for many years. A more challenging task for the audiologist and the otolaryngologist is to distinguish between a cochlear and a retrocochlear lesion. Here too, however, major strides in assessment and diagnosis have been made in recent years, especially since the measurement of brainstem auditory evoked potentials has become a fairly common clinical technique. Progress in the development of tasks for assessing the integrity of the central auditory nervous system (CANS) has not kept pace with the advancements made in identifying and quantifying lesions of the peripheral auditory system. Serious clinical research efforts began 3 decades ago with the classic studies of the Italian investigators (Bocca et al., 1954, 1955). Primarily three reasons account for this slow progress: (1) the dearth of precisely documented CANS lesions in patients tested by audiologists; (2) the lack of sensitivity of conventional auditory test signals for identifying CANS lesions; and (3) most importantly, the resistance of the CANS to exhibit disruption on auditory tasks due to the anatomic and physiologic complexity of the central auditory pathways.

Clinical case reports on hemispherectomized patients provide a dramatic illustration of the difficulty in assessing CANS lesions. Pure tone thresholds and speech recognition (discrimination) scores obtained on such patients with high fidelity monosyllables can be essentially normal in both ears (Goldstein et al, 1956; Goldstein, 1961; Hodgson, 1967). As a consequence, the task of assessing lesions in the central auditory pathways requires that auditory tests be made sufficiently difficult to overcome the combined effects of redundancy of both the auditory system and the acoustic signal. The intrinsic CANS redundancy stems from the bilateral representation of each ear to each side of the brain via the system's multiple network of pathways and crossings, nuclear centers, intertract and interhemispheric connections, and projections to primary and secondary cortical areas. This highly complex system results in multiple mapping or processing of auditory information within the brain. (Refer to detailed description in Chapters 2 and 5.) In addition, auditory signals contain varying degrees of extrinsic redundancy. Both tonal stimuli (e.g., pure tones) and high fidelity speech signals (whether single words or connected discourse) are so redundant that the central auditory system is not taxed in persons with normal peripheral auditory systems. Bocca and his colleagues recognized this problem (Bocca et al, 1954, 1955), and they theorized that disorders of the central auditory system could be detected if the redundancy of speech stimuli was reduced by distorting (degrading) the acoustic properties of the speech test material. They used low-pass filtered, phonetically balanced words and found that word recognition performance by patients with verified lesions of the auditory cortex was reduced substantially in the contralateral compared to the ipsilateral ear. Subsequently, in addition to low-pass filtering, clinical researchers have experimented with reducing speech stimuli redundancy by degrading it in a variety of ways, e.g., periodic interruption, acceleration, or presentation at low sensation levels (Bocca, 1958; Calearo and Lazzaroni, 1957; Matzker, 1959; de Quiros, 1964).

A basic consideration in the construction of auditory tasks using speech stimuli for assessing the integrity of the CANS is the use of several different modes of signal presentation. The signal(s) may be presented in either monaural or binaural listening tasks. Further, under binaural listening conditions, the identical stimuli can be presented simultaneously to both ears (diotic) or a different segment of the message, or different messages, can be delivered to each ear (dichotic). The various types of binaural listening tasks and their applications are described in Chapters 10 and 12.

The principal focus of this chapter concerns the application of monaural central auditory tests to an adult patient population. A detailed discussion concerning the detection and evaluation of central auditory disorders in children is presented by Willeford in Chapter 14. Nevertheless, for the sake of completeness of the present chapter, the discussion of most degraded speech tests includes some mention of the use of such measures with children.

Before beginning a discussion of the various monaural tests, the reader should be alerted to or reminded of certain problems and cautions regarding the use of central auditory tests in general. First, there is the problem mentioned earlier of obtaining auditory test results on patients with *well-documented lesions of the CANS*. While the number of such published reports on adult

patients is limited, similar reports on children are essentially nonexistent. The only literature devoted to this topic in children is focused on efforts to identify and evaluate central auditory processing dysfunction in children typically labeled as "learning-disabled." The rationale for such studies is based on a rather large assumption, namely that auditory perceptual processing disorders in children typically result from "minimal brain dysfunction," which may be attributed to pathology of the central auditory nervous system. The reader should recognize that this method of clinical investigation simply cannot provide anatomical or direct physiological verification of CANS pathology. In commenting on this issue Rintelmann and Lynn (1983) nevertheless acknowledged that:

. . . keeping this limitation in mind, carefully designed and executed clinical studies showing the relationship between performance on a battery of central auditory tests (properly normalized on children) and specific types of learning disabilities should contribute to our understanding of central auditory dysfunction in children (p. 252).

Another critical issue is the importance of having *appropriate normative data* prior to using any testing instrument for clinical assessment of auditory function in children or adults. Obviously, there are numerous variables that can affect the test scores, such as differences in: (1) specific speech material (e.g., syllables, words, sentences); (2) acoustic properties of the talkers' speech; (3) test administration procedures; (4) subject response methods (e.g., open vs closed message sets); (5) scoring methods (e.g., correct-incorrect vs phonemic analysis); and (6) the variables inherent in the specific acoustic test signal used. In the case of degraded speech, the recorded high fidelity signal can be distorted in varying amounts, depending on the method of distortion. This will be considered further later in this chapter as the various degraded speech tests are discussed.

A further serious criticism of much of the literature related to "norms" is that frequently the findings on central auditory tests are reported as abnormal without documenting what constitutes the range of normal behavior on such auditory measures. An equally serious criticism of such clinical investigations is that sometimes normative values are simply stated without giving the reader any information about how the norms were obtained. Moreover, some reports do not even provide a reference(s) to permit the interested reader to ascertain to what age levels such tests should be applied and how they should be properly administered and interpreted. When reading the literature on the application of central auditory tests to both children and adults, the above criticisms and cautions should be kept in mind.

Since the topic of this chapter concerns monaural speech tests, the remainder of this chapter is devoted to a discussion of several types of such measures that have been or currently are used for assessment of the integrity of the CANS. The reader should recognize, however, that while the focus of this chapter is entirely on monaural speech tasks, CANS test batteries typically consist of several different monaural and binaural listening tasks. Moreover, most tasks are comprised primarily of speech stimuli, but some psychoacoustic (behavioral) nonspeech measures (e.g., pure tone masking level difference task, pitch pattern test), plus certain electroacoustic (e.g., acoustic reflex thresholds) and electrophysiologic (e.g., auditory evoked potentials) measures are used also. Each of these measurement methods and their applications to CANS assessment is discussed within this text.

In the interest of historical perspective and in order to emphasize the relative merits of distorted speech over high fidelity speech tests for the assessment of CANS lesions, the application of both of these types of speech signals to monaural listening tasks will be discussed. This chapter is not intended to provide a "step-by-step cook book approach" to test administration procedures. Instead, the goals of this chapter are to present brief descriptions of several monaural speech tests with greater emphasis on those commonly employed, describe the important stimulus parameters of certain tests, and present generalizations concerning test result interpretation. Normative data, when available, are discussed, and the importance of adequate normative data is stressed. Illus-

trative findings from the literature are presented for each of the tests discussed. Also, problems encountered in attempting to identify central auditory disorders in patients with peripheral hearing loss are considered. In the final section of this chapter special attention is devoted to tests for assessing the "central component" of hearing impairment in geriatric patients. Throughout the chapter generalizations are offered concerning the utility of various tests for assessing central auditory disorders based upon our own experiences with certain measures along with findings reported in the literature.

First, high fidelity (undistorted) speech tests will be discussed briefly followed by a more detailed description of several types of distorted speech tasks. The acoustic features of speech that are important to perceptual processing are the temporal, intensity, and frequency parameters of speech stimuli. By definition, for high fidelity or undistorted speech signals none of these three important features are modified in recorded versions of tests; however, the intensity parameter typically is manipulated in decibel sensation level (SL) units, either above the speech reception threshold or above the threshold for a 1000 Hz tone according to the specific test procedure.

UNDISTORTED SPEECH

Conventional measures of speech recognition (discrimination) ability administered in quiet have received limited use in the evaluation of patients suspected of having CANS disorders. Such tests may be administered at a single high or low sensation level or both, or at several sensation levels.

Word Recognition at High and Low Sensation Levels

Findings from undistorted word recognition tests obtained at high (e.g., 40 dB) and/or low sensation levels (e.g., 5 dB) with phonetically balanced words have proven to be of limited value in the detection of central auditory disorders. In a few small sample studies patients with either brainstem or cortical lesions have shown reduced scores on the contralateral compared to the ipsilateral ear for both high and low sensation level test conditions. In general, however, such patients typically achieve normal scores bilaterally on this type of test (Jerger, 1960a and b, 1964; Korsan-Bengtsen, 1973; Lynn and Gilroy, 1972, 1977; Noffsinger and Kurdziel, 1979).

Performance-Intensity Functions

Word recognition scores can be obtained with high fidelity phonetically balanced (PB) words or other types of monosyllables at several sensation levels (SL), ranging from low (e.g., 5 dB SL) to high (e.g., 80 dB SL). With such data a performance-intensity (PI) function can be plotted which graphically displays the listener's change in word recognition over a broad intensity range. Prior to the late 1960s data plotted in this fashion were termed articulation or intelligibility functions. Jerger et al (1968) suggested that performance-intensity functions obtained with PB words (PI-PB) under quiet listening conditions could prove useful in the identification of retrocochlear lesions. Shortly thereafter, in the early 1970s, it was recommended that PI-PB functions be used both as a screening test and as a measure for assessing the extent of a central auditory disorder (Jerger and Jerger, 1971; Jerger, 1973); however, this measure of auditory function has proven more sensitive for detecting nerve VIII lesions than for assessing CANS disorders (Jerger J and Jerger S, 1975).

The PI-PB functions of patients with eighth nerve lesions frequently exhibit a *rollover phenomenon*, that is, successively improved scores (in percent correct) as sensation level is increased until a maximum score (PB Max) is reached, followed by progressively poorer scores (PB Min) at still higher sensation or intensity levels (to a maximum of 110 dB sound pressure level). The amount or magnitude of "rollover" (PB Max-PB Min) considered positive, that is, indicative of a retrocochlear lesion, varies, depending upon the specific word recognition test used. Variables, such as word list difficulty and talker differences, must be considered when deciding how much rollover constitutes a positive result. Hence, normative data must be established for the

specific recorded version of the test to be employed.

A refinement of the rollover computation method was suggested by Jerger and Jerger (1971) based on the observation that the magnitude of rollover may be influenced by the patient's maximum word recognition score, especially in cases of low maximum scores. To correct for this "bias effect" they suggested normalizing the rollover value for each patient by calculating a ratio, that is, by dividing the magnitude of the rollover by the maximum recognition score. This value has been termed the rollover index (RI) ratio and is expressed by the formula:

$$RI = \frac{PB\ Max - PB\ Min}{PB\ Max}$$

The absolute value of the rollover index is also susceptible to all of the variables that affect word recognition test difficulty. To illustrate, Jerger and Jerger (1971) and Dirks et al (1977) used recorded versions of the Harvard Psychoacoustic Laboratory (PAL) PB-50 word lists (Egan, 1948) and found that a rollover index ratio of 0.45 separated retrocochlear from cochlear lesions. Bess (1983), however, used a recorded version of Northwestern University Auditory Test Number 6 (NU-6) (Tillman and Carhart, 1966) and reported that retrocochlear lesions could be distinguished from cochlear lesions using a rollover index cutoff of 0.25. Hence, it is evident that adequate normative data must be obtained on any recorded word recognition test prior to using the test with clinical patients. For further discussion of the application of performance-intensity functions, rollover and rollover index ratios refer to Olsen and Matkin (1979) and Bess (1983) among other sources.

In summary of PI-PB functions, the presence of "rollover" has been observed frequently on the ipsilateral ear of patients with eighth nerve lesions (Jerger and Jerger, 1971; Jerger J and Jerger S, 1975; Dirks et al, 1977; Bess, 1983), but only occasionally on either the contralateral ear or both ears of patients with brainstem lesions, and even less frequently on either the ipsilateral or contralateral ear of patients with temporal lobe disorders. These findings also are consistent with this author's clinical experience of obtaining PI functions on patients with eighth nerve, brainstem, or cortical lesions.

LOW REDUNDANCY DEGRADED SPEECH TESTS

Monaural speech stimuli may be degraded (made more difficult) by electroacoustically modifying the frequency, temporal, or intensity characteristics of the undistorted signal. These parameters may be manipulated singly or in combination. Three different monaural auditory tasks are discussed in this section: (1) filtered speech, (2) interrupted speech, and (3) time-compressed speech.

Filtered Speech

The relationship between the frequency spectrum of speech and speech recognition or perception has been systematically investigated in normal listeners over the past several decades. Licklider and Miller (1951) have thoroughly summarized the findings of the early classic studies on this topic. The normal high fidelity bandwidth for speech can be reduced by about 50% without negatively affecting speech intelligibility. To explain, the speech spectrum encompasses frequencies from below 100 Hz to above 7000 Hz, but only those components between about 250 and 3500 Hz need be transmitted for reasonably good speech understanding. The important facts concerning frequency distortion are: (1) eliminating high frequencies by filtering affects consonant more than vowel recognition, (2) eliminating low frequencies affects vowels more than consonants, and (3) consonant recognition is more critical to speech understanding than vowel recognition.

Hence, speech can be degraded by eliminating a portion of the frequency spectrum via electronic filtering. For example, a word recognition test can be recorded through a low-pass filter to remove a certain amount of high frequency acoustic information normally present. The difficulty of the test, that is, the amount of distortion depends upon the cutoff frequency (e.g., 500 Hz) and the rejection rate (e.g., 18 dB/octave) of the filter. The lower the cutoff frequency and the sharper the rejection rate (slope) of the filter, the more difficult the test becomes due

to increasing amounts of missing high frequency energy. For example, in the often cited early investigation by French and Steinberg (1947) they found that as the low-pass filter cutoff frequency was reduced from 7000 to 1950 Hz (thereby eliminating progressively more high-frequency energy) the average syllable recognition score for normal listeners was reduced from 98 to 69%. Likewise, a similar reduction of syllable recognition scores was achieved by using a high-pass filter to progressively eliminate low frequency energy. As shown in Figure 11.1 French and Steinberg (1947) found that the frequencies both above and below 1900 Hz contributed approximately equally to syllable recognition scores.

Considering the effect of the filter characteristics (cutoff frequency and rejection rate) plus the fact that speech recognition tests vary in difficulty according to both the talker and the test material, normative data must be obtained before a particular filtered speech test can be applied for clinical assessment of patients.

Although speech can be processed through a low-pass, high-pass, or a band- (both low- and high-) pass filter system, most applications of monaural filtered speech tasks used to assess central auditory function have used either low-pass or bandpass filtering. The effect of filtering on the speech recognition scores of young normal adult listeners has been studied by Bocca and Calearo (1963), Kirikae et al, (1964), Korsan-Bengtsen (1973), Teatini (1970), and Willeford (1977) among others. The findings reported have varied, as expected, depending on the filter characteristics (e.g., cutoff frequency, rejection rate) and the speech stimuli used. Normal scores at a high sensation level (e.g., 35 to 50 dB) typically ranged from 60 to 90%. Korsan-Bengtsen (1973) used a bandpass filter system consisting of three coupled ⅓ octave filters with center frequencies of 500, 640, and 800 Hz, respectively, and with rejection rates of 40 dB/octave. She presented filtered sentences at 35 dB SL to a large sample of normal young adult listeners and found a definite practice effect. The average score without practice was 84%, compared to 95% when practice preceded the test session. She reported that the filtered speech task was the only one in her central

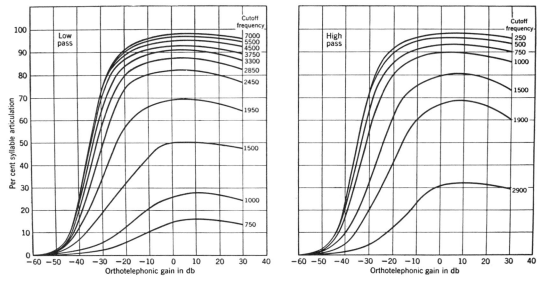

Figure 11.1. Effects of low-pass and high-pass filtering upon mean syllable recognition scores of normal listeners as a function of cutoff frequency. Signal level was expressed in orthotelephonic gain whereby 0 dB is approximately 65 dB sound pressure level at a distance of 1 m in front of the talker. (From French NR, Steinberg JC: Factors governing the intelligibility of speech sounds. *J Acoust Soc Am* 19:90–119, 1947.)

auditory test battery that showed a practice effect.

Several studies have shown that word or sentence recognition for monaurally presented low-pass or bandpass filtered speech is poorer for the ear contralateral to a temporal lobe lesion compared to the ipsilateral side (Bocca, 1958; Bocca et al, 1954, 1955; Hodgson, 1967; Jerger, 1960a and b, 1964; Korsan-Bengtsen, 1973; Lynn et al, 1972; Lynn and Gilroy, 1972, 1977) but is not affected significantly in cases with involvement of the transverse interhemispheric auditory pathways that cross from one hemisphere to the other via the corpus callosum (Gilroy and Lynn, 1974; Lynn et al, 1972; Lynn and Gilroy, 1971, 1972, 1975, 1977; Musiek et al, 1979). Considerably less consistent findings have been obtained with low-pass filtered speech on patients with brainstem lesions (Calearo and Antonelli, 1968; Lynn and Gilroy, 1977). It has been observed that test scores for some patients were abnormal in the ear contralateral to the side of the brainstem primarily involved; in other cases the ipsilateral or both ears showed abnormal results. The level and size of the lesion in the brainstem as well as whether it is extra- or intraaxial are all factors deter-

mining laterality effects (Musiek and Geurkink, 1982). Further, Lynn and Gilroy (1977) pointed out that, because brainstem lesions are often diffuse or bilateral, it is sometimes difficult to establish good correlation between test results and the locus of the brainstem pathology. Hence, the primary usefulness of this test is in identifying lesions of the central auditory system rather than localizing them.

The low-pass filtered speech task has been used also, as part of an auditory test battery, to assess central auditory processing problems in children. The Flowers-Costello Test of Central Auditory Abilities was developed to identify children with auditory problems that cannot be attributed to an intellectual or psychological deficit or a peripheral hearing loss, but Costello (1977) cautioned that this test "... was not designed to locate or specify lesions in the auditory system" (p. 259). After a series of pilot studies which began in the early 1960s the Flowers-Costello Test of Central Auditory Abilities was produced and made available commercially with normative data based on 249 kindergarten-age children (see Flowers et al, 1970). This tape-recorded test consists of two auditory tasks: low-pass filtered speech (24 sentences); and a monaural competing message test with 24 sentences as the primary message and a story recorded by the same talker as the competing signal at a message to competition ratio of 0 dB. A closed message set method of responding is used for both tasks, in that the child points to one of the three pictures (in a set) which completes the sentence. The findings from several studies using the Flowers-Costello test on various samples of children with speech, language, and/or learning problems have been summarized by Costello (1977). She reported that this test has proven useful in identifying many children with central auditory dysfunction.

Willeford (1977) reported preliminary (small sample) normative data for adults and for children between 5 and 9 yr of age on a battery of four central auditory tests including low-pass filtered speech (with a bandwidth from 300 to 500 Hz at a rejection rate of 18 dB per octave) using consonant-nucleus-consonant (CNC) words presented at 50 dB SL re SRT or pure tone average. This low-pass filtered speech task was administered as part of a test battery to 150 learning-disabled children, and 57% showed abnormal findings according to Willeford and Billger (1978).

White (1977) used a duplicated copy of the Willeford tape and established her own local norms for the low-pass filtered speech task on 49 normal children, ranging in age from 6 to 10 yr. She reported that the normal scores at each age were substantially poorer than Willeford's (1977) norms. Further, she found the right ear mean scores were approximately 10% better than left ear mean scores at ages 7 to 10 yr. Based on examination of the individual scores in her normal group, White (1977) believed ". . . differences up to 20% between ears to be normal, and differences of 22–28% to be borderline-normal for the Filtered Speech task" (p. 325). Pinheiro (1977) presented a profile of central auditory test battery results, including low-pass filtered speech, for six children ranging in age from 7 to 14 yr. While reduced performance was shown for certain central auditory tasks, findings on the low-pass filtered speech task could be considered within normal limits for at least four of the six cases illustrated. Musiek and Geurkink (1980) also administered low-pass filtered

speech (500 Hz cutoff at 18 dB/octave) as part of a central auditory test battery to five normal hearing children (8 to 9 yr old) with auditory processing problems. The findings for four of the five children were within normal limits bilaterally. One child exhibited a mild deficit for the right ear only. Also, Martin and Clark (1977) compared the performance of a small group of young normal children to a group of equal size of language learning-disabled children on a monaural low-pass filtered version of the Word Intelligibility by Picture Identification (WIPI) test (Ross and Lerman, 1970). They found that the two groups performed essentially the same on this monaural filtered speech task. They reported, however, that the performance of the two groups could be distinguished when the filtered WIPI test was presented in binaural (diotic and dichotic) modes.

More recently, Willeford (1980) illustrated central auditory test findings for several individual learning-disabled children and found that, while a few exhibited abnormal scores on the low-pass filtered speech test, normal scores were obtained for most of the children. Subsequently, revised norms for the Willeford low-pass filtered speech test (500 Hz cutoff) were presented by Keith (1981) for children from 6 to 10 yr of age based on 40 subjects at each age level. The scores for right and left ears showed a wide range at each age level. Further, no information was given concerning either the subjects or the experimental procedures used to establish these norms. Instead, simply personal communication with Willeford in 1978 was cited as the "basis" for the normative data. The above is a clear illustration of the incomplete and vague information that exists in much of the literature concerning the application of central auditory tests on children.

In summary, children classified as having central auditory processing disorders may or may not exhibit abnormal scores on the monaural low-pass filtered speech task. The sparse and variable findings reported for this low redundancy speech task are not surprising and underscore the need for more complete reporting of normative data in the literature. Further, learning-disabled children do not comprise a homogeneous group and, hence, should not all be expected to demonstrate reduced performance on this task. The monaural low-pass filtered speech test, in its present state of development, should be viewed as a gross screening test for CANS disorders and should not be used without first establishing "local" norms. Findings concerning the relationship between low-pass filtered speech and other central auditory tests applied to children are discussed by Willeford in Chapter 14.

Interrupted Speech

Portions of a speech message can be removed by interruption, that is, by periodically or aperiodically turning the signal on and off by means of an electronic switch. Since most verbal messages are highly redundant, large segments can be removed without negatively affecting understanding. Licklider and Miller (1951) summarized the early pioneering psychoacoustic studies using normal listeners, including their own (Miller and Licklider, 1950), and pointed out that the effect of interruptions upon intelligibility depends upon two variables, i.e., the percentage of time speech is on vs off and the interruption rate. As illustrated in Figure 11.2 these two investigators observed that, if interruption rate is periodic and sufficiently fast, almost all words (Harvard PB 50s) can be understood even at very

low **speech-on-fractions.** Also, for rates slower than 3000 interruptions per second (ips) maximum word recognition reaches a plateau between about 10 and 100 ips. Miller and Licklider (1950) also investigated periodic vs aperiodic interruptions and observed that regular or random interruption has minimal effect on word recognition, provided that the average interruption rate and the average speech-on-time-fraction are held constant. These authors also found that word recognition remained high, even when the silent intervals (interruptions) were filled with intense white noise (e.g., signal to noise ratio −18 dB), provided that the alternation rate between speech and noise was 10 times per second or less. At higher rates of alternation word understanding deteriorated substantially. The psychoacoustic studies by Miller and Licklider (1950) along with later investigations using normal listeners (Bocca, 1958; Calearo and Antonelli, 1963; Teatini, 1970; Korsan-Bengtsen, 1973) helped to establish the foundation for clinical investigations using interrupted speech as a degraded signal for detecting CANS disorders.

As with other degraded speech tests Bocca and his Italian colleagues (Bocca, 1958; Calearo and Antonelli, 1963; and Antonelli, 1970) were among the first investigators to use interrupted speech for testing patients

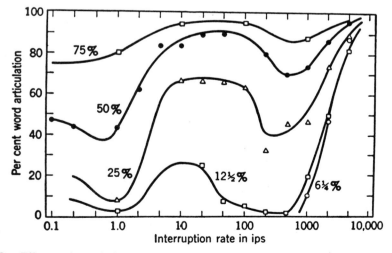

Figure 11.2. Effects of regularly repeated interruptions upon word recognition scores of normal listeners, as a function of the number of interruptions per second and the percentage of time that the signal was on in each interruption cycle. (From Miller GA, Licklider JCR: The intelligibility of interrupted speech. *J Acoust Soc Am* 22:167–173, 1950.)

with CANS pathology. Using both disyllabic words and sentence materials at a message-on-fraction of 50% and from 1 to 40 interruptions per second, Bocca and his associates reported that patients with unilateral temporal lobe lesions showed poorer scores (from 15 to 25%) on the ear contralateral to the lesion compared to the ipsilateral side. The amount of breakdown for interrupted speech scores was observed to be the same for lesions involving either the right or left hemisphere, and the greatest breakdown in performance occurred at 8 to 10 and 20 ips (Calearo and Antonelli, 1963). In patients with brainstem lesions reduced performance on the interrupted speech task was exhibited in either one or both ears (Bocca and Calearo, 1963).

As part of an extensive investigation involving distorted speech audiometry, Korsan-Bengtsen (1973) used Swedish sentences at a constant speech-on-fraction of 0.5 (or 50% on-time) and three rates of interruption: 4, 7, and 10 ips. Prior to testing patients with CANS lesions, Korsan-Bengtsen established normative data using three groups of young adults with normal hearing (N = 85; age range from 17 to 34 yr) and 20 older adults (age range from 50 to 60 yr) and also with normal hearing based on pure tone and spondee thresholds. Performance-intensity functions were obtained for all three interruption rates (4, 7, and 10 ips) by giving the interrupted speech test to 65 of the young adult subjects at five sensation levels (0 to 35 dB SL). The average scores for young normal listeners at 35 dB SL were 96.9% at 10 ips, 95.0% at 7 ips, but were reduced to 80.2% at 4 ips. Interrupted speech scores for the 50 to 60-yr-old subjects at 35 dB SL also remained high (about 95%) at 7 and 10 ips, but average scores for the older group at 4 ips were reduced to 68.9%. Hence, the older normal subjects demonstrated reduced performance compared to the younger adults only at 4 ips.

The interrupted speech test at 7 and 10 ips also was administered by Korsan-Bengtsen (1973) to several small groups of patients, including those with hearing losses of both peripheral and central origin. Findings from peripheral hearing loss cases are discussed later in this chapter. Patients with intracranial lesions were classified into

groups according to the site of the lesion, and the following results were obtained: (1) patients with unilateral temporal lobe lesions involving the auditory cortex displayed striking differences between ipsilateral and contralateral ears with typically poorer scores by 50% or more for the contralateral ear; (2) patients with temporal lobe lesions not involving the auditory cortex showed essentially no difference between ipsi- and contralateral ears; (3) patients with temporal lobe lesions close to the auditory cortex showed differences between ipsi- and contralateral ears with poorer scores via contralateral ears, but differences were smaller than for patients with lesions within the auditory cortex; (4) patients with intracranial tumors not in the temporal lobe (e.g., frontal lobe) revealed essentially normal scores for ipsi- and contralateral ears; and (5) patients with lesions localized primarily to the right side of the brainstem showed markedly poorer scores for the ipsi- compared to the contralateral ear. Based on these findings Korsan-Bengtsen (1973) concluded that the interrupted speech task using sentence materials was quite sensitive for detecting lesions in both the temporal auditory cortex and the brainstem.

In addition to using interrupted speech for testing patients with CANS lesions, this time-distorted speech task also has received some application with elderly adults. A discussion of the findings with older subjects is presented in a later section of this chapter. While this test appears useful in detecting disorders of the CANS in adults, it has received little or no attention from clinical investigators who have concentrated their efforts on assessing central auditory problems in children.

Time-Compressed Speech

As pointed out earlier in this chapter, temporal features of the acoustic signal play an important role in speech perception. Hence, the use of distortion in the time domain of speech has considerable potential as a measure for assessing CANS disorders.

The normal rate of talking varies somewhat according to the speaking habits of the talker and the language used, but it is about 140 words per minute (wpm) for both Italian

(Calearo and Lazzaroni, 1957) and American spoken English (Fairbanks et al, 1957). In general, three different techniques have been used to alter the time characteristics of speech. First, talking rate can be modified somewhat by simply talking faster or slower, but this technique also modifies other dimensions of the speech signal, e.g., vocal pitch and stress, and the speaking rate cannot be controlled precisely. A second and somewhat more controlled approach is to change the rate (speed) of recorded verbal material by simply increasing or decreasing the playback speed of a tape recorder. This method not only changes rate but also produces a frequency shift of the speech signal.

In an effort to avoid the undesirable frequency shifts produced by the fast/slow playback method, Garvey (1953a and b) used a chop-splice procedure whereby certain portions of the recorded signal were manually cut from the tape, and the segments of the signal retained were spliced back together. This (third) method permitted the investigator to systematically vary the temporal features of the recorded message without appreciable distortion of the frequency characteristics of the signal. This technique has received some use (Beasley and Shriner, 1973; Schuckers, et al, 1973; among others), but the chop-splice method was laborious and time-consuming and, hence, has been replaced by more efficient and technically advanced procedures for achieving the same general time-altered effect. An electromechanical time compressor/expander was developed by Fairbanks et al (1954) in order to overcome the problems associated with both the fast/slow playback and the chop-splice techniques. Using this apparatus for "time-compressing" speech, researchers could record and subsequently automatically retain and discard segments of the speech signal. The portions of the signal retained were electromechanically abutted so that there were no silent intervals within the words. Thus, rate can be altered (speeded) without shifting frequency, but, since some acoustic energy is removed, a proportionate amount of acoustic information is discarded also. In the case of expanded speech, acoustic information is not deleted; instead, certain portions of the signal are repeated to accomplish the slower

than normal rate. Based on the principles of the Fairbanks et al (1954) technique, Lee (1972) developed a compressor/expander, consisting of a small tape recorder and a minicomputer. This device has been refined and produced commercially in more than one version and has been the instrument of choice in most studies during the past several years.

For more than 2 decades time- and frequency-altered or time (without frequency)-altered speech has been employed by numerous investigators for a variety of experimental purposes. (For a comprehensive review of various methods used and types of research applications refer to Beasley and Maki, 1976). Among the early investigations concerning the intelligibility of time-compressed speech, it was reported that for normal hearing listeners recognition of spondaic or monosyllabic words may remain as high as 50% when time-compressed by as much as 75%, that is, when the items are presented in 25% of the normal time or rate (Garvey, 1953b; Fairbanks and Kodman, 1957). Sentences were found to be even more resistant than words to time compression (Klumpp and Webster, 1961), and the comprehension of technical connected discourse was observed to be nearly 90% correct when the message time compression was 50%, or 282 wpm (Fairbanks et al, 1957).

Applications of time-altered speech to patients with CANS disorders have been primarily with compressed (accelerated) rather than expanded (slowed) speech. Using the term accelerated speech, Bocca (1958) and his associates (Calearo and Lazzaroni, 1957) used short meaningful sentences at three different rates: 140, 250, and 350 wpm. According to Calearo and Lazzaroni (1957) the different rates of acceleration were accomplished in three ways:

1. By using a speaker having exceptional possibilities of accelerating his speaking rate.
2. By transferring the primitive recording on a magnetic tape which could be rotated at different speeds.
3. By employing a special apparatus which allows a direct acceleration of the message without any alteration of frequency (p. 411).

Hence, the Italian investigators employed each of the methods discussed above for achieving time- and/or frequency-altered speech. Moreover, Calearo and Lazzaroni (1957) claimed that all three methods showed essentially the same results, and, therefore, all three procedures were used in their initial clinical investigations. Later, however, Bocca and his colleagues apparently abandoned the "live-voice" fast talker and taped fast playback techniques in favor of the more precise technique (third general method discussed above). Bocca and Calearo (1963) and Calearo and Antonelli (1968) reported that accelerated speech was accomplished without any frequency shift by use of a special tape recorder with a group of four rotating playback heads. Unfortunately, the experimental procedures employed by the Italian investigators were not well described, and only limited normative data were reported. Calearo and Lazzaroni (1957) found that at a speech rate of 350 wpm five normal hearing subjects achieved the same high sentence recognition scores (100%) as they did at 140 wpm. However, when the speech rate was increased to 350 wpm, the stimulus intensity had to be increased by 10 to 15 dB in order to maintain the same level of speech recognition performance. Similar findings were reported for 20 normal listeners by de Quiros (1964) using the live voice fast talker technique and by Korsan-Bengtsen (1973) for 85 normals using a tape recorder with four movable playback heads, similar to Bocca's system, to avoid changes in the frequency spectrum.

After obtaining varying amounts of normative data, as mentioned above, the aforementioned investigators (Calearo and Lazzaroni, 1957; de Quiros, 1964; Korsan-Bengtsen, 1973; and Quaranta and Cervellera, 1977) employed accelerated speech (usually sentence material) as a means of evaluating central auditory disorders. The findings of these studies suggest that for patients with lesions in the auditory cortex accelerated speech substantially reduces speech recognition in the ear contralateral to the lesion. Patients with diffuse central lesions tend to exhibit decreased scores in both ears. For patients with brainstem involvement, Calearo and Antonelli (1968) found reduced performance in 14 of 23 cases, usually with only one ear affected. Quaranta and Cervellera (1977) found, however, that nine patients with brainstem vascular lesions all showed normal performance on the accelerated speech test.

A collaborative series of studies has been conducted using the Fairbanks et al (1954) method of electromechanically time compressing a monosyllabic word test, Northwestern University Auditory Test Number 6 (NU-6) (Tillman and Carhart, 1966), which was recorded by a male talker (Rintelmann et al, 1974a). The test materials used for each study in the series of investigations were taped copies of the same master tape recording. The goal of this series of investigations was two-fold: (1) to establish normative data for normal listeners and for individuals with peripheral (sensorineural) hearing disorders; and (2) to evaluate and apply this test to patients with central auditory disorders.

In the normative studies word recognition scores were obtained at several senation levels (e.g., 8 to 40 dB in 8 dB steps) for each of several time compression ratios (e.g., 30 to 70% in 10% intervals). The findings with 112 young adult normal listeners (Beasley et al, 1972a and b) demonstrated that word recognition was inversely related to time-compression ratio and directly related to sensation level. In other words, as the percentage of time compression was increased, performance decreased, and scores improved as sensation level was increased. Further, the decrease in word recognition was gradual from 30 to 60%; however, at 70% time compression a dramatic breakdown in performance occurred (see Figs. 11.3 and 11.4). The performance of aged subjects (Konkle et al, 1977) and individuals with noise-induced sensorineural hearing loss (Kurdziel et al, 1975) was also investigated using the same time-compressed version of NU-6. These findings are presented later in the chapter.

Patients with cortical lesions were tested in two investigations (Kurdziel et al, 1976; Rintelmann et al, 1974a) with the above described version of time-compressed monosyllables (NU-6) using 0, 40, and 60% time compression. In both studies patients with diffuse temporal lobe lesions (e.g., cerebral vascular accident cases) showed substantially poorer scores at 60% time compression or less in the contralateral ear, irrespective

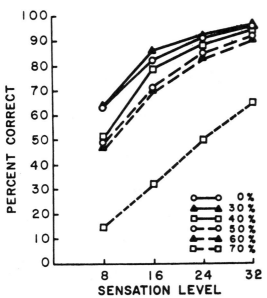

Figure 11.3. Effects of percentages of time compression upon word recognition scores of normal listeners as a function of sensation level. (From Beasley et al: Intelligibility of time-compressed CNC monosyllables. *J Speech Hear Res* 15:340–350, 1972b.)

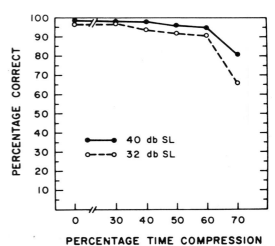

Figure 11.4. Comparison of time-compressed word recognition scores of normal listeners at 32-dB sensation level (Beasley et al, 1972b) to scores at 40-dB sensation level. (From Beasley et al: Perception of time-compressed CNC monosyllables by normal listeners. *J Aud Res* 12:71–75, 1972a.)

of whether the lesion was in the right or left hemisphere. Kurdziel et al (1976) found, however, that for patients with unilateral discrete lesions who had undergone anterior temporal lobe surgery, word recognition scores at 60% time compression generally were equal in both ears and only slightly poorer (about 10%) than scores at 0% time compression. Hence, based on limited data to date, it appears that time-compressed monosyllables may be more sensitive for assessing cerebral lesions that are diffuse or massive than for localized discrete lesions. This conclusion based on our data is in close agreement with the conclusions drawn by Bocca and Calearo (1963) and Korsan-Bengtsen (1973) using Italian and Swedish sentence material, respectively. Nevertheless, this is a tentative conclusion and awaits confirmation after considerably more data have been reported. For example, no data have been reported yet using our technique for patients with brainstem insults.

As stated previously, the interest in time-altered (compressed or expanded) speech has led to the development of improved instrumentation (Lee, 1972) and the use of test materials other than Northwestern University Auditory Test Number 6. The performance of adult normal hearing listeners has been established for the Modified Rhyme Test (Schwartz and Mikus, 1977); for first-order sentential approximations (Freeman and Church, 1977); for the Central Institute for the Deaf (CID) and Revised CID sentence lists; and for third-order sentential approximations (Beasley et al, 1980).

While most studies involving time-altered speech have been concerned with adult subjects, some research has been conducted also with children. The performance of young normal hearing children has been examined for time-compressed versions of the Phonetically Balanced Kindergarten (PBK-50) lists and the Word Intelligibility by Picture Identification (WIPI) test (Beasley et al, 1976). These applications are discussed below.

Sanderson-Leepa and Rintelmann (1976) compared the performance of 60 normal hearing children, divided equally between the ages of 3½, 5½, 7½, 9½, and 11½ yr, on high fidelity (undistorted) tape recorded versions of the WIPI, the PBK-50, and the NU-6 word recognition (speech discrimination) tests. They found that the WIPI test resulted in the highest scores, the PBK-50 was intermediate, and the NU-6 was most difficult. Time-compressed versions of the Sanderson-Leepa and Rintelmann (1976) recordings of both the WIPI and the PBK-50s were constructed by Beasley et al (1976) and administered to young normal hearing children (4, 6, and 8 yr of age). They found that scores improved as a function of increasing age and sensation level and became poorer as a function of greater amounts of time compression. Further, the findings of Beasley et al (1976) supported those of Sanderson-Leepa and Rintelmann (1976) who suggested that the closed message set task of the WIPI was markedly easier for young children than the open message set task of the PBK-50. Hence, the WIPI test appears to be more appropriate for use with young children, while the PBK-50 test can be used effectively with older children. The same recorded version of the time-compressed WIPI test was presented by Orchik and Oelschlaeger (1977) to 48 normal hearing young children (5 and 6 yr of age), who were divided into three groups according to their speech articulation ability. They found significant differences in word recognition scores among the three groups and as a function of the amount of time compression. The authors concluded that children with multiple articulation errors appear to be developmentally delayed in their ability to process time-compressed speech. Ormson and Williams (1975) presented the Beasley et al (1976) time-compressed version of the WIPI test to 40 normal hearing children (6 to 8 yr of age). Thirty of these children exhibited either speech articulatory disorders, reading problems, or both articulatory and reading impairments. Ten children without such learning problems comprised the normal control group. When the findings of this study are viewed in terms of difference scores between 0 and 60% time compression, the time-compressed WIPI test clearly distinguishes normal children from those with specific learning (articulation and reading) problems.

The Beasley et al (1976) time-compressed version of the PBK-50 test was given by Manning et al (1977) to 20 children reported to have auditory perceptual problems. The authors stated that the children with auditory perceptual disorders performed poorer at both 0% (control condition) and at 60%

time compression compared to the normative data of Beasley et al (1976).

Normal hearing children's perception of sentential approximations and temporally distorted meaningful sentences was investigated by Beasley and Flaherty-Rintelmann (1976). They found that as order of sentential approximations was increased to full grammatical sentences, recall accuracy improved, but recall accuracy became poorer as sentence length was increased from three to five words. Also, as the silent interstimulus interval was made longer (from 200 to 400 msec), recall accuracy decreased. In general, as grade level increased (from second to fourth grade), performance improved on all measures. Freeman and Beasley (1978) compared the performance of normal reading to reading-impaired children on a time-compressed version of the Beasley and Flaherty-Rintelmann (1976) stimuli and on the time-compressed WIPI test presented both with and without pictures. They reported that children with reading problems could be differentiated from normal readers based on scores obtained with these auditory tasks.

As discussed above, a limited amount of data for "normal" children is available on time-compressed versions of the WIPI test, the PBK-50 test, and on speech tasks involving sentential approximations. Further, these measures appear to be sensitive to differentiating children with certain specific learning disabilities, e.g., speech articulatory disorders or reading problems. Based on the studies reported to date, the most fruitful application of the various time-compressed speech tasks is to administer these tests at 0 and 60% time compression at a 24-dB sensation level or higher and to compare difference scores (between 0 and 60%) with the comparable values obtained from "normal" children. For example, a normal hearing child who obtains a difference score (0 to 60% time compression) of greater than 10% on the WIPI test given in the usual closed set format at 24 dB SL, according to Beasley and Freeman (1977), ". . .should be followed closely for possible auditory processing difficulties" (p. 160).

In summary, considerable research effort has been devoted to an attempt to establish normative data for both children and adults on time-compressed versions of several different speech recognition tests. The task which remains, however, is to evaluate the various time-compressed test materials mentioned above when used in a patient population having central auditory disorders.

In the preceding sections of this chapter tests have been discussed in which speech signals are distorted by low- and bandpass filtering, periodic interruption, or by time compression. In the two sections to follow a different method is used for degrading the speech stimuli, namely, the so-called competing message task.

COMPETING MESSAGE TESTS

When high fidelity (undistorted) speech stimuli (e.g., words or sentences) are presented monaurally, the difficulty of the listening task can be increased by mixing into a single channel (ear) a primary and a secondary message. The listener's task is to respond to the primary message (e.g., PB words) and ignore the secondary or competing message (e.g., noise, words, sentences, connected discourse, etc.). The difficulty of the competing message test can be varied by manipulating the message to competition (also termed signal to noise) ratio in decibels. This concept will be clarified below in describing two different monaural competing message tests: Speech-in-Noise and Synthetic Sentence Identification with Ipsilateral Competing Message.

Speech-in-Noise

A large body of literature exists describing the effects of broadband and narrow band white noise on the ability of both normal and hearing-impaired listeners to recognize and perceive speech-in-noise. It is beyond the scope of this chapter to review even the most important basic psychoacoustic studies from this extensive literature, but the interested reader is referred to the early classic studies of Kryter (1946), Miller (1947), Licklider (1948), and Hawkins and Stevens (1950), among others. The focus of this section of the chapter is to review briefly the use of monaurally presented speech-in-noise for the assessment of CANS lesions.

A speech-in-noise task has been employed by several investigators for the assessment of retrocochlear lesions (Dayal et al, 1966;

Heilman et al, 1973; Katinsky et al, 1972; Morales-Garcia and Poole, 1972; Noffsinger et al, 1972; Olsen et al, 1975). The primary message for this test is usually monosyllables, which are presented at a high SL (e.g., 40 dB). White noise or speech spectrum noise is presented to the same ear, typically at an overall sound pressure level (SPL) equal to that of the primary message, that is, at approximately a 0 dB signal to noise (S/N) ratio. Normal listeners as well as hearing-impaired patients show wide variability in speech recognition scores obtained in the presence of noise, depending upon the specific primary message, type of noise, and the S/N ratio used. Under the conditions mentioned above, however, normal listeners typically show 20 to 40% poorer scores in noise than in quiet. In evaluating the scores from this task for patients suspected of CANS lesions, the primary comparison is between ipsilateral and contralateral ears in terms of the relative "breakdown" in scores from quiet to noise and the extent to which such breakdown exceeds that of normal listeners.

Abnormal findings have been reported for the speech-in-noise task in ears ipsilateral to eighth nerve lesions (Dayal et al, 1966; Katinsky et al, 1972) and extraaxial brainstem disorders (Dayal et al, 1966), in one or both ears of patients with intraaxial brainstem lesions (Morales-Garcia and Poole, 1972; Noffsinger et al, 1972), in both ears of commissurotomized ("split brain") patients, but with poorer scores on the left compared to the right ear (Musiek et al, 1979) and in ears contralateral to temporal lobe disorders (Heilman et al, 1973; Morales-Garcia and Poole, 1972). Recognizing that no previous investigation had compared the performance of a broad spectrum patient population (e.g., patients with cochlear, eighth nerve, brainstem, or cortical lesions) on a single speech-in-noise test, Olsen et al (1975) conducted a definitive investigation designed to examine this interaction. They employed the NU-6 test at 40 dB SL both in quiet and in white noise (0 dB S/N ratio). They established normative data on a large group of normal listeners and also tested several groups of patients with cochlear, eighth nerve, and CANS disorders. Based on their findings Olsen et al (1975) stated that lesions anywhere in the auditory system from the cochlea through the temporal lobe can exhibit marked reduction in speech recognition scores when measured in the presence of "same ear" white noise. Thus, they concluded that this test "...may have some clinical usefulness in revealing abnormalities in auditory function but not in suggesting a particular site of involvement as being responsible for the dysfunction" (p. 382). This appears to be an appropriate caution regarding the limitation of the speech-in-noise test.

Synthetic Sentence Identification-Ipsilateral Competing Message (SSI-ICM)

Speaks and Jerger (1965) developed the synthetic sentence identification (SSI) test which consists of artificial sentences constructed as approximations to real English sentences based on the rules governing the probabilities of word sequence. Jerger and his associates have found the synthetic sentence identification task presented with an ipsilateral competing message (SSI-ICM) to be useful in assessing CANS dysfunction, especially brainstem lesions (Jerger, 1970a and b; Jerger and Hayes, 1977; Jerger and Jerger, 1974; Jerger J and Jerger S, 1975; Jerger S and Jerger J, 1975). The particular test advocated by Jerger (1973) for evaluating patients with CANS disorders consists of ten third-order approximation sentences. Each sentence has seven words and contains nine syllables (±one syllable). The ten sentences are presented as a closed message set, with a competing message (continuous discourse) presented to the same ear. In general, two methods have been used for presenting this test. In one method, a constant message to competition ratio of 0 dB is used, and the stimulus materials (SSI-ICM) are presented at several SLs, ranging from low to high SL. In the other, more commonly used method, the primary message (synthetic sentences) is given at a constant high SL (e.g., 40 dB), and the intensity level of the competing message (continuous discourse) is varied to achieve message to competition ratios (MCRs) from about +10 to −20 dB in 10 dB steps. Note that in a minus MCR condition the competing message is more intense than the primary message. Both methods described above for administering the SSI-ICM task permit plotting performance-intensity (PI) functions.

According to Jerger (1973) most normal listeners perform at 100% when the message and the competition are at the same level, that is, at an MCR of 0 dB. Normal performance drops to about 80% at an MCR of −10 dB, to about 55% at an MCR of −20 dB, and to about 20% at an MCR of −30 dB. It should be recognized that these normal responses can be expected only for Jerger's recorded version of this test. If another version is used (e.g., different talker or different stimulus items), norms for that version should be established before the test is applied to patients.

Responses on the SSI-ICM task are considered abnormal when the PI functions exhibit marked deficits from expected normal results in one or both ears. Abnormal performance on this task may be exhibited by patients with either brainstem or temporal lobe lesions but occurs more commonly in the former (Jerger and Jerger, 1974; Jerger S and Jerger J, 1975). Brainstem lesions are displayed by depressed performance in either the contralateral ear or in both ears. Temporal lobe lesions produce deficits on the SSI-ICM test also in both ears or, less often, in the contralateral ear only (Jerger J and Jerger S, 1975). The most useful application of the SSI test for differentiating brainstem from temporal lobe lesions is presentation of the competing message in both the ipsilateral and contralateral modes. This latter task is a dichotic test and is discussed in Chapter 12.

Combined Use of Undistorted and Competing Message Tests: PI-PB and SSI-ICM

In an effort to enhance the clinical sensitivity of the performance-intensity function for assessing both peripheral and central auditory disorders, Jerger and Hayes (1977) have advocated comparing the results for two sets of verbal stimuli, phonemically balanced monosyllables (PI-PB) and synthetic sentences (SSI-ICM). They identified three different patterns in patients with cochlear disorders according to the shape of the pure tone audiogram. If the audiometric configuration is flat, the functions will be similar for both types of verbal stimuli; if a high frequency loss is present, the function for the PB words will fall below the function for synthetic sentences; and if the audiometric pattern is rising, the sentence function will fall below the word function. The authors contended that, based on the above described three patterns, site of lesion assessment can be aided in four ways:

1. If the PI functions for both sets of stimuli are consistent with the audiometric configurations and no substantial rollover is found, the probable site of lesion is cochlear.
2. If the relationship between the two PI functions is disproportionate in terms of the amount or shape of the hearing loss and substantial rollover is found for either PI function, a possible site of lesion is the eighth nerve.
3. If the function for the sentences falls below that for the words, and this outcome cannot be attributed to a rising audiometric configuration, a central auditory disorder can be suspected.
4. In presbycusic patients the audiometric contour and the direction and magnitude of difference between the PI functions for words and sentences may demonstrate that the patients have both peripheral and central components to their total auditory disorder.

Hence, the authors propose that by administering both undistorted words and synthetic sentences (with an ipsilateral competing message at 0 dB MCR) at several sensation levels in order to plot PI functions, two of the four possible outcomes described above may assist the clinician in detecting central auditory deficits. This procedure appears to have merit, especially if applied to the presbycusic population. Further discussion of the Jerger and Hayes (1977) test procedure used with elderly patients is presented later in the section on Aging and Central Auditory Tests.

PERIPHERAL HEARING DISORDERS AND CENTRAL AUDITORY TESTS

As stated earlier in this chapter and elsewhere in this text, a patient's performance on central auditory tests typically is interpreted by comparing that individual's scores to normative data derived from a sample of listeners with "normal peripheral auditory mechanisms." This method of interpretation may not be feasible or appropriate for some patients with peripheral hearing impairment. It is well known that conventional (undistorted) speech recognition scores for patients with sensorineural hearing disorders may vary widely, anywhere from close to 0 to 100%, depending upon the etiology or type of disorder and the pure tone audiometric configuration and amount of hearing loss (Bess, 1983). A further complicating factor is that the pure tone audiometric configuration and undistorted speech recognition scores may show substantial ear differences. Hence, one should question the extent to which norms for central auditory tests can be applied to individuals with sensorineural hearing impairment. To illustrate this problem, Miltenberger et al (1978) administered a battery of four central auditory tests to 70 subjects with sensorineural hearing losses. Three of the four tests involved binaural speech tasks. Results of this study demonstrated that while all tasks were affected by certain amounts and configurations of sensorineural hearing loss, the task most negatively affected was the monosyllabic filtered word test. The authors concluded that when central auditory tests are administered to individuals with sensorineural hearing disorders, the results must be interpreted with caution.

Speaks (1980) also has expressed concern over the effect of peripheral hearing loss on the assessment of central auditory deficits. He identified two issues that should receive substantial investigation. Speaks stated:

> The first issue is to determine the extent to which a coexisting peripheral impairment, whether bilaterally symmetric or asymmetric, contaminates the outcome of tests that are intended to tap exclusively central function. The second concern is to determine which test from the central battery is demonstrably least sensitive to the effects of diminished threshold sensitivity. (1980, p. 1854)

Speaks (1980) presented illustrative data on the performance of persons with peripheral hearing loss on both monotic and dichotic listening tasks. He found that patients who obtained 100% performance scores monaurally in both ears on undistorted synthetic sentences demonstrated substantial ear difference scores when the sentences were temporally interrupted. Smaller ear difference scores were exhibited on time-compressed sentences; therefore, limited data suggest that time compression may be less affected by bilaterally symmetric sensorineural hearing loss than temporal interruption.

Early attempts to compare the performance of adult sensorineural hearing-impaired subjects to adult normal listeners on time-compressed word recognition tests were conducted by Luterman et al (1966) and shortly thereafter by Sticht and Gray (1969) using the CID W-22 test. In comparing the relative breakdown in performance between groups as a function of amount of time compression, the investigators of both above cited studies concluded that the time-compressed speech task (as they measured it) did not differentiate normal from sensorineural hearing-impaired subjects. According to Carhart (1965), the speech stimuli (CID W-22) employed by Luterman et al (1966) and Sticht and Gray (1969) might not have been sufficiently difficult to demonstrate differences in performance between normal listeners and sensorineural hearing-impaired subjects. Subsequently, Kurdziel et al (1975) administered time-compressed monosyllabic words (NU-6) to noise-induced sensorineural hearing-impaired subjects. Some variability in performance was found; however, in general, scores for time-compression ratios plotted as a function of sensation level were parallel to those of normal listeners but with lower word recognition scores (see Fig. 11.5). More recently Grimes et al (1984) compared the performance of 28 adult normal listeners to an equal number of subjects with high-frequency sensorineural hearing loss using a commercially available time-compressed version of NU-6. While differences found between the two groups were minimal for speech recognition scores obtained with noncompressed stimuli, performance scores at 60% time compression (32 dB SL) were substantially different. Scores for sensorineural hearing-impaired subjects typically were between 30 and 40%. Scores in this range were 2 SD or more below the normal group mean score. Based on the low time-compressed scores found for sensorineural hearing-impaired subjects, the authors concluded that it would

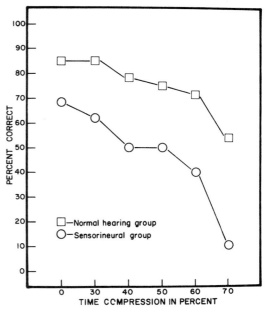

Figure 11.5. Average word recognition scores as a function of time compression, collapsed over sensation level, comparing performance of normal listeners (Beasley et al, 1972b) to sensorineural hearing-impaired subjects. (From Kurdziel S, Rintelmann WF, and Beasley D: Performance of noise-induced hearing impaired listeners on time compressed monosyllables. *J Am Audiol Soc* 1:54–60, 1975. © 1975, Williams & Wilkins, Baltimore.)

be difficult to identify a significant shift when a central disorder coexists with a sensorineural hearing loss.

In order to examine the potential influence of peripheral hearing loss on the interrupted speech task, Korsan-Bengtsen (1973) administered this test with 7 and 10 ips at 35 dB SL to three groups of young adult patients who were reasonably closely equated for pure tone thresholds and also had essentially normal undistorted speech discrimination scores. She reported that cases with conductive hearing loss showed essentially normal results, whereas among patients with cochlear pathology there was a substantial difference between the groups with congenital and acquired hearing losses. Scores for congenital hearing loss patients were nearly normal, but test results for persons with acquired losses (due to Ménière's disease, trauma, or cochlear otosclerosis) were markedly reduced (by about 30%).

Korsan-Bengtsen reasoned that the substantial difference in performance between these two groups could probably be attributed to differences in time of onset of hearing loss. Persons with sensorineural hearing loss from birth may find the additional stress from low redundant speech signals no more taxing than do normal listeners, whereas individuals with acquired hearing loss may experience considerable difficulty in processing distorted speech signals when the distortion imposed by the cochlear lesion is of fairly recent onset.

A central auditory test battery consisting of five dichotic and two monotic tasks was presented by Goldstein (1980) to 33 adults with cochlear hearing loss. She found that tasks using sentence material or spondees were less susceptible than monosyllabic words to the contaminating effects of cochlear pathology upon the subjects' performance on the central auditory tests. Concerning the two monaural tasks used in this investigation, performance for the entire sample was extremely poor on the low-pass filtered speech task at both 50 and 30 dB SL. Goldstein (1980) concluded that performance on this task is substantially affected by cochlear pathology regardless of etiology, audiometric configuration, amount of hearing loss, age, and/or sex. Based on her findings, she stated that the monaural low-pass filtered speech task, as typically employed, has no diagnostic value for patients with cochlear pathology, and she recommended that it not be used with such patients. Regarding the other monaural test Goldstein used, Synthetic Sentence Identification-Ipsilateral Competing Message, her findings suggested that this test could be used with sensorineural hearing loss patients at a 0 dB message to competition ratio (MCR). Goldstein proposed that normal results on this test could help rule out a central auditory disorder, but low scores should not be interpreted as findings suggestive of central auditory dysfunction.

Based on the few studies briefly reviewed above, there is sufficient evidence to suggest that caution must be exercised in using central auditory tests with patients who have peripheral auditory disorders. An obvious conclusion is that norms (preferably *local norms*) should be obtained on young adult listeners (both normals and patients with peripheral hearing impairment) prior to using auditory tasks for assessment of central auditory disorders. Since central test norms should not be contaminated with data from patients who may have coexisting central auditory dysfunction, elderly subjects (approximately age 60 or preferably even younger) should be excluded from normative studies. It is well established that the aging process may result in combined peripheral and central auditory impairment. This topic is considered next.

AGING AND CENTRAL AUDITORY TESTS

Investigators interested in the development of degraded speech tests that are sensitive to the identification and assessment of central auditory disorders have recognized for many years that the geriatric population should be included in such studies. In discussing the application of distorted speech tests Bocca (1958) stated:

The comparative evaluation of the results of our tests in the old age and tumor group of cases is an implicit confirmation that the auditory troubles of old age are mainly cortical in origin, and that insofar as the process of cortical elaboration of the message is concerned, it does not matter whether the cortical lesions are brought about by compression and invasion, or by primary atrophic and degenerative changes (p. 307).

Indeed, Bocca and his colleagues reported that their degraded speech tests frequently showed abnormally low scores in elderly patients, and certain tests (e.g., interrupted speech) even produced substantially poorer responses in aged subjects (over 70 yr old) than in patients with intracranial tumors (Bocca, 1958).

Many investigators who have reported a breakdown in performance by elderly listeners on various degraded speech tests have attributed such reduced performance to age-related atrophic changes involving both the peripheral and central auditory systems (e.g., Antonelli, 1970; Bergman, 1980; Jerger and Hayes, 1977; Kirikae et al, 1964; Konkle et al, 1977; among others). This view has received support from histologic studies of both the temporal bone and the brain (Brody, 1955; Hansen and Reske-Nielsen,

1965; Hinojosa and Naunton, 1980; Kirikae et al, 1964; Samorajski, 1976; Schuknecht, 1964, 1974). A comprehensive yet concise review of the literature concerning atrophic and degenerative changes of both the peripheral and central auditory systems due to aging may be found in Bergman (1980).

Some results exhibited by older adults on the various speech tests discussed in this chapter are presented in the paragraphs below. The information presented here is not intended to be an exhaustive review of the literature, but rather simply an illustration of the types of breakdown in performance that have been observed on certain tests among elderly subjects.

Gaeth (1948) was among the first to observe that some presbycusic subjects displayed speech recognition (discrimination) scores for undistorted PB words that were disproportionately poorer than would be expected based on the amount of hearing loss and the pure tone threshold configuration. Gaeth coined the term "phonemic regression" to label such speech recognition test scores, and his reported observation has been found repeatedly in clinical hearing assessments of the aged in the intervening 30+ yr (Bess and Townsend, 1977; Goetzinger et al, 1961; Orchik and Burgess, 1977; Pestalozza and Shore, 1955; Rintelmann and Schumaier, 1974).

The "rollover" phenomenon, discussed earlier, attributed most often to eighth nerve lesions but also occasionally to cases of CANS disorders, has been displayed in the performance - intensity functions of some presbycusic patients. Such findings, when observed among elderly patients, generally have been considered as retrocochlear or higher central auditory pathway disturbances due to the aging process (Dirks et al, 1977; Gang, 1976; Jerger and Jerger, 1971, 1976; Shirinian and Arnst, 1980).

Elderly subjects also have exhibited abnormally reduced word or sentence recognition scores, typically for both ears, on low redundancy degraded speech tasks. Kirikae et al (1964) compared the performance of older adults (50 to 70 yr) to young normal listeners (20 to 30 yr) on the low-pass filtered (1200 Hz cutoff) speech test using Japanese monosyllables. The two groups were fairly well equated for pure tone thresholds and

undistorted word recognition scores. On the low-pass filtered speech task, the average scores were about 40% for young adults and 25% for the older subjects. Similar findings were obtained by Bergman (1980) who used low-pass filtered speech as one of several measures to study the effects of aging on the perception of speech. He demonstrated that filtering signal energy above 2000 Hz sharply reduced the speech recognition ability of geriatric adults compared to young normal listeners. In contrast, Korsen-Bengtsen (1973) found that older subjects (50 to 60 yr) scored only slightly poorer than young adults on filtered sentences when the two groups were fairly closely equated for pure tone thresholds.

As stated earlier, Bocca (1958) contended that the interrupted speech task was more sensitive to CANS deterioration in the aged than in patients with documented CANS lesions. He reported that the interrupted speech test using PB disyllabic words given at 50 dB SL with a speech on-time fraction of 0.5 at 10 ips produced much poorer responses in aged subjects than in patients with intracranial tumors. Other investigators compared older subjects to young adults, with pure tone thresholds reasonably equated between groups, and used either words or sentence material with interruption rates ranging from 4 to 10 ips. In general, the findings from these studies showed substantially poorer scores for the older compared to the younger subjects (Antonelli, 1970; Bergman, 1971, 1980; Kirikae et al, 1964; Korsan-Bengtsen, 1973).

A comprehensive large scale investigation was reported by Bergman (1980) concerning performance changes on the interrupted speech task as a function of age. Studies were conducted over a period of several years, beginning in 1965 in the United States using English everyday sentences and continuing, after 1974, in Israel with Hebrew sentences. In both studies an interruption rate of 8 ips was used with 50% on time in each interruption cycle. Bergman's findings, shown in Figure 11.6, demonstrate a fairly systematic and substantial reduction in performance of over 400 adult subjects from 20 to 89 yr of age. Scores began to decline sharply after the 4th decade of life. Further, as illustrated in Figure 11.6, the older Israelis

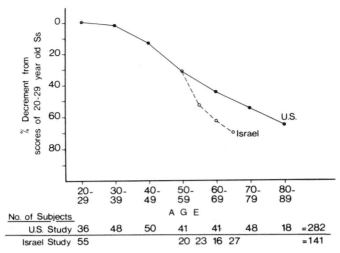

Figure 11.6. Effects of periodic interruptions (50% duty cycle and 8 ips) on average sentence recognition scores as a function of age by decade. Data are from American and Israeli studies using English and Hebrew sentences, respectively. Intermediate Israeli groups include ages 55 to 63 and 64 to 70. Scores are shown as a decrement from the 20- to 29-yr-old group. (From Bergman M: *Aging and the Perception of Speech.* Baltimore, University Park Press, 1980.)

exhibited considerably more breakdown in performance than the Americans of similar age. Bergman (1980) postulated that this finding could perhaps be explained by the fact that the first "native" language of many of the older Israelis was other than Hebrew. The interested reader is referred to Bergman (1980) for the details of this extensive investigation and for other studies concerning speech perception and aging.

Regarding the effect of aging on accelerated speech task performance, Calearo and Lazzaroni (1957) found that when the talking rate of Italian sentences was increased to two and a half times faster than normal speed (from 140 to 350 wpm), persons over 70 yr of age showed substantial breakdown in performance compared to young adults. However, Bergman (1980) also used an acceleration rate of two and a half times faster than normal speed and found only a slight reduction in the understanding of everyday sentences among aged subjects (70 to 89 yr) compared to young (20 to 29 yr) adults. In another study, however, with a more difficult listening task at 50% time compression, Bergman did find substantially reduced scores for the aged compared to young adults. Korsan-Bengtsen (1973) used somewhat slower acceleration (a normal rate of 130 to 290 wpm) and found only slight

reduction in sentence performance scores for subjects 50 to 60 yr old.

Konkle et al (1977) selected aged subjects so that their thresholds for pure tones and speech and their word recognition scores at 0% time compression essentially were equal to normal listeners. Nevertheless, these aged subjects obtained considerably reduced word recognition scores, compared to normals, at all ratios of time compression (20, 40, and 60%). Further, as illustrated in Figure 11.7, the ability to process time-compressed monosyllabic words (NU-6) decreased substantially as a function of age and sensation level. The findings of Konkle et al (1977) are in agreement with the results of an earlier study by Sticht and Gray (1969) who also used monosyllables (CID W-22) and comparable time-compression conditions (36, 46, and 59%). They reported depressed scores for aged compared to young subjects, and the difference between these groups increased as the amount of time compression was increased. Luterman et al (1966), however, used less taxing time-compression ratios (10 and 20%), also with monosyllabic words (CID W-22), and did not find performance differences between young and old adults.

The studies cited above support the conclusion that both the amount of time com-

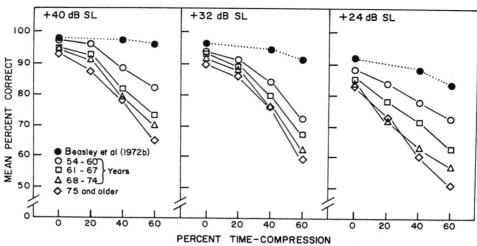

Figure 11.7. Comparison of time-compressed word recognition scores of four groups of elderly subjects to scores of normal listeners at 24- and 32 dB sensation level (Beasley et al, 1972b) and 40 dB sensation level (Beasley et al, 1972a). (From Konkle DF, Beasley DS, Bess F: Intelligibility of time-altered speech in relation to chronological aging. *J Speech Hear Res* 20:108–115, 1977, and © 1977, the American Speech-Language-Hearing Association, Rockville, Maryland.)

pression and the speech test material must be fairly taxing in order to demonstrate CANS impairment in elderly persons.

Concerning the disruptive effects of noise or competing messages on speech understanding among the aged, Bergman (1980) discussed the findings of several studies, including his own. A reasonable generalization from studies of speech-in-noise (e.g., broadband white noise) and competing messages (e.g., connected discourse) is that there is a gradual and fairly linear reduction in performance scores until about the decade of the 60s or 70s, at which time a sharper and more dramatic breakdown in performance occurs. The amount of breakdown and the age when it starts to become severe depend on several factors (e.g., difficulty of the speech task, type of noise, message to competition ratio, etc.).

The aging effect on listener performance on a monaural competing message task was investigated by Orchik and Burgess (1977). They administered the SSI-ICM at five MCRs (+20, 0, −10, −20, and −30 dB) to four groups of subjects with normal hearing categorized by age: 10 to 12, 20 to 29, 40 to 49, and 60 yr and older. Listeners in the two oldest age groups displayed substantial deterioration in performance scores compared to the younger groups. Also, speech recog-

nition became dramatically poorer as the message to competition ratio became more adverse (e.g., −20 and −30 dB MCR). Based on their findings, Orchik and Burgess concluded that an evaluation of an adult hearing-impaired person's understanding of "everyday speech" should not be limited to speech recognition tests in quiet. Further, Orchik (1981) commented later that breakdown in performance scores of older adults under noisy listening conditions may be due to an interaction between peripheral and central auditory deficits.

Similar findings were obtained in the study by Jerger and Hayes (1977) discussed earlier. They plotted mean PB and SSI-ICM maximum scores for 204 patients with sensorineural hearing loss. The subjects were categorized by age groups into eight decades; the youngest group was 10 to 19 years and the oldest was 80 to 89 yr. Results showed that scores on both speech tasks decreased with increasing age by approximately the same amount until the decade of the 60s. Performance scores for the older subjects, aged 60 to 89 yr, deteriorated sharply on the SSI task with an ipsilateral competing message (at 0 dB MCR) compared to their responses to undistorted PB words in quiet. Figure 11.8 displays the findings of Jerger and Hayes (1977) for right ears only. Left

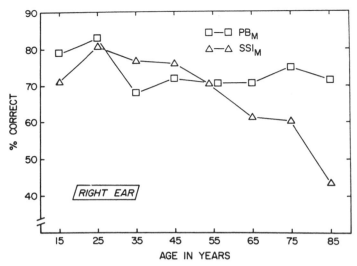

Figure 11.8. Mean PB max and SSI-ICM max by age decade for right ear of 204 patients. Note consistent decreases in SSI max with increasing age. Left ear scores showed similar patterns but somewhat smaller differences between mean PB max and SSI-ICM max. (From Jerger J, Hayes D: Diagnostic speech audiometry. *Arch Otolaryngol* 103:216–222, 1977. Copyright 1977, American Medical Association.)

ear results exhibited similar patterns but somewhat smaller differences between PB max and SSI-ICM max scores. Jerger and Hayes (1977) concluded that by administering PI functions for both of these speech tasks to elderly patients with presbycusis, one can obtain

... a rough estimate of the relative contributions of peripheral and central effects on the patient's total auditory impairment. This factor, the "peripheral-central ratio," may ultimately prove useful in judging the prognosis for successful use of a hearing aid or other rehabilitative measure (p. 222).

The findings of Jerger and Hayes (1977) were supported by those of Shirinian and Arnst (1982) who obtained PI functions for PB words (CID W-22) and the SSI-ICM at 0 dB MCR for 62 aged listeners (60 to 85 yr). Most subjects had a gradually sloping high frequency sensorineural hearing loss typical of presbycusis. Interestingly, a few subjects had normal hearing, but they exhibited an age-related central pattern on the PI-PB and PI-SSI-ICM tasks. Also, some subjects with symmetrical sensorineural hearing loss displayed central findings in one ear only, while others showed central patterns for both ears, but of varying magni-

tudes. Shirinian and Arnst (1982) stressed that a major benefit of being able to identify a possible central component of a presbycusic hearing loss relates to recommendations for hearing aid use. Based on an earlier report by Hayes and Jerger (1979), they reasoned that for aged hearing aid candidates with fairly symmetrical audiometric configurations and undistorted speech recognition scores, the ear of choice for hearing aid fitting should be the one with the least central auditory deficit. They also contended that knowing whether or not an aged patient's sensorineural hearing loss is affected by a central component should permit the clinician to make better predictions about potential benefits from amplification and, hence, to do better counseling and planning of rehabilitation programs for the elderly. Therefore, the ability to identify the central component of hearing loss resulting from aging appears to have merit for both diagnostic and rehabilitative audiology.

Finally, certain cautions should be kept in mind. Concerning studies in which aged listeners are compared to young adults on distorted speech tasks, it is critically important that these two subject groups be equated (as closely as possible) in terms of pure tone thresholds and undistorted speech recognition scores. Otherwise, in the absence of "peripheral patient norms" it is virtually impossible to make meaningful comparisons between aged and young adult performance differences on difficult listening tasks. Also, as Hayes (1981) pointed out: "Aging in the central nervous system may affect intelligence, memory, recall, and learning quite independently of central auditory involvement" (p. 258). As a consequence, findings on behavioral speech tasks, such as those discussed in this chapter, may be contaminated by varying amounts by such non-auditory age-related central nervous system degenerative factors.

In conclusion, the studies reviewed concerning the administration of the various types of monaural undistorted and degraded speech tasks to aged individuals permit the generalization that the more difficult the task, the greater the likelihood that older persons will exhibit poorer performance compared to young adults. Further, reduced performance in the aged, when substantial, probably can be attributed, at least in part, to atrophic and degenerative changes of the central auditory system. For many elderly persons beginning in the decade of the 60s or later, there will be both a peripheral and central clinically significant component to their hearing impairment. Proper selection of a test battery, consisting of both undistorted and distorted speech tasks, may permit the audiologist to grossly determine the relative contributions of the peripheral and central components of the patient's total hearing impairment.

ILLUSTRATIVE CASE FINDINGS

In spite of the large number and variety of tests that have been developed and advocated for use with patients having central auditory dysfunction, no specific battery of tests has received universal acceptance. Clinical investigators still are searching for the most sensitive tasks to both identify and assess central auditory disorders. Hence, testing central auditory function still is in the experimental stage. Each laboratory has its own specific battery of central auditory tests, which typically is comprised of several types of psychoacoustic tasks and electrophysiologic measures. Most clinical investigators use only one or two monaural speech

tasks as part of their test battery. Two, from among the several tests discussed in this chapter, that commonly are used are the low-pass filtered and the time-compressed speech tests. Specific examples of test results for these two tests obtained from patients with central auditory disorders are shown in Figure 11.9. In both cases involving left temporal lobe lesions, the expected finding was observed, that is, substantially reduced performance on the ear contralateral to the lesion compared to the ipsilateral side. Such findings of large differences in performance between ears demonstrate the value of including a monaural speech task as part of the test battery. Also, note that in the example of time-compressed speech test results, normal scores were obtained for both ears at 0% time compression. This finding adds to the significance of the scores obtained at 60% time compression.

CONCLUSIONS

Filtered, interrupted, and accelerated or time-compressed speech tests have been used for nearly 3 decades as low redundancy monaural speech tasks for the identification and assessment of central auditory disorders in adults. Two of these methods, filtered and time-compressed speech tests, have been applied also in an effort to assess central auditory processing deficits in children. In general, all three of these degraded speech tasks are fairly sensitive to identifying massive temporal lobe lesions (e.g., cerebral vascular accidents) in either or both right and left cortical hemispheres. Although the data are sparse concerning the application of these tests to patients with interhemispheric tract or brainstem lesions, conflicting findings have been reported. There is need for more data on these tests with patients having well-documented brainstem or interhemispheric tract lesions. Based on limited available evidence, however, none of these tests are sensitive to distinguishing brainstem from cortical lesions. Nevertheless, all three measures (filtered, interrupted, and time-compressed speech tasks) can serve usefully as screening tests for cortical level lesions. When used as part of a test battery they may assist also in defining the locus of the lesion in some cases. Regarding children with specific learning disabilities (e.g., reading or speech and lan-

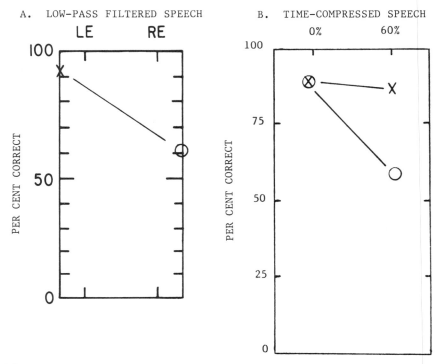

Figure 11.9. (A) Low-pass filtered speech scores (NU-6 with 500 Hz cutoff frequency and 18 dB/octave slope) from a teen-age boy with a left temporal lobe tumor. His pure tone thresholds and undistorted speech recognition scores were normal. (B) Time-compressed speech scores (NU-6 at 0 and 60% time compression) from a middle-aged woman with a left temporal lobe middle cerebral artery aneurysm, postresection. Her pure tone thresholds showed a mild bilaterally symmetrical hearing loss.

guage problems), based on the literature, it appears that time compression is more sensitive than filtering for distinguishing such children from normal listeners.

Two monaural competing message tests that have been employed for identifying central auditory dysfunction in adults are the speech-in-noise task and the synthetic sentence identification test with ipsilateral competing message. The difficulty of both of these tasks is greatly influenced by the message to competition ratio. In general, under adverse listening conditions (e.g., MCR of 0 dB, −10 dB, etc.) the speech-in-noise task can assist in demonstrating central auditory deficits in patients with normal peripheral auditory mechanisms. This task also appears to be most useful as a screening test for central lesions. The SSI-ICM test, however, has been found to be more sensitive for detecting brainstem rather than cortical lesions. Thus, this test may provide informa-

tion about brainstem integrity which the other monaural central tests do not.

Several cautions have been stressed throughout this chapter. The need for the development of norms based on the specific stimulus materials and test procedures employed for both children and adults has been emphasized repeatedly.

Another important concern considered in this chapter is the difficulty in applying central auditory speech tests to patients with peripheral auditory disorders. There remains a need to determine which tests are least affected by coexisting peripheral and central auditory disorders. There is some limited evidence to suggest that the low-pass filtered speech test is substantially influenced by a cochlear lesion, and, hence, may not be an appropriate central test for patients with peripheral lesions. By the same token, time-compressed speech may be less affected by sensorineural hearing loss and, therefore, can be used with such patients, especially those who have a bilaterally symmetrical hearing loss. Such generalizations are based on limited reports, and considerably more clinical research on this topic is needed.

While presbycusis commonly is thought of as a high frequency sensorineural hearing loss, the auditory deficit resulting from aging typically affects both the peripheral and the central auditory systems. Based on the findings of several investigations, each of the low redundancy speech tasks reviewed in this chapter is sensitive to the central component of presbycusis; however, in general, low-pass filtered speech is less effective (for this purpose) than either interrupted or time-compressed speech. Further, comparing performance-intensity functions for undistorted monosyllabic words (e.g., PBs) in quiet vs monaural competing message test (e.g., SSI-ICM) results tends to show substantially greater breakdown in performance on the latter task, typically beginning in the decade of the 60s or later. Such comparative test results can help to identify both a peripheral and central component of an elderly patient's total auditory problem. Finally, such information can have beneficial consequences both for diagnostic and rehabilitative audiology.

References

Antonelli A: Sensitized speech tests in aged people. In Røjskjaer C (ed): *Speech Audiometry* (2nd Danavox Symposium). Odense, Denmark, Danavox Foundation, 1970, pp 66–77.

Beasley D, Bratt G, Rintelmann W: Intelligibility of time-compressed sentential stimuli. *J Speech Hear Res* 23:722–731, 1980.

Beasley DS, Flaherty-Rintelmann AK: Children's perception of temporally distorted sentential approximations of varying length. *Audiology* 15:315–325, 1976.

Beasley DS, Forman B, Rintelmann WF: Perception of time-compressed CNC monosyllables by normal listeners. *J Aud Res* 12:71–75, 1972a.

Beasley DS, Freeman BA: Time-altered speech as a measure of central auditory processing. In Keith RW (ed): *Central Auditory Dysfunction.* New York, Grune & Stratton, 1977, pp 129–176.

Beasley D, Maki J: Time- and frequency-altered speech. In Lass N (ed): *Contemporary Issues in Experimental Phonetics.* New York, Academic Press, 1976, pp 419–458.

Beasley DS, Maki JE, Orchik DJ: Children's perception of time-compressed speech on two measures of speech discrimination. *J Speech Hear Disord* 41:216–225, 1976.

Beasley DS, Schwimmer S, Rintelmann WF: Intelligibility of time-compressed CNC monosyllables. *J Speech Hear Res* 15:340–350, 1972b.

Beasley DS, Shriner TH: Auditory analysis of temporally distorted sentential approximations. *Audiology* 12:262–271, 1973.

Bergman M: Hearing and aging: implications of recent research findings. *Audiology* 10:164–171, 1971.

Bergman M: *Aging and the Perception of Speech.* Baltimore, University Park Press, 1980.

Bess FH: Clinical assessment of speech recognition. In Konkle DF, Rintelmann WF (eds): *Principles of Speech Audiometry.* Baltimore, University Park Press, 1983, pp 127–201.

Bess F, Townsend T: Word discrimination for listeners with flat sensorineural hearing losses. *J Speech Hear Disord* 42:232–237, 1977.

Bocca E: Clinical aspects of cortical deafness. *Laryngoscope* 68:301–309, 1958.

Bocca E, Calearo C: Central hearing processes. In Jerger J (ed): *Modern Developments in Audiology.* New York, Academic Press, 1963, pp 337–370.

Bocca E, Calearo C, Cassinari V: A new method for testing hearing in temporal lobe tumors. *Acta Otolaryngol (Stockh)* 44:219–221, 1954.

Bocca E, Calearo C, Cassinari V, Migliavacca F: Testing "cortical" hearing in temporal lobe tumors. *Acta Otolaryngol* 45:289–304, 1955.

Brody H: Organization of cerebral cortex. III. A study of aging in human cerebral cortex. *J Comp Neurol* 102:511–556, 1955.

Calearo C, Antonelli AR: "Cortical" hearing tests and cerebral dominance. *Acta Otolaryngol (Stockh)* 56:17–26, 1963.

Calearo C, Antonelli AR: Audiometric findings in brainstem lesions. *Acta Otolaryngol (Stockh)* 66:305–319, 1968.

Calearo C, Lazzaroni A: Speech intelligibility in relation to the speed of the message. *Laryngoscope* 67:410–419, 1957.

Carhart R: Problems in the measurement of speech discrimination. *Arch Otolaryngol* 82:253–260, 1965.

Costello MR: Evaluation of auditory behavior of children using the Flowers-Costello test of central auditory abilities. In Keith RW (ed): *Central Auditory Dysfunction.* New York, Grune & Stratton, 1977, pp 257–276.

Dayal VS, Tarantino L, Swisher LP: Neuro-otologic studies in multiple sclerosis. *Laryngoscope* 76:1798–1809, 1966.

de Quiros J: Accelerated speech audiometry, an examination of test results. (Translated by J Tonndorf.) *Trans Beltone Inst Hear Res* 17:48, 1964.

Dirks D, Kamm C, Bower D, Betsworth A: Use of performance-intensity functions for diagnosis. *J Speech Hear Disord* 42:408–415, 1977.

Egan J: Articulation testing methods. *Laryngoscope* 558:955–991, 1948.

Fairbanks G, Everitt W, Jaeger R: Methods for time or frequency compression-expansion of speech. *Transactions of IRE-PGA AU-2*, 1954, pp 7–12.

Fairbanks G, Guttman N, Miron M: Effects of time compression upon the comprehension of connected speech. *J Speech Hear Disord* 22:10–19, 1957.

Fairbanks G, Kodman F: Word intelligibility as a function of time compression. *J Acoust Soc Am* 29:636–644, 1957.

Flowers A, Costello MR, Small V: *Manual for Flowers-Costello Test of Central Auditory Abilities.* Dearborn, MI, Perceptual Learning Systems, 1970.

Freeman BA, Beasley DS: Discrimination of time-altered sentential approximations and monosyllables by children with reading problems. *J Speech Hear Res* 21:497–506, 1978.

Freeman B, Church G: Recall and repetition of time-compressed sentential approximations by normal-hearing young adults. *J Am Audiol Soc* 3:47–50, 1977.

French NR, Steinberg JC: Factors governing the intelligibility of speech sounds. *J Acoust Soc Am* 19:90–119, 1947.

Gaeth J: A Study of Phonemic Regression in Relation to Hearing Loss. Doctoral dissertation, Northwestern University, Evanston, IL, 1948.

Gang R: The effects of age on the diagnostic utility of the rollover phenomenon. *J Speech Hear Disord* 41:63–69, 1976.

Garvey WD: The intelligibility of abbreviated speech patterns. *Q J Speech* 39:296–306, 1953a.

Garvey WD: The intelligibility of speeded speech. *J Exp Psychol* 45:102–108, 1953b.

Gilroy J, Lynn GE: Reversibility of abnormal auditory findings in cerebral hemisphere lesions. *J Neurol Sci* 21:117–131, 1974.

Goetzinger C, Proud G, Dirks D, Embrey J: Study of hearing in advanced age. *Arch Otolaryngol* 73:662–674, 1961.

Goldstein BA: The Effect of Cochlear Dysfunction on Central Auditory Speech Test Performance. Doctoral dissertation, The City University of New York, New York, 1980.

Goldstein R: Hearing and speech in follow-up of left hemispherectomy. *J Speech Hear Disord* 26:126–219, 1961.

Goldstein R, Goodman A, King R: Hearing and speech in infantile hemiplegia before and after hemiplegia. *Neurology* 6:869–875, 1956.

Grimes AM, Mueller HG, Williams DL: Speech audiometry: clinical considerations in the use of time-compressed speech. *Ear Hearing* 5:114–117, 1984.

Hansen C, Reske-Nielsen E: Pathological studies in presbycusis. *Arch Otolaryngol* 82:115–132, 1965.

Hawkins JE Jr, Stevens SS: The masking of pure tones and of speech by white noise. *J Acoust Soc Am* 22:6–13, 1950.

Hayes D: Central auditory problems and the aging process. In Beasley DS, Davis GA (eds): *Aging: Communication Processes and Disorders.* New York, Grune & Stratton, 1981, pp 257–266.

Hayes D, Jerger J: Aging and the use of hearing aids. *Scand Audiol* 8:33–40, 1979.

Heilman KM, Hammer LC, Wilder BJ: An audiometric defect in temporal lobe dysfunction. *Neurology* 23:384–386, 1973.

Hinojosa R, Naunton RF: Presbycusis. In Paparella MM, Shumrick DA (eds): *The Ear. Otolaryngology.* Philadelphia, WB Saunders, 1980, vol 2, pp 1777–1787.

Hodgson W: Audiological report of a patient with left hemispherectomy. *J Speech Hear Disord* 32:39–45, 1967.

Jerger J: Audiological manifestations of lesions in the auditory nervous system. *Laryngoscope* 70:417–425, 1960a.

Jerger J: Observations on auditory behavior in lesions of the central auditory pathways. *Arch Otolaryngol* 71:797–806, 1960b.

Jerger J: Auditory tests for disorders of the central auditory mechanism. In Alford BR, Fields WS (eds): *Neurological Aspects of Auditory and Vestibular Disorders.* Springfield, IL, Charles C Thomas, 1964, pp 77–86.

Jerger J: Development of synthetic sentence identification (SSI) as a tool for speech audiometry. In Røjskjaer C (ed): *Speech Audiometry* (2nd Danavox Symposium). Odense, Denmark, Danavox, 1970a, pp 44–65.

Jerger J: Diagnostic significance of SSI test procedures: retrocochlear site. In Røjskjaer C (ed): *Speech Audiometry* (2nd Danavox Symposium). Odense, Denmark, Danavox, 1970b, pp 163–175.

Jerger J: Audiological findings in aging. *Adv Otorhinollaryngol* 20:115–124, 1973.

Jerger J, Hayes D: Diagnostic speech audiometry. *Arch Otolaryngol* 103:216–222, 1977.

Jerger J, Jerger S: Diagnostic significance of PB word functions. *Arch Otolaryngol* 93:573–580, 1971.

Jerger J, Jerger S: Auditory findings in brainstem disorders. *Arch Otolaryngol* 99:324–350, 1974.

Jerger J, Jerger S: Clinical validity of central auditory tests. *Scand Audiol* 4:147–163, 1975.

Jerger J, Jerger S: Comments on "The effects of age on the diagnostic utility of the rollover phenomenon." *J Speech Hear Disord* 41:556–557, 1976.

Jerger J, Speaks C, Trammell J: A new approach to speech audiometry. *J Speech Hear Disord* 33:318–328, 1968.

Jerger S, Jerger J: Extra- and intra-axial brainstem auditory disorders. *Audiology* 14:93–117, 1975.

Katinsky S, Lovrinic J, Buchheit W: Cochlear findings in VIIIth nerve tumors. *Audiology* 11:213–217, 1972.

Keith RW: Audiological and auditory-language tests of central auditory function. In Keith RW (ed): *Central Auditory and Language Disorders in Children.* Houston, College-Hill Press, 1981, pp 61–76.

Kirikae I, Sato T, Shitara T: A study of hearing in advanced age. *Laryngoscope* 74:205–220, 1964.

Klumpp RG, Webster JC: Intelligibility of time-compressed speech. *J Acoust Soc Am* 33:265–267, 1961.

Konkle DF, Beasley DS, Bess F: Intelligibility of time-altered speech in relation to chronological aging. *J Speech Hear Res* 20:108–115, 1977.

Korsan-Bengtsen M: Distorted speech audiometry: a methodological and clinical study. *Acta Otolaryngol [Suppl] (Stockh)* 310:7–75, 1973.

Kryter KD: Effects of ear protective devices on the intelligibility of speech in noise. *J Acoust Soc Am* 18:413–417, 1946.

Kurdziel S, Noffsinger D, Olsen W: Performance by cortical lesion patients on 40% and 60% time-compressed materials. *J Am Audiol Soc* 2:3–7, 1976.

Kurdziel S, Rintelmann WF, Beasley D: Performance of noise-induced hearing impaired listeners on time-compressed CNC monosyllables. *J Am Audiol Soc* 1:54–60, 1975.

Lee F: Time compression and expansion of speech by the sampling method. *J Audio Eng Soc* 20:738–742,

1972.

Licklider JCR: The influence of interaural phase relations upon the masking of speech by white noise. *J Acoust Soc Am* 20:150–159, 1948.

Licklider JCR, Miller GA: The perception of speech. In Stevens SS (ed): *Handbook of Experimental Psychology.* New York, Wiley, 1951, pp 1040–1074.

Luterman DM, Welsh OL, Melrose J: Responses of aged males to time-altered speech stimuli. *J Speech Hear Res* 9:226–230, 1966.

Lynn GE, Benitez JT, Eisenbrey AB, Gilroy J, Wilner HI: Neuro-audiological correlates in cerebral hemisphere lesions: temporal and parietal lobe tumors. *Audiol J Aud Commun* 11:115–134, 1972.

Lynn GE, Gilroy J: Auditory manifestations of lesions of the corpus collosum. *ASHA* 13:566, 1971.

Lynn GE, Gilroy J: Neuro-audiological abnormalities in patients with temporal-lobe tumors. *J Neurol Sci* 17:167–184, 1972.

Lynn GE, Gilroy J: Effects of brain lesions on the perception of monotic and dichotic speech stimuli. In Sullivan MD (ed): *Central Auditory Processing Disorders.* Omaha, University of Nebraska, 1975, pp 47–83.

Lynn GE, Gilroy J: Evaluation of central auditory dysfunction in patients with neurological disorders. In Keith RW (ed): *Central Auditory Dysfunction.* New York, Grune & Stratton, 1977, pp 177–221.

Manning WH, Johnston KL, Beasley DS: The performance of children with auditory perceptual disorders on a time-compressed speech discrimination measure. *J Speech Hear Disord* 42:77–84, 1977.

Martin FN, Clark JG: Audiologic detection of auditory processing disorders in children. *J Am Audiol Soc* 3:140–146, 1977.

Matzker J: Two new methods for the assessment of central auditory functions in cases of brain disease. *Ann Otol Rhinol Laryngol* 68:1185–1197, 1959.

Miller GA: The masking of speech. *Psychol Bull* 44:105–129, 1947.

Miller GA, Licklider JCR: The intelligibility of interrupted speech. *J Acoust Soc Am* 22:167–173, 1950.

Miltenberger GE, Dawson GJ, Raica AN: Central auditory testing with peripheral hearing loss. *Arch Otolaryngol* 104:11–15, 1978.

Morales-Garcia C, Poole JO: Masked speech audiometry in central deafness. *Acta Otolaryngol (Stockh)* 74:307–316, 1972.

Musiek FE, Geurkink NA: Auditory perceptual problems in children: considerations for the otolaryngologist and audiologist. *Laryngoscope* 90:962–971, 1980.

Musiek FE, Geurkink NA: Auditory brain stem response and central auditory test findings for patients with brain stem lesions: a preliminary report. *Laryngoscope* 92:891–900, 1982.

Musiek FE, Wilson DH, Pinheiro ML: Audiological manifestations in "split-brain" patients. *J Am Audiol Soc* 5:25–29, 1979.

Noffsinger PD, Kurdziel SA: Assessment of central auditory lesions. In Rintelmann WF (ed): *Hearing Assessment.* Baltimore, University Park Press, 1979, pp 351–377.

Noffsinger D, Olsen WO, Carhart R, Hart CW, Sahgal V: Auditory and vestibular aberrations in multiple sclerosis. *Acta Otolaryngol [Suppl] (Stockh)* 303:1–

63, 1972.

Olsen WO, Matkin ND: Speech audiometry. In Rintelmann WF (ed): *Hearing Assessment.* Baltimore, University Park Press, 1979, pp 133–206.

Olsen WO, Noffsinger D, Kurdziel S: Speech discrimination in quiet and in white noise by patients with peripheral and central lesions. *Acta Otolaryngol (Stockh)* 80:375–382, 1975.

Orchik DJ: Peripheral auditory problems and the aging process. In Beasley DS, Davis GA (eds): *Aging Communication Processes and Disorders.* New York, Grune & Stratton, 1981, pp 243–255.

Orchik DJ, Burgess J: Synthetic sentence identification as a function of the age of the listener. *J Am Audiol Soc* 3:42–46, 1977.

Orchik DJ, Oelschlaeger ML: Time-compressed speech discrimination in children and its relationship to articulation. *J Am Audiol Soc* 3:37–41, 1977.

Ormson K, Williams D: Central auditory function as assessed by time-compressed speech with elementary school children having articulatory and reading problems. Paper presented at the convention of the American Speech and Hearing Association, Washington, DC, Nov 1975.

Pestalozza G, Shore I: Clinical evaluation of presbycusis on the basis of different tests of auditory function. *Laryngoscope* 65:1136–1163, 1955.

Pinheiro ML: Tests of central auditory function in children with learning disabilities. In Keith RW (ed): *Central Auditory Dysfunction.* New York, Grune & Stratton, 1977, pp 223–256.

Quaranta A, Cervellera G: Masking level differences in central nervous system diseases. *Arch Otolaryngol* 103:482–484, 1977.

Rintelmann WF, Beasley D, Lynn G: Time-Compressed CNC Monosyllables: Case Findings in Central Auditory Disorders. Paper presented to the Michigan Speech and Hearing Association, Detroit, 1974a.

Rintelmann WF, Lynn GE: Speech stimuli for assessment of central auditory disorders. In Konkle DF, Rintelmann WF (eds): *Principles of Speech Audiometry.* Baltimore, University Park Press, 1983, pp 231–284.

Rintelmann WF, Schumaier DR: Experiment III: factors affecting speech discrimination in a clinical setting: list equivalence, hearing loss, and phonemic regression. Six experiments on speech discrimination utilizing CNC monosyllables. *J Aud Res* 2(suppl):12–15, 1974.

Ross M, Lerman J: A picture identification test for hearing-impaired children. *J Speech Hear Res* 13:44–53, 1970.

Samorajski T: How the human brain responds to aging. *J Am Geriatr Soc* 24:4–11, 1976.

Sanderson-Leepa ME, Rintelmann WF: Articulation functions and test-retest performance of normal-hearing children on three speech discrimination tests: WIPI, PBK-50, and N.U. Auditory Test No. 6. *J Speech Hear Disord* 41:503–519, 1976.

Schuckers GH, Shriner TH, Daniloff RG: Auditory reassembly of segmental sentences by children. *J Speech Hear Res* 16:116–127, 1973.

Schuknecht HF: Further observations on the pathology of presbycusis. *Arch Otolaryngol* 80:369–382, 1964.

Schuknecht HF: Disorders of growth, metabolism and aging. In: *Pathology of the Ear.* Cambridge, MA,

Harvard University Press, 1974, ch 10, pp 351–410.

Schwartz DM, Mikus B: Performance of normal hearing listeners on the time-compressed modified rhyme test. *J Am Audiol Soc* 3:14–19, 1977.

Shirinian MJ, Arnst DJ: PI-PB rollover in a group of aged listeners. *Ear Hearing* 1:50–53, 1980.

Shirinian MJ, Arnst DJ: Patterns in the performance-intensity functions for phonetically balanced word lists and synthetic sentences in aged listeners. *Arch Otolaryngol* 108:15–20, 1982.

Speaks C: Evaluation of disorders of the central auditory system. In Paparella MM, Shumrick DA (eds): *The Ear. Otolaryngology.* Philadelphia, WB Saunders, 1980, vol 2, pp 1846–1860.

Speaks C, Jerger J: Method for measurement of speech identification. *J Speech Hear Res* 8:185–194, 1965.

Sticht TG, Gray BB: The intelligibility of time compressed words as a function of age and hearing loss. *J Speech Hear Res* 12:443–448, 1969.

Teatini GP: Sensitized speech tests (SST): results in normal subjects. In Røjskjaer C (ed): *Speech Audiometry* (2nd Danavox Symposium). Odense, Denmark, Danavox Foundation, 1970, p 37.

Tillman T, Carhart R: An Expanded Test for Speech Discrimination Utilizing CNC Monosyllabic Words: N.U. Auditory Test No. 6. Technical Report SAM-TR-66-65, USAF School of Aerospace Medicine, Aerospace Medical Division (AFSC), Brooks Air Force Base, TX, 1966.

White EJ: Children's performance on the SSW test and Willeford battery: interim clinical data. In Keith RW (ed): *Central Auditory Dysfunction.* New York, Grune & Stratton, 1977, pp 319–340.

Willeford JA: Assessing central auditory behavior in children: a test battery approach. In Keith RW (ed): *Central Auditory Dysfunction.* New York, Grune & Stratton, 1977, pp 43–72.

Willeford JA: Central auditory behaviors in learning-disabled children. *Semin Speech Lang Hear* 1:127–140, 1980.

Willeford JA, Billger JM: Auditory perception in children with learning disabilities. In Katz J (ed): *Handbook of Clinical Audiology,* ed 2. Baltimore, Williams & Wilkins, 1978, pp 410–425.

CHAPTER 12

Dichotic Speech Tests in the Detection of Central Auditory Dysfunction

FRANK E. MUSIEK, Ph.D.
MARILYN L. PINHEIRO, Ph.D.

The technical and procedural aspects of dichotic tests are presented by Drs. Musiek and Pinheiro. Binaural integration and binaural separation tasks are discussed as well as the results of clinical research on patients with brainstem lesions, cortical/ hemispheric damage, and interhemispheric (corpus callosum) pathology.

Dichotic speech testing, introduced by Broadbent (1954), requires the simultaneous presentation of a different speech signal to each of the ears. Since its inception, this procedure has garnered considerable interest as a research and clinical tool (Berlin and McNeil, 1976). It has primarily been used either to measure hemispheric asymmetry (Kimura, 1961a) or to indicate brain dysfunction (Kimura, 1961b).

This chapter will consider the use of dichotic speech tests as a tool in the detection of lesions of the central nervous system (CNS). It will describe technical and procedural aspects to be considered when using these tests: use and preservation of tapes, acoustics, and normative data. It will describe the two major dichotic listening tasks and the tests falling within each category and will then review the dichotic speech findings on subjects with lesions of the central nervous system (CNS). The chapter will conclude with a brief mention of other types of dichotic testing.

TECHNICAL AND PROCEDURAL ASPECTS

Use and Preservation of Dichotic Tapes

High quality magnetic tape must be used for the recording of dichotic speech stimuli. The tape recorder should be a quarter- or half-track instrument. Both are viable for dichotic materials; however, the half-track instrument has a slightly better signal to noise ratio. Acoustic difficulties can arise when half-track tape is played on a quarter-track recorder (see Berlin and Cullen, 1975 for more details).

The heads of a tape recorder should be cleaned often and their alignment checked. If the heads are not in good working order, unwanted noise and acoustic distortion can occur.

In using tapes on which complex materials are recorded, such as dichotic and other central auditory test materials, these writers find a reel-to-reel recorder played at 7½ ips superior to a cassette tape recorder played at a slower rate. To maintain acoustic fidelity, tapes should be stored "tails out" at comfortable room temperatures.

Acoustics

Acoustics are an important consideration in the clinical application of dichotic testing. This section reviews a few prominent acoustical factors in dichotic listening.

Onset-Offset-Alignment

The recording of dichotic speech requires careful attention to time alignment (Cutting, 1976). In some tests onsets for items on each channel are closely matched, while other tests have considerable differences in onset times of the dichotic items. Generally, the closer the onset times, the more difficult the task and the more prominent the ear advantage. One of many other factors (Berlin and Cullen, 1975) is the length of the dichotic token. Dichotic words are generally easier to recognize than consonant/vowel (CV) syllables because their length allows more acoustic, temporal, and linguistic cues. Offset alignment is also a factor in dichotic listening. If a phoneme lags in a dichotic presentation, it is more accurately reported than the competing (leading) phoneme. This lag effect, documented by Berlin et al (1973), may not be present in individuals with brain disorders (Berlin et al, 1975b).

Intensity

The intensity level of a speech stimulus affects its intelligibility. If speech materials are not presented at high enough levels, performance will suffer (Roeser et al, 1972). Asymmetries in intensity between two channels may bias a dichotic test. Though there is evidence that small differences may be inconsequential, it is worthwhile to acoustically check and compare the intensity levels (Berlin and Cullen, 1975).

Phonemic Considerations

In speech, natural characteristics of some phonemes make them more perceptible than others. For example, voiceless stops such as "p" are perceived better than voiced stops such as "b" (Studdert-Kennedy et al, 1972; Berlin and Cullen, 1975). If these effects are not counterbalanced, they may bias a dichotic paradigm.

Signal to Noise Ratio

The signal to noise ratio affects the accuracy of speech perception. The poorer the ratio, the poorer the intelligibility for speech. In dichotic listening each channel should have an equally good ratio. If this is not the case, the dichotic results may be biased (Berlin and Cullen, 1975).

Listening Strategies

Depending upon the dichotic task, the subject often develops a listening strategy that helps in completing the task. These strategies vary from person to person and undoubtedly have an effect on performance in dichotic listening. (For more discussion of strategies in dichotic listening see Weiss and House, 1973.)

Normative Data

Normative data must be carefully established before tests are used clinically. The normative sample should represent subjects in a wide range of vocations, social and economic environments, and age groups. Hearing sensitivity in conventional speech discrimination measures should be symmetrical and within normal limits bilaterally.

In normal subjects a right ear advantage (REA) has been reported consistently (Kimura, 1961a; Bryden, 1963; Dirks, 1964; Berlin et al, 1973), with the REA greater as the stimuli are more closely aligned (Berlin et al, 1975b). Though this REA is commonly accepted, Efron (in Chapter 9) raises some interesting views which should cause one to question the basis of this tenet. He claims that symmetrical hearing cannot be assumed even if thresholds are similar. At suprathreshold levels, hearing abilities may be poorer for one ear than the other, and this difference could bias dichotic results. He points out that inferring hemispheric specialization on rather weak and variable ear advantages (such as for speech and music) may be inappropriate and tenuous. He questions the averaging of scores, earphone reversal for counterbalancing, acoustic coupling effects, and the assumption of symmetrical brainstem pathways as viable notions in dichotic listening research. His chapter calls attention to some commonly overlooked variables in dichotic listening which need further investigation and consideration and which bear directly on the establishment of normative data.

In selecting and establishing norms for dichotic speech tests, it is advantageous to use a task on which normal subjects do well.

This allows a greater range over which abnormal scores may be differentiated from normal scores. If the task is relatively easy, variability is often (but not always) reduced. Mediocre scores with a large standard deviation make it difficult to differentiate the abnormal performance of a patient.

Subcortical Asymmetry (Peripheral Hearing)

There are subcortical asymmetries that may bias dichotic listening results (see Chapter 9). One of the most common is hearing loss. Conductive losses primarily affect only the intensity aspect, but sensory deficits may be associated with recruitment, tolerance problems, poor frequency, intensity, temporal resolution, and other such factors. All of these may affect the dichotic speech test results.

Roeser et al (1976) have clearly demonstrated how dichotic CVs and digit results are affected by sensorineural hearing loss. Normal hearers performed better than hearing-impaired subjects. Also, normal hearers showed a REA on both tests, while the hearing-impaired group did not. Individual ear preferences increased as hearing loss increased for digits and CVs. There also appeared to be a relationship between monaural speech discrimination tests (W-22) and performance on dichotic speech tasks.

Based on Roeser's study, it seems critical to evaluate pure tone sensitivity and monaural speech discrimination ability before dichotic testing. This allows documentation of normal sensitivity and speech discrimination and permits consideration of possible effects on dichotic listening when these measures are neither normal nor bilaterally symmetrical.

If one employs dichotic speech tasks to assess cortical function, both the auditory periphery and brainstem pathways should be symmetrical and normal. Brainstem asymmetries, like peripheral asymmetries, can serve to bias dichotic results (see Chapter 9, and the latter part of this chapter).

DICHOTIC SPEECH TASKS

We will consider two major kinds of dichotic listening tasks: binaural integration and binaural separation. A description is

given for the more popular tests falling within each category.

Binaural Integration Tasks

Binaural integration tasks require the subject to respond to the stimuli presented to both ears, that is, if the words "back" and "run" are dichotically presented, the subject must repeat both words. Three types of binaural integration tasks will be discussed: dichotic digits and words, staggered spondaic words (SSW), CVs (nonsense syllables).

Dichotic Digits and Words

In reviewing the literature it becomes apparent that the majority of dichotic studies have used digits or words. There are a variety of ways dichotic digits or words can be administered. A common approach is mentioned in some of the authors' work (Musiek et al, 1979; Musiek and Wilson, 1979; Musiek, 1983). This procedure calls for the presentation of two digits to each ear simultaneously. (For example, the digits 8,1 are presented to the left ear and 2,9 to the right ear.

LE: 8,1
RE: 2,9

They are naturally spoken and placed on tape. All digits from one through ten are used with the exception of seven. The digits are presented at a 50 dB sensation level (SL) in reference to the subject's spondee threshold or pure tone average. Onset alignments and other acoustic details of the test items are reported elsewhere (Musiek, 1983). Forty digits (20 pairs) are presented to each ear. The subject repeats all the digits heard in any order (free recall). A percentage correct is derived for each ear. This version of the dichotic digits requires little time to administer and is easily scored (Musiek, 1983).

Other procedures have also been used with these stimuli in an attempt to detect CNS dysfunction. Kimura (1961b) used three digits to each ear as her dichotic stimulus in examining subjects with temporal lobe damage. This approach, or a highly similar one, has been used by a variety of other investigators in testing brain-damaged subjects (Shankweiler, 1966; Netley, 1972; Bakker et al, 1973; Siegenthaler and Knellinger, 1981).

Many investigators used a modification of this approach to measure selected parameter effects on brain-damaged subjects. Roeser and Daly (1974) used three digit pairs but performed an intensity function as digits were presented at intensities from 10 to 70 dB SL. Other investigators changed the number of digits in the dichotic pair, with some using one or two (Mazzuchi and Parma, 1978; Sparks et al, 1970; Petit and Noll, 1979; Niccum et al, 1981) and others four or five (Bryden and Zurif, 1970; Schulhoff and Goodglass, 1969). The rate of digit presentation was varied by some authors (Bryden and Zurif, 1970; Oxbury and Oxbury, 1969). Though most studies used free recall, Bryden and Zurif (1970) required an ordered recall. The subject was asked to repeat the digits to the left ear first, then those to the right ear, or vice versa. Tsunoda and Oka (1971) reported yet a different dichotic digit task. They asked their subjects to add the two digits presented to each ear, i.e.,

LE: $4 + 3 = 7$
RE: $2 + 4 = 6$

Fewer approaches have been used with dichotic word presentation. The most traditional one is reported by Sparks and Geschwind (1968) and Sparks et al (1970). They presented monosyllabic words (animal names), one to each ear. These words were presented at 44 dB above the pure tone average for each ear. There were 20 words presented to each ear (total = 40 words). The subject simply repeated all the words heard (free recall). Hutchinson (1973), in his report on aphasics, used a similar approach, but the initial consonant in his monosyllabic word pairs was the same. Niccum et al (1981), like Hutchinson, used dichotic monosyllables, but also used words in which only the initial phoneme was different (e.g., fan, man). This is similar to the rhyme test of Wexler and Hawles (1983); however, in this task the words are synthetic. Niccum also used high contrast words (e.g., cloud, book) to assess auditory function of aphasics. Bisyllabic (Mazzuchi and Parma, 1978) and even trisyllabic words (Damasio and Damasio, 1979) have been used in dichotic assessment of brain dysfunction.

Staggered Spondaic Words (SSW)

Another distinct and unique modification of dichotic word tests was reported by Katz in 1962. This test was named the Staggered Spondaic Word (SSW) test and has since become perhaps the most widely used central auditory test in audiology (Katz, 1977).

The SSW is composed of two spondees with a staggered onset. The last half of the first spondee and the first half of the second spondee are presented dichotically, while the remaining spondee segments are presented in isolation to opposite ears. The following is an example of one test item:

```
        (LNC)   (LC)
LE:     race    horse
RE:             street    car
                (RC)     (RNC)
```

Abbreviations used are LNC, left noncompeting; LC, left competing; RC, right competing; RNC, right noncompeting. The subject is required to repeat all the words presented. The 40 test items are presented at 50 dB SL (re: SRT). Katz has developed some rather extensive scoring and interpretational methods which can be only briefly mentioned here (for details see Brunt, 1978). In addition to monitoring errors in the competing (dichotic) and noncompeting (isolated words) condition, Katz recommends checking for a response bias. These include reversals and ear and order effects. Reversals (of which there are several kinds) mean the order of the words is repeated incorrectly. For example, the subject may say streetcar, racehorse when he should say racehorse, streetcar. Since lead items are alternated between ears, it is possible to compare the number of errors for the lead spondee for the left and right ear. If one ear has at least five errors more than the other, it is termed an "ear effect." Order effects compare errors for first vs second presented spondees, with a difference of five considered significant. The SSW also attempts to account for peripheral hearing loss by subtracting the percent error for speech discrimination from the SSW raw score in each of the four conditions. There also is a classification for degree of deficit on the test, ranging from a mark of normal to severely depressed. To use this classification, one combines the scores from each ear in the competing and noncompeting condition and divides by two. In addition, the most extreme ear score, right or left (usually the most errors), and the condition (either LNC, LC, RC, RNC) is used in this classification. See Brunt (1978) for more detailed information on the administration and scoring of the SSW.

CV's (Nonsense Syllables)

Consonant-vowels, such as ba, da, ga (voiced) and pa, ta, ka (unvoiced), have made their way from an entirely experimental procedure into the clinical domain. Shankweiler and Studdert-Kennedy (1967) and Berlin et al (1968) composed some of the early paradigms for this procedure as well as for single phonemes (vowels). In their early work, synthetic speech was used, and durations were approximately 200 msec. Onset alignments were close to simultaneous (Shankweiler and Studdert-Kennedy, 1967; Lowe et al, 1970). This was the experimental "state of the art" until Berlin et al (1973) introduced the "lag" procedure using CVs. Berlin and his colleagues studied the effect of lagging the CV presented to one ear in reference to the other. Onsets were at 15-, 30-, 60-, and 90 msec time lags, and the presentation level, often poorly defined in earlier studies, was 78 dB SPL (re: 1 kHz).

Subjects usually responded in a free recall strategy (Berlin et al, 1973), indicating the appropriate CV through either verbal report, written report, or selection from multiple choices (closed set) (Niccum et al, 1981; Porter et al, 1976; Oscar-Berman et al, 1975; Berlin et al, 1973).

Berlin's tape has 60 pairs of CVs at 0-, 30-, 60-, and 90 msec time lags. The writers of this chapter feel that it is clinically feasible to employ a maximum of 60 to 120 CV pairs per test session, and we have noted higher scores when using a closed set (circling a correct response from six alternatives) instead of a verbal report.

Binaural Separation Tasks

In a binaural separation task, the subject responds to only the words presented to a designated ear and ignores the other words in the opposite ear. Three types of binaural separation tasks will be discussed: the Com-

peting Sentence Tests, the Northwestern University Number 20 Test (NU 20, previously NU 2), and the Synthetic Sentence Identification with Contralateral Competing Message (SSI-CCM) test.

Competing Sentences

Dichotically presented sentences have been used for some time in most of the early research dealing with attention and selective listening in normal subjects (Moray, 1959; Treisman and Geffen, 1968). In 1968 Willeford (see Willeford, 1977), along with his graduate students, developed a Competing Sentence Test, which has become the most clinically popular test of this type (see also Chapter 14). The test is composed of 25 pairs of simple sentences that are 6 or 7 words in length. The sentences are presented dichotically, with one at 35 dB SL and the other at 50 dB SL (re: SRT). The lower intensity sentence is the *target*, and the higher intensity sentence serves as the *competition*. The subject is to repeat only the target sentence and ignore the competing sentence. One ear receives ten target sentences, while the other is presented ten competing sentences; then this arrangement is reversed. These writers use the five additional sentences as practice, though some investigators use them as a dichotic integration task (Pinheiro, 1977).

Guidelines for scoring the Competing Sentence Test do not seem to be well-detailed in the literature. It is these writers' understanding from discussion and unpublished data from Willeford that the intent of the test is to measure the meaning the sentences carry and not the identification of each word in the sentence. Hence, this format allows variability for interpretation. (In Chapter 14 Willeford discusses this test's usage with children.) Our scheme for scoring the Competing Sentence Test is as follows:

1. Each correctly repeated target sentence is worth 10%. A correct response requires that the content/meaning of the target sentence is not compromised; however, the sentence does not have to be repeated verbatim.
2. Each sentence which is not correct is assigned a 0, 2.5, 5, or 7.5% value, depending upon how much meaning

is lost when the subject repeats the primary sentence (i.e., if one-half the meaning is maintained, 5% credit is given).

Synthetic Sentence Identification with Contralateral Competing Message (SSI-CCM)

The SSI-CCM is the counterpart of the SSI-ICM discussed earlier in Chapter 11. The SSI-ICM uses third order approximations of English sentences which are presented to one ear. The SSI-CCM has the same material, but the meaningful connected discourse is presented to the contralateral ear (Jerger, 1970). The primary message is introduced at a moderate SL (40 dB), while the competing message is varied to produce message to competition ratios ranging from 0 to 40 dB.

The response procedure is a closed set, with the patient pointing to or verbally reporting the number of the sentence that he has heard. The same ten sentences can be used at various SLs; however, their order is randomized for the various lists (Jerger, 1973). An answer sheet allows rapid scoring.

Northwestern University Test No. 20 (NU 20)

The NU 20 was originally developed as a procedure for evaluation of hearing aids (Olsen and Carhart, 1967). Subsequently, however, it has been clinically used as a dichotic speech test for central lesions (Noffsinger et al, 1972). An earlier test, called the NU 2, was also employed as a central test (Jerger, 1964). The main difference between the NU 2 and the NU 20 is the use of different monosyllables (Rintelmann and Lynn, 1983).

The dichotic NU 20 has a carrier phrase, with an NU 6 monosyllable on one channel which is presented to one ear (primary message) while a competing sentence from the Bell Telephone Intelligibility List is presented to the other ear. The alignment is such that the competing sentence begins before the carrier phrase and ends after the monosyllabic word.

Example:

LE: Say the word *pool*.
       (primary message)
RE: What training is given boy scouts?
       (competing sentence)

Based on Jerger's (1964) early work, it has been recommended that the NU 20 (and NU 2) be administered at a −10 dB primary to competing message ratio, with the primary message presented at 40 to 50 dB SL (re: SRT, Noffsinger and Kurdziel, 1979). For the NU 20 the subject's task is to repeat the monosyllabic word(s) and ignore the competing sentence(s). Generally, 50 items are presented to each ear, and a percentage correct is derived. The NU 20 can and has been administered as a monotic test (Musiek, 1977), but more clinical research must be done to ascertain its value in this test condition.

There is one additional binaural separation task that deserves brief mention, although there was only one article published about it to these authors' knowledge. Dobie and Simmons (1971) published a dichotic procedure which employed the CVs, pa, ta, and ka. The subjects were instructed to attend to only one ear (right or left) and report the CV presented to that ear. The attended items were presented at +15 dB, 0 dB, −15 dB, −25 dB, and −35 dB in reference to the unattended items, which were kept at a constant 75 dB SPL. Twenty CV pairs were presented at each intensity level for a total of 100 pairs. Those interested in this test are directed to the Dobie and Simmons' article.

DICHOTIC SPEECH FINDINGS IN LESIONS OF THE CENTRAL NERVOUS SYSTEM

The following section of this chapter embraces the main issue in dichotic speech tests—their value in detecting disorders of the central nervous system. A review of dichotic speech results in patients with brainstem, hemispheric, and interhemispheric lesions is presented.

Brainstem Lesions

There is a paucity of data on dichotic speech tests and brainstem disorders. This is due to two factors: the strong precedent set for the use of dichotic testing as a procedure for cortical/hemispheric evaluation and the difficulty in recruiting brainstem-lesioned subjects simply due to the nature of their problem.

Binaural Integration Tasks

Dichotic Digits. Although dichotic digits have been used primarily in cortical/hemispheric and interhemispheric disorders, they also appear to be of value in brainstem lesions. Stephens and Thornton (1976), using Kimura's form of the dichotic digit test, resported that 5 of 13 patients with brainstem pathology yielded abnormal results. Of the five subnormal findings, three subjects demonstrated unilateral deficits and two bilateral deficits. Siegenthaler and Knellinger (1981) reported dichotic digit results in a subject with a brainstem vascular disorder and three subjects with brainstem neural degeneration. The subject with a vascular disorder demonstrated a severe right ear deficit and essentially normal left ear performance. The mean dichotic scores for the remaining subjects were similar for right and left ears and only slightly below the mean normal scores.

Musiek and Geurkink (1982) reported that seven of ten subjects with brainstem involvement demonstrated abnormal results on the dichotic digit test. Four of these seven subjects showed bilateral abnormalities, while three were unilateral. Musiek (1983), in an extension of the study just mentioned, reported 9 of 12 brainstem subjects with abnormal dichotic digit results.

SSW. Katz (1970) reported a case of left-sided low brainstem tumor. The SSW in this case demonstrated normal performance for the right ear and a severe deficit for the left competing and noncompeting conditions. In the same article, a left-sided high brainstem lesion also showed a left ear deficit in the competing condition.

Jerger and Jerger (1975) compared SSW results on ten patients with intraaxial brainstem lesions to ten normal subjects. The pathological group revealed 44 and 16% (mean) poorer scores for the ear contralateral and ipsilateral to the side of the lesion, respectively. Stephens and Thornton (1976) administered the SSW to 14 patients with brainstem disorders. Six of these fourteen patients yielded abnormal results, with four demonstrating unilateral and two bilateral deficits. Pinheiro et al (1982) reported SSW findings on a patient with a specific gunshot wound to the right side of the pons. Tests showed a mild-moderate (70% correct) left ear deficit in the competing condition and a significant order effect. Rintelmann and Lynn (1983) reported two brainstem tumor cases with SSW results. One was a bilateral pontomesencephalic lesion, which yielded a slight left ear competing condition deficit. The other case was a left-sided pontomedullary lesion, which also showed a severe left ear deficit on SSW. In this latter case, though, pure tone sensitivity was good, and speech discrimination in quiet was very poor for the left ear.

Musiek and Geurkink (1982) and Musiek (1983) reported abnormal SSW results on approximately 60% of their subjects with brainstem disorders. The majority of those who demonstrated only unilateral brainstem lesions showed ipsilateral or bilateral ear abnormalities.

Dichotic CVs. Only one report to these writers' knowledge has been filed on dichotic CVs in a brainstem lesion. Berlin et al (1975a) reported on a patient with a lesion in the area of the right medial geniculate. This patient demonstrated practically complete suppression of the CVs presented to the left ear. Right ear scores were grossly normal.

Binaural Separation Tasks

Competing Sentences. Musiek and Geurkink (1982) and Musiek (1983) have reported abnormal competing sentence test results in about one-half of their subjects with brainstem lesions. In these studies, scores on this test seemed to indicate either very good or extremely poor performance for brainstem-involved subjects. The majority of subjects showed unilateral deficits in the ears ipsilateral to the lesion.

Rintelmann and Lynn (1983), in the two subjects mentioned earlier, reported normal competing sentence results in a patient with a bilateral, high brainstem lesion. However, a patient with a low left-sided brainstem tumor yielded a 0% score on that side and a 100% score contralaterally. Pinheiro et al (1982), in her patient with a right pontine lesion, reported a marked left ear deficit on competing sentences.

The NU 20 or NU 2. Jerger (1964) filed one of the first reports on the performance of subjects (n = 7) with brainstem lesions (rostral to cochlear nuclei) using the forerunner to the NU 20, the NU 2. Jerger showed lower mean scores for the ear contralateral (53%) to the side of the brainstem lesion than for the ear ipsilateral (70%) to the lesion. Noffsinger et al (1972) employed the NU 20 with 54 patients with multiple sclerosis; 12 yielded abnormal scores. It should be understood, however, that multiple sclerosis doesn't exclusively affect the brainstem; some cortical or interhemispheric disruption may also exist in this disease. Noffsinger et al (1975) reported a brainstem case involving the pontomedullary area which yielded scores approaching normal bilaterally on the NU 20.

SSI-CCM. It is clear the SSI-ICM, counterpart to the SSI-CCM, is the appropriate test for assessing brainstem lesions (see Chapter 11). As Jerger (1973) and Jerger and Jerger (1974, 1975) have shown, the dichotically presented SSI-CCM is generally unaffected by brainstem lesions. However, as their 1974 article shows, occasionally abnormal results will be found on the SSI-CCM in brainstem disorders. Because the SSI-ICM is an excellent tool for detecting brainstem involvement and the SSI-CCM is essentially unaffected by these lesions but is sensitive to cortical lesions, these tests complement each other nicely.

Laterality Effects

Many test findings seem unclear and contradictory in relation to brainstem lesions because the brainstem is so compact and intricate and can be affected in a wide variety of ways by a given insult. In dichotic speech tests as well as other central tests, laterality findings and trends are quite variable. Many reports, incuding some from these writers, indicate that ipsilateral and binaural deficits are most common in brainstem lesions (Katz, 1970, 1978; Calearo and Antonelli, 1968; Musiek and Geurkink, 1982; Musiek, 1983). However, Jerger and Jerger (1974, 1975) claim contralateral and binaural deficits are the most common. Jerger and Jerger (1974) bring out an important point concerning intra- vs extraaxial lesions. They

comment that often extraaxial lesions mimic eighth nerve lesions yielding an ipsilateral effect, while intraaxial lesions (above the cochlear nuclei) show contralateral ear effects. Certainly, given the anatomical data about auditory fiber crossover at the brainstem, lesions located lower in the brainstem may be more apt to yield an ipsilateral deficit, while higher lesions may yield a contralateral one. However, all of the views just mentioned do not accommodate every situation. The multiple effects of a given lesion and the neurophysiological complexity of the brainstem disallow clear interpretation of laterality in dichotic test results at this time.

General Comments

Determination of the value of dichotic tests in the detection of brainstem lesions requires further study. There are a variety of case reports, but only a few major studies in this area. Reliable trends and indices are difficult to observe. The dichotic integration tests appear more sensitive to brainstem disorders than the dichotic separation tests; however, even the former demonstrate only moderate detection rates for brainstem lesions. Given the excellent capability of auditory brainstem response (ABR) and other tests such as masking level difference (MLD) for detecting brainstem disorders, dichotic tests may be unnecessary; more data are needed to give support to this viewpoint.

Cortical/Hemispheric Lesions

The greatest effort in the use of dichotic speech tasks has been in measuring hemispheric asymmetry and/or specialization. Dichotic listening tasks have been used to test individuals with various kinds of brain disorders (Fig. 12.1). If one hemisphere is damaged and is dominant for a specific type of function, then procedures which test that particular function should show abnormal results. A preponderance of theoretical, clinical, and experimental data indicates that the right and left hemispheres are dominant for different functions in normal individuals. Table 12.1 provides a description of these differing functions.

An interhemispheric summation is needed for functions requiring both sides of the brain in order to decode and respond most appropriately to a given stimulus. This requires good communication between left and right hemispheres. Thus, in attempting to measure auditory function at the cortical level one must be concerned not only with the capabilities of each hemisphere but also with interhemispheric interaction. Some dichotic speech studies are able to measure intra- and interhemispheric dysfunctions.

Binaural Integration Tasks

Dichotic Digits and Words. Kimura (1961b) was one of the first to employ dichotic digits in testing brain-damaged subjects. Several important findings evolved

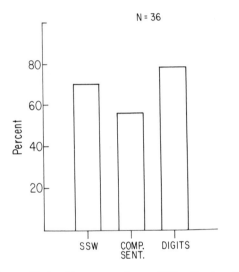

Figure 12.1. The percentage of 36 patients with CNS lesions with abnormal results on the SSW, competing sentences, and dichotic digits. All these patients demonstrated either normal hearing or a mild hearing loss bilaterally. All patients had excellent speech discrimination ability bilaterally. Twelve patients had brainstem involvement, and 24 had cortical/hemispheric lesions.

from this now classic study. Kimura's subjects had undergone partial removal of the anterior midtemporal lobe for control of cortical seizure activity. After surgery, deficits were noted in the ear contralateral to the operated hemisphere. In many cases, when a portion of the left temporal lobe was excised, deficits were noted in both ears. This did not occur when the right temporal lobe was involved. In six patients who had Heschl's gyrus removed, a greater deficit was noted than for any of the other lesion sites. Kimura did not note any impairment on dichotic digits for a number of patients with frontal lobe excisions.

Based on her findings, Kimura developed a model for dichotic perception. The model, which also has a physiologic base (Rosenweig, 1951), states that the contralateral input from cochlea to cortex is stronger than the ipsilateral input. In a situation where there is monaural input, either pathway is able to initiate the appropriate neural function to allow accurate perception of a speech signal. However, in the dichotic situation the contralateral pathway dominates (Fig. 12.2). The greater number of neural elements in this pathway may, in the dichotic condition, result in a suppression of the ipsilateral fibers. In a dichotic situation there may be competition for the same neural tissue, with the stronger (contralateral) pathway winning the competition. Hence, when one hemisphere is damaged, the effect is most readily seen in the contralateral ear (Fig. 12.3). Kimura's model and pathological findings have generally been supported by many others using a variety of dichotic tasks (Berlin et al, 1972a, 1973; Sparks et al, 1970; Musiek and Sachs, 1980; Speaks et al 1975; Studdert-Kennedy and Shankweiler, 1970; and others). Alternative models and considerations have been discussed and have

Table 12.1
Description of the Types of Functions Attributed to the Cerebral Hemispheres

Left hemisphere	Right hemisphere
Speech (language)	Music
Sequencing (temporal ordering)	Spatial/artistic
Detailed	General
Analytic	Gestalt
Reading, writing	Figure and facial recognition
Controlled	Emotional
Concrete	Abstract
Active	Receptive

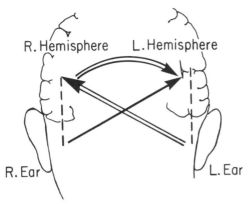

Figure 12.2. The auditory routes to the cortex. This also shows the basis for the left ear deficit for dichotic speech tests in split-brain patients. That is, given that ipsilateral pathways are suppressed in the dichotic mode contralateral inputs become highly dominant. In the dichotic situation, the stimulus presented to the right ear goes directly to the left hemisphere; hence, a verbal report can be made for this stimulus. However, left ear stimuli go to the right hemisphere. If the corpus callosum is compromised there cannot be transfer to the left hemisphere; hence, there is inability to verbally report left ear speech stimuli. (From Musiek F, Sachs E Jr: Reversible neuroaudiologic findings in a case of right frontal lobe abscess with recovery. *Arch Otolaryngol* 106:280–283, 1980. Copyright 1980, American Medical Association.)

merit (Speaks et al, 1975; Siditis, 1982), but the Kimura model remains the most popular.

Subsequent to Kimura's 1961 article, a variety of other studies using dichotic digits or words generally supported her findings in brain-damaged subjects (Schuloff and Goodglass, 1969; Goodglass, 1967; Oxbury and Oxbury, 1969; Netley, 1972; Tsunoda and Oka, 1971; Zurif and Ramier, 1972; Mazzuchi and Parma, 1978; Niccum et al, 1981; Musiek, 1983). Some of these reports added new information or served to generate new ideas about dichotic testing approaches and central auditory dysfunction. For example, Oxbury and Oxbury (1969) showed that the order in which the digits were reported was affected by the side of the lesion. Essentially, the digits presented to the ear contralateral to the lesion (temporal lobectomy) were repeated after the digits presented to the ear contralateral to the healthy hemisphere.

Mazzuchi and Parma (1978) reported that

in subjects (temporal lobe epileptics) with unilateral brain damage, contralateral ear presentation of digits was subjectively preferred to ipsilateral ear presentation. Speaks (1975) used the dichotic digit test on two patients with temporal lobe lesions and reported marked contralateral ear deficits in both subjects. At that time Speaks commented that, although his experience was limited, he felt the digit test was one of the better clinical tests. Niccum et al (1981) used a variety of dichotic tests on 16 aphasic patients with unilateral left hemisphere damage. These subjects showed a mean left ear advantage ranging from approximately 37 to 44% for these tests. On the digits, eight patients scored 50% or less for the ear contralateral to the lesion, while all subjects scored 85% or better for the ipsilateral ear.

Musiek (1983), using the version of the dichotic digit test described earlier, tested 21 subjects with intracranial lesions (9 brainstem, 12 hemispheric). Eighteen of these subjects showed abnormal findings in at least one ear. Contralateral mean ear scores were significantly poorer than ipsilateral ear mean scores for the subjects with cortical lesions. This report emphasized the test's clinical feasibility. It was easily scored and

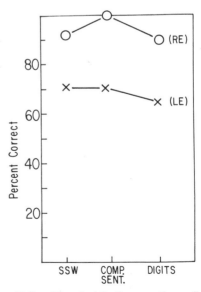

Figure 12.3. Classical findings on three dichotic speech tests for a middle-aged patient who suffered a mild CVA of the right cerebral cortex. Pure tone thresholds indicated symmetrical borderline normal hearing bilaterally with excellent speech discrimination ability bilaterally.

required approximately 4 min to administer. In a companion study (Musiek, 1983), the dichotic digit test was compared to the SSW and competing sentence test for 12 subjects with brainstem lesions and 18 subjects with cortical/hemispheric lesions. The dichotic digit test yielded slightly more abnormal findings for both groups than either the SSW or competing sentences.

SSW. Katz's initial articles on the SSW (Katz, 1962, 1970; Katz et al, 1963) showed case examples of subjects with brain damage and abnormal SSW results. Generally, the lowest scores were for the ear contralateral to the damaged hemisphere. Katz, in a 1968 article, showed a close correspondence between neurological judgment as to the cerebral site of lesion and the SSW findings for 17 patients with cerebral disorders.

Lynn and Gilroy (1972) reported on five patients with anterior and five patients with posterior temporal lobe tumors. According to Brunt's (1978) interpretation of the results of this study, all ten had abnormal SSWs. However, those patients with posterior lesions demonstrated lower scores than those with anterior lesions. Lynn and Gilroy (1975) reported similar results on a larger population of patients with posterior and anterior temporal lobe lesions. McClellen et al (1973), as cited by Brunt (1978), reported SSW results on 15 patients with left hemispheric lesions and 15 with right hemispheric lesions. Both of these groups demonstrated significantly poorer results than a group (N = 15) of normal subjects. In this study, the ears contralateral to the brain lesions yielded lower mean scores, but this was not as evident for left hemisphere lesions as for right. Katz and Pack (1975) clearly showed greater "contralateral" deficits for 13 patients with lesions of the auditory reception area, while mean SSW scores for 17 patients with CNS lesions in other areas of the brain were normal. Similar findings were reported later (Katz 1977). Lynn and Gilroy (1977) showed similar contralateral ear performance on the SSW for right (N = 11) and left (N = 11) hemispheric lesions.

There are several studies which have compared the SSW with other central tests on patients with cortical/hemispheric lesions. Jerger and Jerger (1975) found the SSW to be perhaps the most sensitive to temporal lobe lesions of a group of tests (SSI-ICM, SSI-CCM, performance intensity function

with phonetically balanced words (PI-PB)). However, Olsen and Kurdziel (1978) found an excess number of errors on the SSW in only 4 of 22 patients with cortical lesions, while (Berlin's) dichotic CVs detected far more abnormalities in this group. Collard et al (1982) showed similar performance on the SSW, dichotic digits, and dichotic CVs for subjects who were temporal lobectomy candidates. Approximately one-half of the subjects showed abnormal scores on these tests. In addition, there was not a strong trend for contralateral ear deficits in this group of subjects.

Musiek (1983), as mentioned earlier, compared SSW, competing sentences, and dichotic digits on subjects with brainstem (N = 12) and hemispheric lesions (N = 18).

Dichotic CVs. One of the first reports on using dichotic CVs with central auditory nervous system (CANS) damaged patients was by Berlin et al (1972b). They demonstrated that normal subjects obtained better scores for the trailing stimulus when the CV presented to one ear was delayed in time (i.e., 30 to 90 msec). This was termed the "lag effect." In four temporal lobectomy patients this lag effect was lost, and deficits were noted in the ear contralateral to the damaged hemisphere. A subsequent report by Berlin et al (1975b) showed similar results for temporal lobectomies. However, in tests of four hemispherectomy patients, the ear contralateral to the lesion yielded poor CV scores, while the ipsilateral ear scores were higher (near 100%) than data obtained from normal subjects. Berlin et al (1975) interpreted this latter finding as indicating that hemispherectomy patients have neither phonetic nor acoustic competition between the two auditory channels in the brain.

Zurif and Ramier (1972), in one of their early studies, employed dichotic CVs on 20 left and 20 right brain-damaged subjects as well as on a group of normal controls. The right brain-damaged group showed a contralateral ear deficit, but the left brain-damaged subjects revealed similar findings for each ear.

It seems that when the contralateral ear deficit is shown in central nervous system (CNS) disorders, it requires much more intensity to that ear to offset the suppressive effect of the other ear (auditory channel). Berlin et al (1972a) showed that 20 to 40 dB greater intensity was required for the "weak ear" (contralateral to the lesion) to perform as well as the "strong ear" for dichotic CVs.

Speaks et al (1975) showed extremely depressed scores for the ear contralateral to the side of the brain lesion in all ten patients tested with dichotic CVs. Interestingly, even the CVs in a monotic condition were poorer for the ear contralateral to the lesion.

Olsen (1977) reported on CV results in 40 patients with temporal lobectomy. These findings were compared with results from 50 normal subjects. The results are constructed in Table 12.2. Overall, 31 of 40 patients revealed decreased scores in one or both ears for dichotic CVs. In a later study Olsen and Kurdziel (1978) reported dichotic CV scores on 20 of 22 patients with temporal lobe lesions. Olsen and Kurdziel compared these results to findings on SSW for the same group of patients and found the CV test to be more sensitive.

Niccum et al (1981) employed the CV test (and other measures) with 14 aphasic patients with only left hemispheric involvement. A mean left ear advantage of 22% was noted. Eleven patients showed right ear scores below 50%, while five showed left ear scores below the same level. In comparison to dichotic digits and low and high contrast dichotic words the CVs seem to have slightly more potential in detecting overall abnormality. However, the other measures showed greater ear differences and were clinically more usable.

As mentioned earlier, Collard et al (1982) reported that approximately one-half of the temporal lobectomy candidates demonstrated abnormal performance on dichotic CVs. This result was similar to dichotic digits and SSW findings.

Binaural Separation Tasks

Competing Sentences. The competing sentence test has been employed more with learning-disabled children than with neurologically impaired adults. A group of studies done at Wayne State University School of Medicine provides much of the early information on the competing sentence tests and CANS involvement (Lynn and Gilroy, 1972, 1975, 1977). More specifically, in six patients with posterior temporal lobe involvement a 0% score was obtained from the ear contralateral to the lesion, while a 100% score was noted for the ipsilateral ear (Lynn and Gilroy, 1972). However, four of five patients with lesions of the anterior temporal lobe revealed normal findings on competing sentences according to Lynn and Gilroy (1972). Lynn and Gilroy (1977) reported competing sentence results on 11 left and 11 right temporal lobe tumors. Mean scores showed approximately a 40 to 45% poorer score for the ear contralateral to the lesioned hemisphere.

In comparing the competing sentence test and the SSW, strikingly similar results have been shown on the same neurological populations (Lynn and Gilroy, 1972, 1975, 1977). However, for these studies the SSW was scored differently than advocated by Katz (Brunt, 1978). In a study by Musiek (1983) the competing sentence test, SSW, and dichotic digit test were administered to 12 subjects with brainstem lesions and 18 subjects with hemispheric lesions. As mentioned earlier, the competing sentence test did not fare as well as the dichotic digits or SSW. For a unilateral brainstem group it did demonstrate the lowest mean score of the three tests; yet, 6 of 12 subjects with brainstem lesions performed within the normal criteria. Collard et al (1982) reported abnormal results on the competing sentence test for 72% of their temporal lobectomy candidates. This yielded a greater percentage of abnormalities than the SSW, dichotic CVs, and dichotic digits

Northwestern University 20 (or 2). Jerger

Table 12.2
Pattern of Results[a]

RE	LE	Left temporal lobectomy (n = 21)	Right temporal lobectomy (n = 19)
Normal	Normal	6	3
Decreased	Decreased	4	1
Normal	Decreased	6	11
Decreased	Normal	5	4

[a] From Olsen W: Performance of Temporal Lobectomy Patients with Dichotic CV Test Materials. Presented at the ASHA Convention, Chicago, Nov 1977.

(1964) was perhaps the first to evaluate the clinical capability of the NU 2 (now NU 20) in patients with lesions of the CANS. In six patients with lesions that affected Heschl's gyrus, the mean scores were 69 and 24% for the ears ipsilateral and contralateral to the lesion, respectively. Burke and Noffsinger (1976) used the NU 20 with 21 patients with right and 21 patients with left temporal lobe lesions. Mean scores for the ear contralateral to the brain lesion were about 44 and 33% lower than ipsilateral scores for right and left cortical lesions, respectively. Noffsinger and Kurdziel (1979) also presented several case illustrations in which the NU 20 results were similar to the two studies just mentioned for subjects with CANS lesions.

Although there is a paucity of clinical research data on the NU 20, the work that has been done has shown it to be a potentially viable test for central auditory lesions.

Synthetic Sentence Identification with Contralateral Competing Message (SSI-CCM). The SSI-CCM has been shown to be of value in detecting cerebral lesions since the early 1970s (Jerger, 1970, 1973). The Jerger and Jerger article in 1975 provides the best perspective as to results on the SSI-CCM. In this study ten patients with a variety of temporal lesions were administered the SSI-CCM. The average deficit was 20% for the ear contralateral to the lesioned hemisphere. This was about 17% more of a deficit than in the ipsilateral ear. Normal findings for the average SSI-CCM scores were noted for brainstem and nonauditory CNS lesion groups, indicating that the SSI-CCM may be valuable in differential diagnosis.

Subsequent reports on the SSI-CCM have demonstrated similar findings on patients with temporal lobe disorders (Keith, 1977; Jerger and Jerger, 1981).

Interhemispheric Lesions (Corpus Callosum)

In 1968, two important studies appeared in the literature concerning dichotic listening in split-brain patients. Sparks and Geschwind (1968) and Milner et al (1968) showed that these patients performed poorly for digits or words presented to the left ear. Right ear performance was essentially normal for the split-brain subjects in these studies.

These initial studies showed the importance of auditory interhemispheric interaction and how it may be evaluated. The split-brain subject is extremely rare but can provide information on brain function that generally cannot be obtained in any other manner. Dichotic speech tests have often been employed with split-brain subjects or patients with lesions of the corpus callosum because they generally show a marked effect. On the other hand, monaural speech tests generally do not show any deficit for split-brain subjects. As mentioned, the deficit for split-brain subjects is for the left ear. This deficit is often complete in that the split-brain subject cannot verbally report any of the speech stimuli presented to the left ear in a dichotic situation (Musiek et al, 1979; Musiek and Wilson, 1979). However, the performance of these subjects depends on a number of factors, such as test materials and the patient's verbal capacity of each hemisphere. For example, slightly poorer left ear scores are demonstrated on the dichotic digit test (Musiek and Kibbe, 1985) than the SSW; however, both show marked left ear dysfunction (Fig. 12.4).

The basis for the left ear deficit is shown

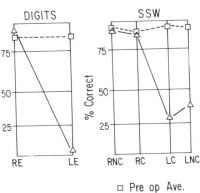

Figure 12.4. Average dichotic digits and SSW results for four right-handed patients who had undergone complete commissurotomy, with the anterior commissure left intact (*RNC*, right noncompeting; *RC*, right competing; *LC*, left competing; *LNC*, left noncompeting conditions for SSW). All patients demonstrated normal pure tone thresholds and excellent speech discrimination ability pre- and postoperatively. (From Musiek F, Kibbe K: An overview of audiological test results in patients with commissurotomy. In Reeves A (ed): *Epilepsy and the Corpus Callosum.* New York, Plenum Press, 1985.)

and described in Figure 12.2. One of the important aspects of the model of interhemispheric interaction is that it may have multiple applications for detecting and analyzing lesions of the corpus callosum and left hemisphere.

Sparks et al (1970) used dichotic digits and words in their evaluation of 20 left and 20 right brain-damaged adult subjects. Results from both of these tests showed the classic "contralateral" ear deficit for both the left and right brain-damaged subjects. However, Sparks et al also showed that the ipsilateral scores for the right brain-damaged group were considerably higher than those for the left brain-damaged group. Damasio et al (1976) reported complete left ear extinction for dichotic digits and words on two patients with deep brain lesions affecting the corpus callosum. One of these patients had primarily a left hemisphere lesion. Damasio and Damasio (1979), using dichotic words, showed severe left ear deficits for eight patients with lesions near the lateral wall of the lateral ventricle at the level of the trigone. Damasio and Damasio concluded that the immediate neural outflow of the auditory fibers of the corpus callosum leaves the posterior region and courses around the lateral ventricle to the auditory cortex.

The SSW and competing sentence tests showed left ear deficits for left parietal lobe lesions in several patients reported by Lynn and Gilroy (1977) and Rintelmann and Lynn (1983). This finding could indicate that the corpus callosum fibers had been compromised.

Right hemisphere lesions can also compromise the corpus callosum, but it is difficult to separate the classic contralateral ear effect from actual interhemispheric transfer problems, in that both of these conditions can yield the same kind of dichotic results (Musiek and Sachs, 1980; Damasio and Damasio, 1979).

Geschwind (1982) has reported that the fibers of the corpus callosum and fibers which connect to the corpus callosum are compromised in a surprisingly high proportion of hemispheric lesions. If this is the case, it has strong implications for dichotic speech test results in many instances.

Compromise of the auditory fibers of the corpus callosum may give various degrees of left ear deficit. As pointed out in the studies just mentioned, an ipsilateral ear rather than contralateral ear deficit is noted if the lesion is in the left brain. Many reports prior to the Sparks et al (1970) article showed poor ipsilateral dichotic scores for left hemisphere lesions but did not entertain the possibility of dysfunction of the corpus callosum (Kimura, 1961b; Goodglass, 1967; Schulhoff and Goodglass, 1969). In these writers' opinion this type of dysfunction affects central auditory test results far more often than is generally realized. In left hemisphere lesions, where there is some deficit in the left ear on dichotic listening tasks, one should consider involvement of the corpus callosum.

The interhemispheric lesion, agenesis of the corpus callosum, demonstrates different findings. Bryden and Zurif (1970) employed dichotic digits in assessing one case of agenesis of the corpus callosum. More recently, Lortie et al (1981) used dichotic words and CVs in assessing five subjects with callosal agenesis. Results from both of these studies demonstrated similar performance for both left and right ears on the dichotic tests mentioned. These findings were markedly different from dichotic test results on patients with surgical section of the callosum mentioned earlier. The agenesis of the corpus callosum perhaps allows the development in each hemisphere of functions that are usually dependent on interhemispheric interaction, such as speech and speech-related functions (Bryden and Zurif, 1970). This type of brain plasticity probably is manifested in the early years of development.

OTHER TYPES OF DICHOTIC TESTING

Acoustic stimuli other than speech have been used in dichotic listening tests. Efron in this book (Chapter 9) discusses some of his dichotic nonspeech procedures. However, dichotic tests involving melodies or some type of musical stimuli slightly different from Efron's work are relatively common in the literature.

Kimura (1964) showed that when brief melodies were presented dichotically, better performance was noted for the left ear. This implied that the right hemisphere might better process this type of acoustic material than the left. Other studies have demonstrated that when there is right hemisphere damage, left ear deficits are noted for the perception of dichotic melodies or similar musical segments (Shankweiler, 1966). However, it has been suggested that it may not be music, but rather the components of music, for which the right hemisphere/left ear is dominant (Siditis, 1981). (For an excellent review of this subject see Gates and Bradshaw, 1977.)

SUMMARY

This chapter reviewed dichotic speech findings in patients with CNS lesions (Table 12.3). It emphasized the importance of acoustical factors in testing and the collection of good normative data before employing dichotic speech tests with a clinical population. Two categories of dichotic speech tasks, binaural integration and binaural separation, were defined. Binaural integration tasks discussed were dichotic digits/words, SSW, and dichotic CVs. Binaural separation tasks presented were Competing Sentences, Northwestern University Test 20, and the SSI-CCM.

In reviewing the literature on dichotic speech tasks and brainstem lesions it appears that binaural integration tasks are of more value than separation tasks. Binaural effects are often noted with brainstem involvement, but it remains debatable whether the ear ipsilateral or contralateral to the side of the lesion is most affected. Factors such as site of the lesion in the brainstem (high or low) as well as whether it is an intra-or extraaxial

lesion should be considered in determining laterality effects.

Hemispheric/cortical lesions classically show deficits for dichotic speech tests in the ear contralateral to the involved hemisphere. There are, however, exceptions to this. The most notable occurs when there is compromise of auditory fibers of the corpus callosum from a deep left hemisphere lesion. In this situation, as in split-brain subjects, a left ear deficit is noted. Hence, the deficit is ipsilateral.

It is difficult to ascertain the exact level of clinical validity of the dichotic tests discussed in this chapter because there are few studies. Although more work must be done, dichotic speech testing still remains a valuable and interesting manner of measuring central auditory dysfunction.

References

Bakker DJ, Smink T, Reitsma P: Ear dominance and reading ability. *Cortex* 9:301–312, 1973.

Berlin C, Cullen J: Acoustical problems in dichotic listening tasks. In: *Brain and Language Development.* New York, Academic Press, 1975.

Berlin C, Cullen J, Berlin H, Tobey E, Mouney D: Dichotic Listening in a Patient with a Presumed Lesion in the Region of the Medial Geniculate Bodies. A paper presented at the 90th Meeting of the Acoustical Society of America, San Francisco, Nov 7, 1975a.

Berlin CL, Cullen JK Jr, Hughes LF, Berlin JL, Lowe-Bell SS, Thompson CL: *Acoustic Variables in Dichotic Listening.* Proceedings of a Symposium on Central Auditory Processing Disorders, Univ of Nebraska Medical Center, Omaha, 1975b.

Berlin C, Lowe S, Thompson L, Cullen J: The construction and perception of simultaneous messages. *ASHA* 10:397, 1968.

Berlin C, Lowe-Bell S, Cullen J Jr, Thompson S, Loovis C: Dichotic speech perception: an interpretation of right-ear advantage and temporal offset effects. *J Acoust Soc Am* 53:699–709, 1973.

Berlin C, Lowe-Bell S, Cullen J, Thompson L, Stafford M: Is speech special? Perhaps the temporal lobectomy patient can tell us. *J Acoust Soc Am* 52:702–705, 1972a.

Berlin C, Lowe-Bell S, Jannetta P, Kline D: Central auditory deficits after temporal lobectomy. *Arch Otolaryngol* 96:4–10, 1972b.

Berlin C, McNeil M: Dichotic Listening. In Lass N (ed): *Contemporary Issues in Experimental Phonetics.* New York, Academic Press, 1976.

Broadbent DE: The role of auditory localization in attention and memory span. *J Exp Psychol* 47:191–196, 1954.

Brunt M: The Staggered Spondaic Word Test. In Katz J (ed): *Handbook of Clinical Audiology.* Baltimore, Williams & Wilkins, 1978.

Bryden MP: Ear preference in auditory perception. *J*

Table 12.3
Expected Dichotic Speech Results for Various Sites of Lesion in the CNS

Site of lesion	Probable dichotic speech results[a]
Low brainstem	Ipsilateral ear deficit (3)
High brainstem	Contralateral ear deficit (2)
	Bilateral ear deficit (2)
	Ipsilateral ear deficit (1)
Cortex/hemispheric	Moderate contralateral ear deficit (3)
Interhemispheric (corpus callosum)	Severe left ear deficit (3)

[a] 3, high probability of occurrence; 2, moderate probability of occurrence; 1, low probability of occurrence.

Exp Psychol 16:291–299, 1963.

Bryden MP, Zurif EB: Dichotic listening performance in a case of agenesis of the corpus callosum. *Neuropsychologia* 8:443–450, 1970.

Burke M, Noffsinger D: Dichotic Performance by Cortical Lesion Patients Utilizing Meaningful and Meaningless Competition. Presented at the ASHA Convention, Houston, Nov 1976.

Calearo C, Antonelli A: Audiometric findings in brainstem lesions. *Acta Otolaryngol* 66:305–319, 1968.

Collard M, Lesser R, Luedere H, Rothner A, Erenberg G, Hahn J, Dinner D, Cruse R: Results of Four Dichotic Speech Tests for Temporal Lobectomy Candidates. Presented at Academy of Neurology, Washington, DC, April 22, 1982.

Cutting J: Auditory and linguistic processes in speech perception: influence from six fusions in dichotic listening. *Psychol Rev* 83:114–140, 1976.

Damasio H, Damasio A: Paradoxic ear extinction in dichotic listening: possible anatomic significance. *Neurology* 29:644–653, 1979.

Damasio H, Damasio A: Castro-Caldas A, Ferro J: Dichotic listening pattern in relation to interhemispheric disconnexion. *Neuropsychologia* 14:247–250, 1976.

Dirks DD: Perception of dichotic and monaural verbal material and cerebral dominance for speech. *Acta Otolaryngol* 58:73–80, 1964.

Dobie RA, Simmons FB: A dichotic threshold test: normal and brain-damaged subjects. *J Speech Hear Res* 14:71–81, 1971.

Gates A, Bradshaw J: Role of the cerebral hemispheres in music. *Brain Lang* 4:403–431, 1977.

Geschwind N: The Frequency of Callosal Syndromes in Neurological Practice. Presented at a Symposium on Epilepsy and the Corpus Callosum, Hanover, NH, July 14, 1982.

Goodglass H: Binaural digit presentation and early lateral brain damage. *Cortex* 3:295–306, 1967.

Hutchinson BB: Performance of aphasics on a dichotic listening task. *J Aud Res* 13:64–70, 1973.

Jerger J: Auditory Tests for Disorders of the Central Auditory Mechanism. In Fields WS (ed): *Neurological Aspects of Auditory and Vestibular Disorders.* Springfield, IL, Charles C Thomas, 1964.

Jerger J: Development of the synthetic sentence identification (SSI) as a tool for speech audiometry. In Rojskjaer C (ed): *Speech Audiometry.* Odense, Denmark, Danavox, 1970.

Jerger J: *Modern Developments in Audiology.* New York, Academic Press, 1973, pp 75–115.

Jerger J, Jerger S: Auditory findings in brainstem disorders. *Arch Otolaryngol* 99:342–350, 1974.

Jerger J, Jerger S: Clinical validity of central auditory tests. *Scand Audiol* 4:147–163, 1975.

Jerger J, Jerger S: *Auditory Disorders: A Manual for Clinical Evaluation.* Boston, Little, Brown, 1981.

Katz J: The use of staggered spondaic words for assessing the integrity of the central auditory system. *J Aud Res* 2:327–337, 1962.

Katz J: The SSW test: an interim report. *J Speech Hear Disord* 33:132–146, 1968.

Katz J: Audiologic diagnosis: cochlea to cortex. *Menorah Med J* 1:25–38, 1970.

Katz J: The Staggered Spondaic Word test. In Keith R (ed): *Central Auditory Dysfunction.* New York, Grune & Stratton, 1977.

Katz J (ed): *Handbook of Clinical Audiology.* Baltimore, Williams & Wilkins, 1978.

Katz J, Basil RA, Smith JM: A staggered spondaic word test for detecting central auditory lesions. *Ann Otol Rhinol Laryngol* 72:906–917, 1963.

Katz J, Pack G: New developments in differential diagnosis using the SSW test. In Sullivan H (ed): *Proceedings of a Symposium on Central Auditory Processing Disorders.* Omaha, University of Nebraska Medical Center, 1975.

Keith R: *Central Auditory Dysfunction.* New York, Grune & Stratton, 1977.

Kimura D: Cerebral dominance and the perception of verbal stimuli. *Can J Psychol* 15:166–171, 1961a.

Kimura D: Some effects of temporal lobe damage on auditory perception. *Can J Psychol* 15:157–165, 1961b.

Kimura D: Left-right difference in the perception of melodies. *Q J Exp Psychol* 16:355–358, 1964.

Lortie J, Lassonde M, Ptito M: Dichotic Listening in Callosal Agenesis. Presented at the Society for Neuroscience Meeting, Los Angeles, October 18, 1981.

Lowe S, Cullen J Jr, Berlin C, Thompson C, Willett M: Perception of simultaneous dichotic and monotic monosyllables. *J Speech Hear Res* 13:812–822, 1970.

Lynn G, Gilroy J: Neuroaudiological abnormalities in patients with temporal lobe tumors. *J Neurol Sci* 17:167–184, 1972.

Lynn G, Gilroy J: Effects of brain lesions on the perception of monotic and dichotic speech stimuli. In Sullivan H (ed): *Proceedings of a Symposium on Central Auditory Processing Disorders.* Omaha, University of Nebraska Medical Center, 1975, pp 47–83.

Lynn G, Gilroy J: Evaluation of central auditory dysfunction in patients with neurological disorders. In Keith R (ed): *Central Auditory Dysfunction.* New York, Grune & Stratton, 1977.

Mazzuchi A, Parma M: Responses to dichotic listening tasks in temporal epilepics with or without clinically evident lesions. *Cortex* 14:381–390, 1978.

McClellen M, Wertz R, Collins M: The Effects of Interhemispheric Lesions on Central Auditory Behavior. Presented at the ASHA convention, Detroit, 1973.

Milner B, Taylor S, Sperry R: Lateralized suppression of dichotically presented digits after commissural section in man. *Science* 161:184–185, 1968.

Moray N: Attention in dichotic listening: affective cues and the influence of instructions. *Q J Exp Psychol* 11:56–60, 1959.

Musiek F: New Clinical Implications of the NU 20 Test Tapes. Presented at the ASHA Convention, Chicago, Nov 3, 1977.

Musiek F: Assessment of central auditory dysfunction: the dichotic digit test revisited. *Ear Hear* 4:79–83, 1983.

Musiek F: The results of three dichotic speech tests on subjects with intracranial lesions. *Ear Hear*, 1983.

Musiek F, Geurkink N: Auditory brainstem response (ABR) and central auditory test (CAT) findings for patients with brainstem lesions: a preliminary report. *Laryngoscope* 92:891–900, 1982.

Musiek F, Kibbe K: An overview of audiological test results in patients with commissurotomy. In Reeves A (ed): *Epilepsy and the Corpus Callosum.* New York, Plenum Press, 1985.

Musiek F, Sachs E Jr: Reversible neuroaudiologic findings in a case of right frontal lobe abscess with recovery. *Arch Otolaryngol* 106:280–283, 1980.

Musiek F, Wilson D: SSW and Dichotic Digit results pre- and postcommissurotomy: a case report. *J Speech Hear Disord* 44:528–533, 1979.

Musiek F, Wilson D, Pinheiro M: Audiological manifestations in split-brain patients. *J Am Aud Soc* 5:25–29, 1979.

Netley C: Dichotic listening performance of hemispherectomized patients. *Neurophychologia* 10:233–240, 1972.

Niccum N, Rubens A, Speaks C: Effects of stimulus material on the dichotic listening performance of aphasic patients. *J Speech Hear Res* 24:526–534, 1981.

Noffsinger D, Kurdziel S: Assessment of central auditory lesions. In Rintelmann W (ed): *Hearing Assessment*. Baltimore, University Park Press, 1979, pp 351–377.

Noffsinger D, Kurdziel S, Applebaum E: Value of special auditory tests in the latero-medial inferior pontine syndrome. *Ann Otol Rhinol Laryngol* 84:384–390, 1975.

Noffsinger D, Olsen W, Carhart R, Hart C, Sahgal V: Auditory and vestibular aberrations in multiple sclerosis. *Acta Otolaryngol [Suppl] Stockh* 303, 1972.

Olsen W: Performance of Temporal Lobectomy Patients with Dichotic CV Test Materials. Presented at the ASHA Convention, Chicago, Nov 1977.

Olsen W, Carhart R: Development of test procedures for evaluation of binaural aids. In: *Bulletin of Prosthetic Research: Prosthetic and Sensory Aids Service.* Washington, DC, Veterans Administration, 1967, pp 22–49.

Olsen W, Kurdziel S: Berlin Dichotic and Katz SSW Test Results for Temporal Lobe Lesion Patients. Paper presented at the ASHA Convention, San Francisco, 1978.

Oscar-Berman M, Zurif EB, Blumstein S: Effects of unilateral brain damage on the processing of speech sounds in two languages. *Brain Lang* 2:345–355, 1975.

Oxbury J, Oxbury S: Effect of temporal lobectomy on the report of dichotically presented digits. *Cortex* 5:3–14, 1969.

Petit J, Noll J: Cerebral dominance in aphasia recovery. *Brain Lang* 7:191–200, 1979.

Pinheiro M: Tests of central auditory function in children with learning disabilities. In Keith R (ed): *Central Auditory Dysfunction*. New York, Grune & Stratton, 1977, ch 7.

Pinheiro M, Jacobson G, Boller F: Auditory dysfunction following a gunshot wound of the pons. *J Speech Hear Disord* 47:296–300, 1982.

Porter R, Troendle R, Berlin C: Effects of practice on the perception of dichotically presented stop-consonant-vowel syllables. *J Acoust Soc Am* 59:679–682, 1976.

Rintelmann W, Lynn G: Speech stimuli for assessment of central auditory disorders. In Konkle D, Rintelmann W (eds): *Principles of Speech Audiometry*. Baltimore, University Park Press, 1983.

Roeser R, Daly D: Auditory cortex disconnection associated with thalamic tumor: A case report. *Neurology* 24:555–559, 1974.

Roeser RJ, Johns DF, Price LL: Effects of intensity on dichotically presented digits. *J Aud Res* 12:184–186, 1972.

Roeser R, Johns D, Price L: Dichotic listening in adults with sensorineural hearing loss. *J Am Audiol Soc* 2:19–25, 1976.

Rosenweig M: Representation of the two ears at the auditory cortex. *Am J Physiol* 167:147–158, 1951.

Schulhoff C, Goodglass H: Dichotic listening, side of brain injury and cerebral dominance. *Neuropsychologia* 7:149–160, 1969.

Shankweiler D: Effects of temporal lobe damage on perception of dichotically presented melodies. *J Comp Physiol Psychol* 62:115–119, 1966.

Shankweiler D, Studdert-Kennedy M: Identification of consonants and vowels presented to left and right ears. *Q J Exp Psychol* 19:59–63, 1967.

Siditis J: The complex tone test: implications for the assessment of auditory laterality effects. *Neuropsychologia* 19:103–112, 1981.

Siditis J: Predicting brain organization from dichotic listening performance: cortical and subcortical functional asymmetries contribute to perceptual asymmetries. *Brain Lang* 17:287–300, 1982.

Siegenthaler B, Knellinger L: Dichotic listening by brain-injured adults: observation of divergent test responses. *J Commun Disord* 14:399–409, 1981.

Sparks R, Geschwind N: Dichotic listening in man after section of neocortical commissures. *Cortex* 4:3–16, 1968.

Sparks R, Goodglass H, Nichel B: Ipsilateral versus contralateral extinction in dichotic listening resulting from hemisphere lesions. *Cortex* 6:249–260, 1970.

Speaks C: Dichotic listening: A clinical or research tool? In Sullivan H (ed): *Proceedings of a Symposium on Central Auditory Processing Disorders*. Omaha, University of Nebraska Medical Center, 1975.

Speaks C, Gray T, Miller J, Rubens A: Central auditory deficits and temporal-lobe lesions. *J Speech Hear Disord* 40:192–205, 1975.

Stephens S, Thornton A: Subjective and electrophysiologic tests in brainstem lesions. *Arch Otolaryngol* 102:608–613, 1976.

Studdert-Kennedy M, Shankweiler D: Hemispheric specialization for speech perception. *J Acoust Soc Am* 48:579–594, 1970.

Studdert-Kennedy M, Shankweiler D, Pisoni D: Auditory and phonetic processing in speech perception: evidence from a dichotic study. *Cognit Psychol* 3:455–466, 1972.

Treisman AM, Geffen G: Selective attention and cerebral dominance in perceiving and responding to speech messages. *Q J Exp Psychol* 79:139–150, 1968.

Tsunoda T, Oka M: Cerebral hemisphere dominance test and localization of speech. *J Aud Res* 11:177–189, 1971.

Weiss M, House A: Perception of dichotic vowels. *J Acoust Soc Am* 53:51–58, 1973.

Wexler B, Hawles T: Increasing the power of dichotic methods: the fused rhymed words test. *Neuropsychologia* 21:59–66, 1983.

Willeford J: Assessing central auditory behavior in children: a test battery approach. In Keith R (ed): *Central Auditory Dysfunction*. New York, Grune & Stratton, 1977, pp 43–73.

Zurif EB, Ramier AM: Some effects of unilateral brain damage on the perception of dichotically presented phoneme sequences and digits. *Neuropsychologia* 10:103–110, 1972.

CHAPTER 13

Sequencing and Temporal Ordering in the Auditory System

MARILYN L. PINHEIRO, Ph.D.
FRANK E. MUSIEK, Ph.D.

Drs. Pinheiro and Musiek explore the history and present status of research in auditory sequencing, temporal ordering, and temporal patterns. Applications of these tasks to normal and pathological populations are discussed in relation to assessment of central auditory dysfunction.

INTRODUCTION

All functions of the central auditory system are influenced by time in some way because acoustic events occur in time. Within the system the pattern of neural activity is strongly mediated by temporal information precise to within a few microseconds. Cells in all of the auditory nuclei as well as in auditory cortex have been shown to be sensitive to the effects of time. Even a single sound may depend on time for its localization in space which may be determined by the differing time of arrival of the sound waves at each ear (Chapters 5 and 10). Other aspects of temporal processing in the central auditory nervous system are discussed in other chapters of this book.

This chapter will present a particular aspect of temporal function in the central auditory system, i.e., temporal or serial ordering, or temporal sequencing. This function involves the perception and/or processing of two or more auditory stimuli in their order of occurrence in time. This function is usually measured by a judgment of order or the behavioral sequencing of the stimuli. More complex series of acoustic stimuli are often called temporal patterns. This chapter will consider the importance of temporal ordering ability and the many variables affecting it, its relationship to language, relevant research, theories on the coding of temporal sequences, possible clinical applications of serial ordering tasks in assessment of this function in humans, and conclusions based on present knowledge of the subject.

Temporal sequencing is undoubtedly one of the more basic and important functions of the central auditory nervous system. Furth (1964) and Furth and Youniss (1967) postulated that the discrimination of sound sequences preceded the development of language. Lashley (1951), Neff (1964), and Hirsh (1967) pointed to the relationship between the sequential analysis of patterned temporal stimuli and the perception and production of speech. The latter author concluded that the speaking and understanding of language, surely the most complex function of the human central nervous system, depended on the ability to deal with sound sequences. Eisenson (1968) wrote that speech consists of sound elements and combinations of sound elements (linguistic events) that are temporal and sequential. Thus, even the comprehension of a single word often depends on accurate perception of the temporal order of the sound elements in that word. For example, perception of the /s/ sound *before* the /t/ differentiates the word "fist" from the word "fits" in which the /s/ sound is perceived to be *after* the /t/. Sequence has been found to be vital to speech perception at even more fundamental levels. In studies using synthetic speech Delattre et al (1955) discovered that the order or sequence of frequencies from high to low, or low to high, in frequency glides into vowel formants was used to identify the stop consonants.

After describing a number of tests of central auditory function, Berlin and Lowe (1972) concluded that temporal sequence was a highly significant factor in any tests that produced meaningful results. They postulated that the impairment of sequencing ability demonstrated in patients with brain lesions might be basic to dysfunction on tasks of both sound localization and lateralization and on tests using either filtered or dichotic speech. A discussion of temporal ordering studies of brain-damaged subjects later in this chapter will illustrate the effects of cortical lesions on sequencing tasks and further demonstrate the relationship between language and temporal sequencing.

Another important consideration in the relationship of temporal sequencing ability to both speech comprehension and speech production is that language processing is required in certain temporal ordering tasks when the elements or components in the sequences must be reproduced serially by either a verbal or manual response.

PSYCHOPHYSICAL VARIABLES IN TEMPORAL SEQUENCING

Temporal sequencing has many different and important aspects, and the results of research in this area are affected by many psychophysical variables, so that comparisons between studies are often difficult. A discussion of the more important variables follows.

Subject Training

Some studies have used trained subjects, while others have used naive subjects in their investigations of temporal ordering abilities. It is obvious that learning can affect results unless subjects are trained to certain criteria. The amount of training necessary depends on both the complexity of the stimuli and the difficulty of the psychophysical task. Warren (1974) felt that training of subjects was not necessary for sequences in which the components had a duration of at least 200 msec each on some temporal ordering tasks. Efron (1963) pointed out that a naive subject performs significantly more poorly than a trained normal subject on certain temporal ordering tasks. Whether or not subjects should be trained may depend on the type of data that is being collected. Psychophysical data for descriptions and measurements of basic human auditory functions and the capacity of the central auditory nervous system to process certain information should be approached by controlling as many of the variables as possible. In such a case a well trained subject should give a more even and accurate performance. However, the normative data to be used as a basis for clinical procedures might best be established on a naive population, since generally time is not available for more than the most elementary training of patients in a clinical setting. If one is comparing the performance of a naive clinical population with the performance of trained subjects, one must be aware that differences, even significant ones, may be expected, even though both groups are composed of so-called "normal" subjects. Also, one must be careful of comparing brain-damaged patients with trained normal subjects, unless the brain-damaged patients are given the same or a greater amount of training. Almost certainly a brain-damaged individual cannot be trained to the same criteria as a normal subject, although most patients with brain lesions improve their performance on certain tasks with training, just as normal naive subjects do.

Stimuli for Temporal Ordering Tasks

Type of Stimuli

Many different types of stimuli have been utilized in studies of temporal ordering by different investigators. Noise, tones, clicks, speech or speech-like sounds, or a combination of some of these have served as stimuli. The auditory signals in a sequence used to investigate the function of temporal ordering should not require the basic function of discrimination between or among acoustic cues not under study. In other words, if there is any difference among the signals in frequency, intensity, or duration, the subject should be able to distinguish between them easily in isolation. Tones used in studies of temporal sequencing have varied in their frequencies. The frequency range as well as the frequency relationship or separation between tones in such a task has been found to be important (Bregman and Campbell, 1971). Divenyi and Hirsh (1974) reported that a frequency separation of less than one-third to two-thirds of an octave decreased the accuracy of subject responses, while Thomas and Fitzgibbons (1971) observed that temporal order was identified more readily when the tones were within a musical fourth. Divenyi and Hirsh (1974) also noted that a simple harmonic relationship among components of a sequence facilitated temporal order judgments. The position of certain frequencies within a sequence has also been found to influence results (Watson et al, 1975).

Number of Components

Sequences of stimuli have been composed of two, three, four, or more components. The number of components in a sequence obviously influences the difficulty of the psychophysical task. The task of ordering three elements is different from that of ordering only two elements or from that of ordering more than three elements. In fact, it is possible that the number of stimuli affect the manner of processing in a temporal ordering task.

Duration of Components

The duration of the individual components in a sequence also affects perception of the sequence and the task of ordering it. Some studies have used very brief components as short as 10 msec or less, whereas other investigators have used components of several hundred milliseconds in duration. Several researchers have noted that the perception of very brief elements in a sequence is qualitatively different from that of the perception of longer elements. Divenyi and Hirsh (1974) summarized duration requirements for the components of a contiguous sequence necessary for judgments of temporal order. They reported that in repeated sequences of four contiguous components each component must be of 125 to 700 msec duration. (A naive subject required 700 msec for such a task.) If the four component sequence was presented only once, each component had to be 200 msec in

duration (Warren et al, 1972). For sequences of three components, each component needed a duration of 50 msec (Peters and Wood, 1973). If the subject had to judge which of two components came first, each component required a duration of 20 msec (Hirsh, 1959). In order to discriminate between two separate sequences, each component needed to be 90 msec in duration (Leshowitz and Hanzi, 1972). Absolute identification of the temporal order of four different contiguous sounds required a duration of at least 200 msec for each sound (Warren, 1972). The above data refer only to sequences with contiguous components and do not take into account sequences in which the individual components are separated by silent intervals. The type of stimuli used also influences the duration individual components must have for judgments of temporal order. Also, the type of temporal order judgment required affects the necessary duration of sequential components.

Rate and Manner of Presentation

Rate and manner of presentation of the stimuli also influence the judgement of temporal order. Very brief stimuli presented at a rapid rate are thought to be judged by spectral differences, whereas longer components presented at a slower rate are usually perceived as individually different or separate sounds (Nickerson and Freeman, 1974). Very rapid rates of presentation do not permit actual temporal ordering of the stimuli, although rapid rates have been used for other types of temporal ordering tasks that employ simpler judgments needing less cognitive processing. The manner of presentation interacts with the rate of presentation. Many studies have used stimuli presented successively or contiguously with no silent intervals between components of the sequence. Some studies have presented these contiguous components with abrupt changes between components. Others have used a glide from one component to the next (Dannenbring, 1971).

Other Variables

In still other investigations the components of sequences, or the sequences themselves, or both (when more than one is presented for discrimination) have been separated in time by silent intervals, and performance has been improved (Neisser, 1972; Thomas et al, 1971; Warren, 1972). The duration of this silent interval also has been found to be important (Peters and Wood, 1973; Handel and Yoder 1975). Some researchers have used overlapping stimuli with different onset times.

Some sequences used in studies of temporal ordering ability have varied along only one acoustic dimension, i.e., intensity, frequency, or duration of components, while others have varied a number of acoustic dimensions. Investigators have employed patterns that were binary, and others have presented sequences in which all components differed. Some sequences have been unidirectional in tonal presentation, while others have not. Some sequences have been presented in pairs, some presented only once, and some repeated continuously on a tape loop. Sequential stimuli have also been presented to subjects monaurally, binaurally, diotically, dichotically, in alternating ears, and in sound field.

Investigators have noted that some sequences have a "certainty" (Watson and Kelly, 1981) or "goodness" (Garner and Clement, 1963; Royer and Garner, 1970) of pattern that makes them easier to order than other patterns (Neisser, 1972; Warren and Obusek, 1972; Divenyi, 1978).

Finally, speech and speech-like sounds have been found to be sequenced into temporal order more easily than nonspeech stimuli (Warren et al, 1969; Thomas et al, 1970).

Temporal Order Judgments

The type of temporal order judgment the subject is asked to make also influences results of studies in temporal sequencing (Warren and Obusek, 1972). Some responses require a higher level of cognitive processing than others. In some investigations subjects have been required to determine whether overlapping stimuli were simultaneous or successive in onset times. In other investigations subjects have had to decide which of a pair of overlapping sounds began first in time. Subjects have been asked to judge whether two sequences were the same or different. Some workers have used

tracking procedures in which the subjects tried to respond to or identify each component of a sequence as it occurred. In some studies subjects have been required to identify a particular pulse in a series of pulses as different or changed. Another method used was to have the subject adjust the frequency of one component in the second sequence of a pair of sequences to match the same component in the first sequence. Some judgments required matching a sequence pictured on a response button to the sequence heard. The most difficult type of judgment of temporal order appears to be a description of the sequence or actual ordering of the components by labeling them verbally or pointing to or pressing buttons in a sequence that matches the sequence heard, or repeating the actual order of the components of the sequence in some other form of response (Preusser, 1972). The actual temporal ordering of components in a sequence apparently involves language processing when either verbal or manual responses are required of the subject. Hummed responses for tonal sequences or pitch patterns have also been investigated and found to be an imitative type of response involving less cognitive processing than a verbal or manual response (Pinheiro and Tinta, 1977; Pinheiro, 1978).

Attention and Recall

It is difficult to separate the variables of attention and recall because the attention of the subject obviously affects recall of the sequence. Recall is a powerful variable in all types of judgments of temporal order, since the response must follow the stimulus after some brief period of time, whatever the psychophysical procedure. In tracking responses the subject has to recall only one component at a time. In other response paradigms the subject has to remember pairs of sequences or a single sequence with several or more components. If recall is inaccurate, not even the simplest type of temporal order judgment can be made correctly.

Shulman and Greenberg (1971) felt that the division of attention between memory (recall) and perception interfered with perceptual processing. Attention and recall are both variables not only difficult to control, but also difficult or impossible to measure.

In some studies attention has been encouraged by having the subject himself initiate the stimulus so that he listened to it only when he felt most ready to listen and attend. Subjects have also been rewarded for participation in studies, or according to their levels of performance, encouraging as high a degree of attention and accuracy as possible. Training has been shown to improve recall also as the stimuli become more familiar, although overtraining might decrease attention to stimuli that are no longer novel. Miscik and colleagues (1972) reported that retention of auditory sequences was a combined function of stimulus duration, interstimulus interval, and encoding techniques the subject used for processing his response.

Other Factors in Temporal Ordering

Instrumentation has varied from one research laboratory to another, and this must be taken into account when studies of temporal ordering are compared. A few investigators have used loud speakers for presentation of stimuli, although most have employed earphones. Some workers have tested subjects using tape loops, while others have generated the signals as they were presented.

The intensity level or sensation level at which the auditory sequences are presented may also influence results. This psychophysical variable has not been adequately investigated. Ptacek and Pinheiro (1971) and Pinheiro and Ptacek (1971) reported that lower levels of presentation decreased performance for sequences of three noise or tone bursts involving a frequency or intensity difference within the sequence.

All of these variables must be considered when comparing results of studies or designing research on temporal ordering. Many of the variables interact and also affect the manner of coding the subject uses to process his response.

Research on Temporal Sequencing: Normal Subjects

A number of important variables that influence temporal sequencing ability have been treated in different ways in the studies summarized below, so that it is difficult to compare them. Although a discussion of these variables preceded this review of the literature, an attempt has been made to organize this part of the chapter according to some similarities in the psychophysical procedures and types of response employed in the tasks reported.

Some of the studies have used *overlapping stimuli*, requiring that the subject discriminate between them. Patterson and Green (1970) found that pairs of brief wave forms with the same energy spectra (Huffman sequences) appeared qualitatively different when the onset times of the stimuli in a pair were separated by only 1.5 to 2.0 msec. Efron's work (1973) confirmed this finding; his well trained subjects distinguished the difference between two micropatterns with onset asynchronies of 2 msec. He further determined that the last stimulus element in each micropattern dominated the perceived pitch of the pattern and that subjects used this qualitative difference on which to base their same/different judgments. These studies employed very brief stimuli which overlapped in time, and it is difficult to determine whether this type of discrimination is actually based on temporal order information conserved by the central auditory system, as suggested by Efron, or solely on qualitative information as proposed by Nickerson and Freeman (1974), or on both of these factors.

In 1959 Hirsh tested the ability of trained normal subjects to judge which of two overlapping tones started first, i.e., a high tone or a low tone. He found that a 20 msec difference in onset times was necessary for a 75% success rate in performing this task. Thus, reporting the actual temporal order of two stimuli took ten times longer than a decision about the separateness of the sounds, which required only 2 msec. He found that this time factor of 20 msec applied to reporting temporal order, independent of whether the pairs of acoustic stimuli were two tones, tone and wide band noise, tone and click, or two clicks. Hirsh and Sherrick (1961) extended these findings, discovering that the same time factor held for temporal order judgments in all sensory modalities and across modalities. Efron (1973) also noted that the reporting of temporal order took ten times longer than a same/different judgment in the discrimination of two micropatterns. However, when subjects were not trained, both Efron (1963) and Hirsh and Fraisse (1964) found that a 60 msec onset asynchrony between overlapping stimuli was necessary for the same temporal order judgment. When Efron trained naive subjects, performance improved until it reached Hirsh's original figure of 20 msec.

Homick and colleagues (1969) found that the judgment of temporal order for a tone presented before or during a noise was less difficult when the frequency of the tone was lower than the centerband frequency of the noise. Tones of low intensity increased the difficulty of temporal order judgments.

Judgments between simultaneity and successiveness are based on the perception that two or more sounds occur either at the same time or follow one another. Without some successiveness of stimuli, there is no temporal order. Exner (1875) was the earliest worker to describe this phenomenon when he found that the clicks of a Savart wheel were perceived as successive only when the interval between clicks was about 2 msec. When clicks were delivered separately to the two ears, a separation interval of 64 msec was necessary for the subject to perceive successiveness.

A number of investigators have assessed temporal sequencing ability in normal subjects using patterns of successive, *contiguous stimuli.* Nickerson and Freeman's subjects (1974) could make a same/different judgment between patterns of contiguous components with durations as brief as 5 msec (a rate of 200 per second). These results supported similar work reported earlier by Wilcox et al (1972).

In 1981 Watson and Kelly summarized a series of experiments on temporal ordering carried out by their group. They determined the just detectable increment in frequency, intensity, or duration of a single component in one of a pair of patterns that enabled subjects to make a same/different judgment or use a method of adjustment to make the two patterns the same. They also employed contiguous tonal patterns about half a second in duration (similar to the duration of a spoken word) with each component of a pattern (10 contiguous components) approximately 40 msec in duration (similar to the duration of one of the shorter English phonemes). Trained subjects found that

early or low frequency components in the patterns were difficult to resolve, whereas late and high frequency components were resolved as easily as the same components presented in isolation. Results indicated that an overall factor of 50 was necessary for a detectable increment in frequency. The necessary increment in intensity was only 3 to 4 dB. A detectable change in duration was in the order of 50 to 60%. Their results also were influenced strongly by the certainty or uncertainty associated with the patterns in a given task. In minimum uncertainty experiments, when the change occurred in the same component of the same pattern on each trial, accuracy was high. In stimulus conditions of very high uncertainty in which pattern components varied in frequency, intensity, duration, and position within the pattern on each trial, subject performance was poor. The type of judgment required in these studies differed from a response in which actual temporal order is reported.

Other investigators have also used contiguous sequences of stimuli for temporal ordering tasks. Warren et al (1969) employed a continuously repeating sequence of three different sounds (1000 Hz tone, broadband noise, and a 600 Hz tone), each of 200 msec duration. Subjects could accurately differentiate the sounds but could not temporally order them. In a further study Warren and Obusek (1972) used four different repeating contiguous sounds (1000 Hz tone, 2000 Hz octave band of noise which sounded like a hiss, 796 Hz tone, and a 40 Hz square wave buzz) with the same results. However, subjects were able to make the discrimination between pairs of these patterns for a same/different response, even though they could not name the order of the sounds. Trained subjects (Warren, 1974) could make same/different judgments for pairs of sequences made up of three or four contiguous sounds of 5 to 10 msec duration for each component. Warren concluded that direct identification of temporal order for repeating contiguous sequences was determined by the maximum rate at which verbal labels could be mentally attached to successive nonrelated components as they occurred in real time. A component duration of 170 msec was needed for numbering an item, while components of 250 msec could be named by matching them with cards during the repeating sequence. For a verbal temporal order response, each component in a single nonrepeating sequence had to be 450 to 670 msec in duration.

Divenyi and Hirsh (1974) and Divenyi (1978) reported that trained subjects could identify a sequence of three different contiguous tones with durations as brief as 10 msec or less for each component. Unidirectional sequences were the easiest to recognize.

Bregman and Campbell (1971) studied repeating sequences of six different 100 msec contiguous tones. Three of the tones were in the high frequency range, and three were in the low frequency range. Performance on writing down the components was better within either the high frequency range or the low frequency range of the sequence than between the two ranges. Subjects usually wrote down the triplet within one frequency range first and then filled in the labels for tones within the other range. In other words, listeners appeared to organize components of the sequence into two separate subjective "streams," one for each frequency range. Subjects were scored on the triplets within each range, and the level of success within a stream was about 70% for labeling of the tones in any order within a range. Thus, this experiment did not require accurate temporal ordering.

Thomas and Fitzgibbons (1971) also investigated continuously repeating sequences of pure tones with all components within a musical fourth. A duration of 125 msec for each of the contiguous components was sufficient for temporal ordering, but longer component durations were necessary when the contiguous tones were more widely spaced in frequency, depending on their specific distribution within the pattern.

Royer and Garner (1966, 1970) reported a series of studies using continuous sequences of eight or nine contiguous sounds in a binary pattern, presented in sound field. Subjects tracked the sequences with buzzers corresponding to the two different tones within the sequence as well as to their location at left or right speakers. Written responses were also investigated. Garner and Gottwald (1968) repeated the study, requiring verbal responses at the termination of the sequence.

A number of researchers found that performance on temporal ordering tasks was improved when *silent intervals* were inserted *between successive components* of a sequence or between sequences or both (Thomas et al, 1971; Neisser, 1972; and Warren and Obusek, 1972). Peters and Wood (1973) presented three different pulsed tones separated in time, and the subject either judged the order of the tones or identified the position of a single component within a sequence. Handel (1973) and Handel and Yoder (1975) used repeating auditory patterns which were also segmented. The subject listened continuously until he could identify the pattern. Increasing the intensity of a single pattern component improved performance over uniform presentation, although increasing the silent interval between two or more of the eight pattern components improved it even more.

Work by Pinheiro (1977a and b, 1978), Pinheiro and Ptacek (1971), Pinheiro and Andrews (1973), Pinheiro and Tinta (1977), and Pinheiro et al (1977) employed temporally spaced triplets of sounds with a difference or change in the frequency, intensity, or duration of one of the three pattern components. Thus, intensity patterns were made up of "loud" and "soft" elements. Duration patterns had "long" and "short" bursts, and frequency or pitch patterns were composed of "high" and "low" tones. Various durations of components (150 to 500 msec) and silent intervals (50 to 300 msec) were studied. Subjects had short training periods with no improvement in performance observed after the first 20 to 25 sequences. Patterns composed of tones were easier to order than patterns with noise burst components. Pitch pattern sequences were temporally ordered more easily than sequences in which either intensity or duration was the variable (Fig. 13.1). Performance by normal subjects on tonal patterns in which the duration of only one component was varied was strongly influenced by the length of the silent interval between components rather than by the duration of either the "long" or "short" pattern elements. Duration patterns, in which time was the only factor, seemed to be processed differently from either pitch or intensity patterns. Adult subjects reached a performance level close to 100% when pitch pattern components and the interburst silent intervals had durations of 150 to 200 msec, with a total pattern duration of about 900 msec.

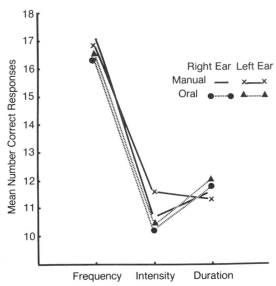

Figure 13.1. Normal subjects: means for correct responses to 18 tonal sequences in each ear for two different response modes, manual and oral (verbal) and for three different types of tonal patterns. Frequency patterns were made up of "high" (1000 Hz) tones and "low" (600 Hz) tones. Intensity patterns had a 10 dB difference between "soft" (45 dB SL) and "loud" (55 dB SL) 1000 Hz tones. Tones for both these types of patterns were 150 msec in duration with a 100 msec silent interval between tones. Duration patterns were composed of 150 msec "short" tones and 200 msec "long" tones of 1000 Hz. Silent intervals were 100 msec. All patterns were presented at 55 dB SL relative to the subject's 1000 Hz threshold for each ear. Only the "soft" tone in the intensity patterns was less intense. Note that performance on frequency (pitch) patterns was significantly better than for either intensity or duration patterns. There were no significant differences between response modes or between ears.

Normal children of 9 years of age could perform as well as adults, but younger children required longer durations of pattern components (see Chapter 14). Performance decreased with age for children of less than 9 years.

Different response modes were also investigated (Pinheiro and Tinta, 1977), i.e., manual, verbal, and hummed, but all responses except the latter, which was imitative, required actual temporal ordering of a sequence presented a single time. There were no differences among response modes for normal subjects (Fig. 13.2). The only pitch pattern study in which a difference between the two ears reached significance was one in which pattern components alternated randomly between ears. Sequences that began in the right ear were more readily put into the correct temporal order. There was no significant deterioration in performance of normal subjects when pitch patterns were presented with either competing piano music or competing discourse at equal sensation level (SL) in the same or opposite ear (Pinheiro et al, 1977). There was no difference between right and left hands on manual performance after the brief practice period. DeFosse (1978) and DeFosse and Pinheiro (1978) also studied dichotic pitch patterns in musicians and nonmusicians, with the expected finding that the former performed better across different response modes and report conditions. In addition, the two groups seemed to process the stimuli differently, i.e., nonmusicians were left ear-dominant, whereas musicians performed equally well for both ears.

When individual pattern triplets were an-

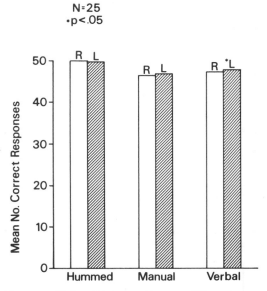

Figure 13.2. Pitch patterns—different response modes. Normal adult subjects showed no differences among three different response modes (manual, verbal, or hummed). There were no significant differences between ears for any response modes or for ears across response modes.

alyzed in several of the studies, it was found that normal subjects scored better on some combinations of pitch pattern components than on others, depending on the position of frequency components within the pattern or the location(s) of change from one frequency to the other. In other words, subjects demonstrated individual pitch pattern biases consistent with data published by Efron and Yund (1975). Similar individual pattern biases were also demonstrated in pattern research using components of two different intensities or two different durations (Figs. 13.1 and 13.2).

A number of investigators have found that speech and speech-like sounds are more easily put into their correct temporal order than nonspeech sounds (Warren et al, 1969; Thomas et al, 1970). The latter researchers used continuously repeating sequences of four temporally spaced vowels and concluded that each component required a duration of 125 msec for correct judgments of temporal order. Thomas and colleagues (1971) also studied the temporal ordering of four continuously repeating vowels. Silent intervals between components facilitated performance. Miscik et al (1972) found that recall of temporal order of three- or four-digit sequences was improved by increasing either digit duration or interdigit interval duration.

Several of the speech tests which have been developed to measure the capacity of the central auditory system involve the temporal ordering of speech stimuli (words, digits, or sentences). However, the sequencing of speech stimuli probably depends on somewhat different central processes than the temporal ordering of nonspeech stimuli. These tests are discussed in other chapters of this book.

Coding of Temporal Order Information

Theories

A number of theories relating to the coding of sequential and patterned auditory stimuli by the central nervous system have been proposed. Any relevant theory must be consistent with our knowledge of psychoacoustics and the neuroanatomy (Chapter 2) and neurophysiology (Chapters 3 and 5) of the central auditory nuclei, neural pathways,

interhemispheric and cortical function. In general, the theories of coding of temporal order information suggest the presence of some central mechanism which may determine, in one way or another, the precision of temporal order judgments, after the variables previously discussed in this chapter are taken into account.

Hirsh and Sherrick (1961) proposed a time-organizing mechanism central to and independent of sensory mechanisms. Swisher and Hirsh (1972) reported that results of their study indicated that auditory cortex is important in organizing and maintaining the sequence of neural events that represent the appropriate order of the acoustic stimuli. Neff et al (1975) studied pattern discrimination in animals and summarized their discussion by positing that "auditory cortex appears to be essential for behavioral discrimination in which the effects of neural activity set off by acoustic stimuli must be maintained in the brain in some form for short intervals" (p. 345). In other words, the components of a sequence or pattern elicit neural events that interact so that the sequence or pattern can be recognized to form the basis of a comparison for pattern discrimination or any other type of response that involves temporal ordering. Animal and human research on temporal sequencing supports this conclusion, since cortical ablations in animals and cortical lesions in humans have impaired this ability. Teuber (1960), however, expressed his belief that the afferent sensory systems are also implicated in the interaction of concomitant and successive stimuli, resulting in the patterning of perception at the cortical level. A similar suggestion was made by Massaro (1972) who postulated a "preperceptual image" to preserve sequential information after the stimulus sequence is presented so that it can be "read out" later for processing by the central mechanism. Bever (1975) described a "template" of the sequence which was preserved for analysis by the central mechanism. These theories are not incompatible, and further discussion of the basis for these theories will be included later in this chapter.

A number of investigators have applied the figure/ground theory to temporal ordering. Teuber (1960) felt that this principle had analogues in other sensory systems. For example, it has been used to explain visual phenomena. Royer and Garner (1966, 1970) also proposed the figure/ground effect, at least for rapid rates of presentation of binary sequences (sequences involving only two different components). Bregman and Campbell's (1971) theory of "sensory stream segregation" appears to be another way of describing the same process, with the only difference a semantic one. Royer and Garner, while adhering to the figure/ground theory, also concluded that the perceived pattern was a temporal Gestalten or unit. These authors felt that holistic organization of a sequence was important to its coding because they found that their subjects became aware of the entire pattern presented to them before selecting a "preferred" organization. Divenyi (1978) also compared temporal ordering of auditory patterns to gestalt, form, or shape in the visual system. Pinheiro observed that subjects perceived a pattern of three temporally spaced tones as a whole before they could label the first tone alone as a "high" or "low" pitch; they could easily recognize and label either frequency heard in isolation. Leeuwenberg (1971) and Handel (1973) also described the perception of patterns as units, and Bever (1975) agreed that sequences could be organized holistically. Vitz and Todd (1969) described the coding of patterns in units in their model. Warren (1974) reported that the perception of longer sequences occurred in "temporal groupings," while Miscik and colleagues (1972) and Preusser (1972) used the term "chunking." None of these theories of the perception and coding of sequences (figure/ground, holistic, temporal grouping, or chunking) is actually contradictory to any of the others. Shorter sequences may be perceived as units, while longer sequences may be organized perceptually into two or more units or groupings or chunks. The units or groupings may be organized according to the figure/ground relationship of the components; this would seem to be the same as "sensory stream segregation."

The above theories relate to the internal structure of the sequence or temporal pattern which Pollack (1968) described as crucial to its perception. Hirsh (1959) pointed out the importance of change within the internal structure of a sequence. This idea relates directly to the fact that neurons in the central nervous system respond more frequently to change in a stimulus than to its steady state. Handel (1973) and Pinheiro and Ptacek (1971) also discussed the relationship of changes in the internal structure of a sequence to its perception.

A somewhat different approach to coding of temporal order information was suggested by Efron in 1973. He observed that his subjects judged which of two brief stimuli with different onset times began first by transforming the auditory stimuli into a spatial dimension. Pinheiro's subjects also frequently reported that they perceived three-tone binary pitch patterns as if they occurred in a spatial dimension, with the higher frequency perceived as "up" and the lower frequency perceived as "down."

Several investigators in the area of auditory temporal processing have postulated two different manners of coding, depending on the requirements of the behavioral task. Broadbent and Ladefoged (1950), Patterson and Green (1970), and Nickerson and Freeman (1974) theorized that perception of rapid sequences of brief stimuli depended on recognition of a difference in quality between the stimuli. In other words, when the individual components were presented so rapidly that the subject could not hear a distinct separation between components or perceive an actual successiveness in the sequence, coding of the temporal information might have been handled by an analysis of pitch or spectral differences, whereas coding of more slowly presented sequences could be based on the temporal information itself. Warren et al (1972) also proposed a two-stage process for the coding of certain types of sequential information. He thought that rapidly presented sequences of brief stimuli were recognized as a whole pattern; then the order of the components was inferred from a previously learned rule describing their internal arrangements. Components presented at slower rates (with durations of individual components of approximately 200 msec) could have verbal labels attached to them as they occurred in time.

Neisser (1972) suggested that a behavioral response which involved the actual temporal ordering or reporting of a sequence first required an "analog" of the sequence. The analog would consist of a set of distinctive features of the pattern or sequence. Although the analog itself could be used without further processing to determine a same/different response in comparing two rapid sequences of brief components, a second stage of processing the analog into a "string" would be necessary when verbal labels of the components were required. The string would consist of the verbal signs isomorphic to the components themselves with respect to their order.

Bever (1975) and Handel (1973) also felt that there had to be two different and separate steps in coding temporal order information.

Anatomical/Physiological Bases

Both the anatomy and the physiology of the central auditory system have been described in Chapters 2, 3, and 5 of this book. Therefore, only a brief discussion of the points relative to temporal ordering will be reviewed here.

It is evident that there exists a hierarchy of functions in all sensory systems, and it has been demonstrated that cells in every central auditory nucleus, up to and including cortex, respond to the temporal patterning of stimuli in various ways. Some neurons begin firing at the onset of an auditory stimulus and cease firing when the stimulus ceases. Other neurons begin firing when a stimulus ends. The firing pattern of a neuron may change as there occurs a change in the stimulus. The most important brainstem area for the coding of temporal information may be the superior olivary complex. Cells in the medial superior olivary nuclei have been shown to be extremely sensitive to temporal factors.

Feature-sensitive elements in the auditory brainstem nuclei also respond to the frequency and intensity and/or other characteristics of the stimulus, and feature extraction takes place. Cortical neurons also have analytical characteristics (Evans, 1974). The pattern of a sequence is probably enhanced by interaction between afferent and efferent auditory systems and, at a more basic level, between excitatory and inhibitory neurons. This contrast enhancement has been observed in the visual system (Campbell, 1981) and is believed to exist in the auditory system also (Evans and Whitfield, 1964). Such contrast information would be important in

perceiving the relationship among sequence components (Suga, 1965, 1972; Wollberg and Newman, 1972).

Teuber (1960) proposed that all sensory perception was patterned and depended on the interaction of concomitant and successive processes in the central nervous system, and Efron has postulated that processing in the subcortical auditory nuclei may be responsible for what others have interpreted to be hemispheric specialization (Chapter 9). Data from the brainstem nuclei are passed on to cortex for further processing of temporal order.

Most investigators have concluded that the actual conscious perception of temporal order necessary to any sort of behavioral response and the processing of that response occur at the cortical level (Sternberg and Knoll, 1973). In the auditory system the cortical areas involved in perception of the sequential stimuli are located in the temporal lobes of the brain, primarily in the transverse gyri of Heschl. The processing of the information and the behavioral response involve much wider areas of cortex, and these areas may be found in either one or both temporal lobes with perhaps some involvement of the inferior parietal lobule and frontal cortex as well, depending on the manner of coding and the type of response required of the subject. Ablation studies of temporal ordering in animals (Diamond and Neff, 1957; Goldberg et al, 1957; Neff, 1961; Diamond et al, 1962; Colavita et al, 1974; Colavita and Weisberg, 1977) and studies of humans with brain dysfunction (Milner, 1962; Shankweiler, 1966; Leftoff, 1981; and others) support this conclusion. Verbal or manual response to an auditory sequence may require intact cortical language areas (Lomas and Kimura, 1976), such as the left supramarginal and angular gyri of the left inferior parietal lobule in most right-handed and some left-handed individuals. The output of these responses also may involve frontal cortex close to the central fissure where initiation of motor activity occurs. The tracts of white matter (nerve fibers) underlying the cortex intrahemispherically and interhemispherically may be involved also in the processing and in transmission from one region to another. Therefore, from the initial perception of a temporal sequence through its processing to an overt response of some kind, it is obvious that large sections of cortex are activated. Damage to any of the involved areas may result in impairment of temporal ordering ability, making it difficult or impossible to specify any one area of the brain in humans as responsible for this ability. In cats Colavita and Weisberg (1977) implicated insular-temporal cortex.

Beyond the initial reception of the stimulus information in the primary areas of the temporal lobes, little is actually known about how an auditory sequence is processed. It seems necessary that some storage or short-term memory be involved, since a sequence cannot be recognized as such or processed until it is completed over time. The location in the brain for sequential memory is unknown. It may be bilateral, located in different areas for different sensory systems, and even for different stimuli in the same sensory system. DeRenzi and colleagues (1977) reported that patients with left hemisphere damage could recall the serial order of visual information but could not use a verbal memory code.

In several animals, such as birds and monkeys, neural units have been observed with special sensitivity to patterns of sounds which are meaningful or significant to that particular organism (Konishi, 1970; Funkenstein and Winter, 1973). Man probably has this same special neural capacity attuned to sequences involving speech or perhaps some other very meaningful learned patterns.

Sequences are made up of different components, so that it is possible that a temporal pattern may become spatially represented by cortical neurons, even though its components are sequential. If there are differences in the spectral characteristics of the components, different neurons could respond to the different components. It is known that "frequency maps" exist in every nucleus throughout the auditory system (Chapters 2 and 5), so that components of different frequencies would activate neural units in different areas of central auditory nuclei. This physiological "spatial" response may contribute to pattern recognition and temporal order processing. Pinheiro (1971) found that subjects showed improved performance for frequency or pitch patterns over patterns in which only the intensity of components or only the duration of components was manipulated.

Hemispheric Dominance

Some investigators concluded from their studies that the left hemisphere is dominant for temporal sequencing in most individuals (Efron, 1963; Carmon and Nachshon, 1971; Krashen, 1972; Halperin et al, 1973; Lackner and Teuber, 1973; Papcun et al, 1974). Still other researchers have proposed that the right hemisphere is more important for discriminating tonal sequences (Milner, 1962), unfamiliar melodies presented dichotically (Shankweiler, 1966), recorded bird songs presented binaurally (Milner et al, 1965), and dichotic tonal sequences (Schuloff and Goodglass, 1969). Karaseva (1972) and Lhermitte and colleagues (1971) reported that patients with either unilateral or bilateral lesions of temporal lobe had difficulty in discriminating rhythmic patterns of clicks. It is possible that the different psychophysical methods used in these different studies led the authors to interpret their results in different ways. Considering the above citations it may be possible that both hemispheres of the brain are involved in temporal sequencing. The general function of the left hemisphere has been described as analytical and, therefore, important to serial ordering of temporal information (see references below). It may compare or analyze the interrelationships among the components of a sequence. The left hemisphere in most right-handed individuals and in some left-handed individuals is also dominant for language processing. Many temporal ordering judgments require language processing, even when the actual response is not verbal. The right hemisphere has been described as dominant for holistic functions (Levy-Agresti and Sperry, 1968; Semmes, 1968; Halperin et al, 1973; Papcun et al, 1974; Bever and Chiarello, 1974; and Bever, 1975). This function is also important to temporal sequencing, and the right side of the brain may be active in determining the contours, overall pattern, or Gestalt of a sequence. Thus, there may well be interhemispheric interaction in temporal ordering, even when the stimulus sequence is not made up of speech elements.

Work by Musiek and colleagues (1980) and Musiek and Kibbe (1984) with split-brain patients appears to support this conclusion. These studies demonstrated that patients with surgical sections of their interhemispheric commissures could hum an imitative response to an auditory sequence presented monaurally to either ear, but they could not give a verbal or manual response to the same monaural stimulus. These results appear to indicate that some right hemispheric processing was involved and that this information could not be transferred to the left hemisphere when a response involving language processing was required. Although the left hemisphere could readily initiate speech, it could not give a verbal or manual response to a sequence, even when that sequence was presented to the right ear.

Bever (1975) observed that naive listeners processed a muscial sequence by focusing on its gestalt or overall contour (right hemisphere), whereas trained listeners were prone to process the stimulus sequence by observing and analyzing the relationships among components (left hemisphere). In contrast, a study of Papcun and colleagues (1974) concluded that naive subjects processed dichotic Morse code signals in the left hemisphere, while trained subjects used the right side of the brain. In many years of clinical examinations of brain-damaged patients with Pitch Pattern Sequences, Pinheiro did not find any consistent differences between ears in normal or brain-damaged subjects, although performance tended to be poorer for the contralateral ear in patients with cerebral lesions, whichever side of the brain was impaired. Her results did not seem to implicate either side of the brain as more specialized than the other in temporal ordering for the type of sequences and responses required in her studies (cited in this chapter).

A review of all these findings suggests that whether or not it appears that one hemisphere of the brain is specialized for a certain temporal ordering task may depend on the type of sequence employed, the kind of behavioral judgment required of the subject, and the manner of coding the information and processing the response.

TEMPORAL ORDERING TESTS AVAILABLE FOR CLINICAL USE

A number of speech tests used in the clinical assessment of the central auditory nervous system involve aspects of sequencing, i.e., Competing Sentences, Staggered Spondee Words, Digits, etc., discussed in Chapters 12 and 14.

In school settings the Auditory Sequential Memory subtest of the Illinois Test of Psychological Abilities (ITPA) and the verbal sequences of the Developmental Learning Materials are often used to assess reading skills or employed as therapeutic tasks for children with learning, language, and/or reading problems. However, these tests usually are not applied in the audiology clinic where central auditory evaluations are conducted.

This chapter will consider only the nonverbal sequencing tasks. Unfortunately, at present there is no one such test in routine clinical use, although a number of procedures of this type have been studied in clinical populations. Among these are the Seashore Test of Tonal Memory (Milner, 1962), dichotic melodies (Kimura, 1964; Shankweiler, 1966), pulsed Doppler sequences (Pollack, 1968), and musical chords (Gordon, 1970). Other tasks employing sequences have been documented, and some of these studies were discussed earlier in this chapter. None of these tasks has wide clinical application.

One test of temporal ordering ability which is available for clinical use is the Pitch Pattern Sequence Test developed by Pinheiro. There are two separate versions available, one for adults and one for children (described in Chapter 14). The adult version consists of 120 test pattern sequences. Each sequence is made up of three tone bursts, two of one frequency and one of a second frequency, arranged in six possible combinations. The "high" tone is 1430 Hz and the "low" tone is 880 Hz. Duration of each tone is 200 msec, and there is a silent interval of 150 msec between tones, so that the total duration of each sequence is 900 msec. The test is preceded by a practice session during which the clinician ascertains whether the patient can distinguish between "high" and "low" tones presented in pairs. This discrimination task is followed by a practice session on 20 randomized sequences before the actual test is begun. The presentation level is 50 dB above the 1000 Hz threshold for each ear. The test may be administered monaurally (Fig. 13.3) or binaurally under earphones or in sound field with similar results. Verbal, manual, and/or hummed responses may be required, depending on the capabil-

L= Low Frequency (880Hz)

H= High Frequency (1122Hz)

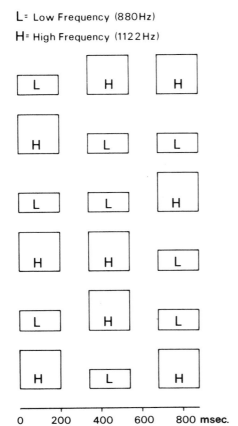

Figure 13.3. Block diagram example of monaural pitch patterns in the six possible combinations of the two frequencies used to make up the sequences.

ity of the patient and the data desired by the clinician. A comparison of either verbal or manual responses with hummed responses is valuable in differentiating an impairment in perception from an impairment in processing the auditory sequences. This type of task offers several advantages in central auditory assessment. The sequential stimuli are nonverbal; the task is a very easy one for normal adults; and various response methods may be tailored to the ability of the patient to respond. Patients with lesions in auditory cortex in either hemisphere or patients with interhemispheric dysfunction have shown impairment on this task. However, test results do not "localize" the lesion. It is recommended that this test be used as part of a central auditory test battery.

CLINICAL EVIDENCE OF IMPAIRMENT IN TEMPORAL SEQUENCING ABILITY IN BRAIN-DAMAGED PATIENTS

Variables involved in investigations of temporal ordering ability in patients with brain dysfunction are numerous and difficult or impossible to control. Some of these include differences in site, size, and type of lesion. Pathological populations of subjects with similar brain insults are usually small. Damage that is unilateral may produce bilateral deficits. Duration of the brain injury and amount of recovery may differ from patient to patient. Results may depend on whether or not the patient is stable. Also, age, years of education, and intelligence level influence results in these patients even more than in the normal population, since these variables strongly affect recovery.

The relationship between the auditory function of temporal ordering and injury to the brain has been studied by numerous investigators in both animals and man.

In human subjects even small areas of brain damage seem to be detrimental to the ability to sequence auditory stimuli, especially nonspeech patterns. Milner (1962) reported that patients with temporal lobectomies performed poorly on the Seashore Test of Tonal Memory. Two sequences of three to five tones each were presented in succession, with one tone in the second sequence differing from the same tone in the first sequence. The patient had to identify the tone that was different. Patients with right temporal lobectomies made more errors than patients with left temporal lobectomies. In 1965 Milner and associates reported similar findings on patients with right and left temporal lobectomies for recorded bird songs presented binaurally. Shankweiler (1966) reported similar results for dichotic melodies on a similar group of patients.

Efron (1963) found that aphasic patients required up to 1 sec to judge the temporal order of two brief 10 msec sounds. Patients with lesions of the dominant temporal lobe required 150 to 600 msec for the task. Hirsh (1967) reported similar results on aphasic patients, but found no correlation between the severity of the aphasia and the sequencing difficulty. Jerger and coworkers (1969) reported that a patient with bilateral temporal lobe lesions needed 300 to 500 msec difference in onset times of two tones in order to judge whether the first tone was high or low in pitch. A normal subject made the same judgment in 10 to 25 msec. Swisher and Hirsh (1972) also found that their patients with lesions in either the right or left hemisphere required greater differences between the onset times of two auditory signals than normal subjects for making judgments of temporal order. Fluent aphasics were the most impaired in performance, while patients with right hemisphere damage had greater deficits when the successive tonal stimuli were presented to separate ears. Lackner and Teuber (1973) also reported that cortically damaged patients needed longer silent intervals than normal subjects between stimuli to perceive separation.

Schuloff and Goodglass (1969) used dichotic materials to test patients with either right or left hemisphere lesions. They concluded that the left hemisphere was dominant for sequencing digits, whereas the right hemisphere was dominant for the temporal ordering of tone sequences. However, the deficits in performance were always greater for the ear contralateral to the lesion. Lhermitte and associates (1971) reported that patients with bilateral temporal lobe damage could recognize intensity and frequency differences but could not discriminate between two different temporal sequences. Karaseva's (1972) patients with unilateral damage to the auditory projection areas of the temporal lobe were impaired in the discrimination of rhythmic patterns of clicks in the ear contralateral to the lesion. Hemiplegics examined by Belmont and Handler (1971) always reported that the ear contralateral to the lesion was stimulated last when pairs of 500 Hz tones of 200 msec duration were separated by 20, 50, or 80 msec in onset times, with one tone presented to one ear and the second tone to the other ear. DeRenzi and his colleagues (1977) found that brain-damaged subjects could not use a verbal memory code to recall serial order information. Carmon and Nachson (1971) noted that patients with left hemisphere lesions were severely impaired in pointing to the locations in correct order for a sequence of three to five bimodal stimuli (colored light bulbs and tones) presented in a temporal

series. Patients with right hemisphere lesions performed as well as normal subjects.

Pinheiro (1976) and Pinheiro and associates (1977) observed that patients with lesions in either hemisphere of the brain performed more poorly than normal subjects in sequencing auditory patterns composed of three temporally spaced noise or tone bursts. There was little difference between pathological groups or between ears within each group (Fig. 13.4). When piano music or discourse competed with the pitch pattern sequences in either the ipsilateral or contralateral ear at equal SLs there were no differences among listening conditions in com-

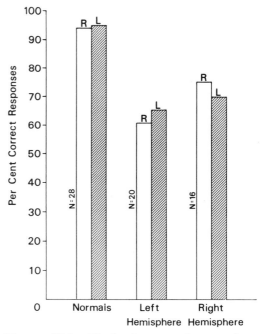

Figure 13.4. Block diagram of manual responses to pitch patterns by normal subjects and subjects with right and left hemisphere lesions. Subjects with brain lesions performed significantly more poorly than normal subjects, and the ear contralateral to the lesion in either hemisphere tended to have lower scores. When scores for ears contralateral to the lesions were compared, there were no significant differences. However, the performance on patterns presented to the right ear was significantly poorer for the left brain-damaged group than for the right brain-damaged group. All subjects had normal pure tone thresholds to 4000 Hz and normal speech discrimination scores.

paring performances for contralateral ears or ipsilateral ears. There was a significant difference between ears within both the right hemisphere (RH) group and the left hemisphere (LH) group when pitch patterns were presented to one ear and competing music to the other ear. In this case, the ear opposite the lesioned hemisphere was better. The only significant difference between the two groups of brain-damaged patients was observed for the pitch pattern/competing discourse condition; RH patients surprisingly scored better for the left ear.

The following variety of individual case studies may further illustrate the fact that lesions in either hemisphere of the brain seem to affect performance on pitch patterns almost equally in both ears. Although the site and size of the lesion within a hemisphere does not appear to result in differences between ears, they do affect performance. These patients had normal hearing for pure tones and speech. A 27-yr-old patient who had a right anterior temporal lobectomy for a seizure disorder scored only 35% correct for each ear. In contrast, a 59-yr-old patient with a left anterior temporal lobe astrocytoma achieved 100% on pitch patterns in both ears prior to any surgery. A 16-yr-old patient being treated for seizures and a behavioral disorder was found to have a large glioma in the left thalamus, invading the left hemisphere, after he performed at 0% on pitch patterns for both ears. (This patient also scored poorly on several other central auditory tests. See Fig. 10.1, p. 162.) A 49-yr-old patient with right hydrocephalus scored only 18% for both ears. Figure 13.5 illustrates a similar bilateral deficit on pattern performance in a patient with a right temporal lobe epileptic focus.

In a large group of patients with multiple sclerosis, the wide individual variability prohibited any general conclusions relative to pitch pattern performance. However, the level ranged from 60 to 100%, and these scores were significantly better than scores for patients with other right and left hemisphere lesions. Musiek and colleagues (1982) reported that their patient with Charcot-Marie-Tooth disease achieved 15% correct for the right ear and 2% for the left ear; these scores were at chance level.

Musiek et al (1980) reported that split-brain patients performed at approximately

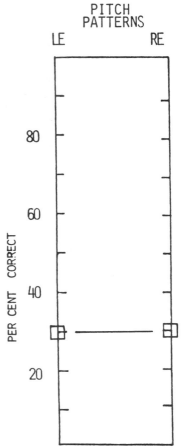

Figure 13.5. Frequency (pitch) pattern results for a 22-yr-old, right-handed male who had a right-sided temporal lobe epileptic focus. Pure tone thresholds were normal bilaterally, and speech discrimination ability was excellent in both ears. It is interesting to note the bilateral deficit for a lesion limited to one hemisphere (normal performance = 75% or better).

chance level on both frequency and intensity patterns when they were required to verbally repeat the sequence of the tones. Right ear performance tended to be poorer. These same patients were able to hum the tonal patterns normally. Musiek and Kibbe (1984) further confirmed these findings recently on a series of patients who underwent commissurotomies for intractible epilepsy (Fig. 13.6).

It may still be too early to determine how brainstem lesions affect performance on temporal sequencing tests, such as the sequencing of patterns. In a rare case of sur-

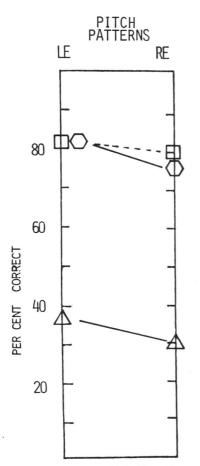

PITCH PATTERNS

Figure 13.6. Frequency (pitch) pattern results pre (□) and post (△) complete commissurotomy for a young adult right-handed male. The ability to hum the patterns postsurgery is indicated by (○). Pure tone thresholds were normal bilaterally, and speech discrimination ability was excellent for both ears (normal performance = 75% or better).

vival of a penetrating wound of the right pons Pinheiro et al (1982) found a difference between ears; right ear performance was approximately normal at 88%, whereas left ear performance was at chance level at 15%. Musiek and Geurkink (1982) found that seven patients with brainstem lesions performed normally on patterns for both ears. However, three patients gave abnormal performance, one for both ears, one for the right ear, and one for the left ear. In a patient with an extraaxial brainstem tumor pattern performance was normal for both ears (Musiek et al, 1983).

CONCLUSION

It is evident that temporal ordering or sequencing is an important central auditory function that should be assessed in any evaluation of the central auditory nervous system. It is a process which may underlie other auditory and language deficits observed in individuals with suspected or confirmed brain dysfunction.

Results of both experimental and clinical research reported in this chapter and in Chapter 9 by Efron indicate that this is a worthwhile area for further investigation. It is also clear that much research is still needed in the development of a viable clinical procedure.

References

Belmont I, Handler A: Delayed information processing and judgment of temporal order following cerebral damage. *J Nerv Ment Dis* 152:353–361, 1971.

Berlin CI, Lowe SS: Differential diagnostic evaluation: central auditory function. In Katz J (ed): *Handbook of Clinical Audiology.* Baltimore, Williams & Wilkins, 1972, ch 15, pp 280–312.

Bever TG: Cerebral asymmetries in humans are due to the differentiation of two incompatible processes: holistic and analytic. *Ann NY Acad Sci* 263:251–262, 1975.

Bever TG, Chiarello RJ: Cerebral dominance in musicians and nonmusicians. *Science* 185:537–539, 1974.

Bregman AS, Campbell J: Primary auditory stream segregation and perception of order in rapid sequences of tones. *J Exp Psychol* 89:244–249, 1971.

Broadbent DE, Ladefoged P: Auditory perception of temporal order. *J Acoust Soc Am* 31:1539, 1950.

Campbell FW: The physics of visual perception. In Pompeiano O, Marsan CA (eds): *Brain Mechanisms of Perceptual Awareness and Purposeful Behavior.* International Brain Research Organization Monograph Series. New York, Raven Press, 1981, vol 8, pp 101–132.

Carmon A, Nachshon I: Effect of unilateral brain damage on perception of temporal order. *Cortex* 7:410–418, 1971.

Colavita FB, Szelgio FV, Zimmer SD: Temporal pattern discrimination in cats with insular-temporal lesions. *Brain Res* 79:153–156, 1974.

Colavita FB, Wiesberg DH: Spatio-temporal pattern discrimination in cats with insular-temporal lesions. *Brain Res Bull* 3:7–9, 1977.

Dannenbring G: The effect of continuity on auditory stream segregation. Master's thesis, McGill University, Montreal, 1971.

DeFosse CO: Effects of report order and response mode on dichotic pitch pattern scores of musicians and nonmusicians. Ph.D. thesis, University of Toledo, Toledo, OH, 1978.

DeFosse CO, Pinheiro ML: Perception of Dichotic Pitch Patterns by Musicians and Nonmusicians. Presented at a meeting of the American Speech Hearing Association, San Francisco, November, 1978.

Delattre PC, Liberman AM, Cooper FS: Acoustic loci and transitional cues for consonants. *J Acoust Soc Am* 27:769–773, 1955.

DeRenzi E, Faglioni P, Villa P: Sequential memory for figures in brain-damaged patients. *Neuropsychology* 15:43–49, 1977.

Diamond IT, Goldberg JM, Neff WD: Tonal discrimination after ablation of auditory cortex. *J Neurophysiol* 25:223–225, 1962.

Diamond IT, Neff WD: Ablation of temporal cortex and discrimination of auditory patterns. *J Neurophysiol* 20:300–315, 1957.

Divenyi PL: Some figural properties of auditory patterns. *J Acoust Soc Am* 64:1369–1385, 1978.

Divenyi PL, Hirsh IJ: Identification of temporal order in three-tone sequences. *J Acoust Soc Am* 56:144–151, 1974.

Efron R: Temporal perception, aphasia, and déjà vu. *Brain* 86:403–424, 1963.

Efron R: Conservation of temporal information by perceptual systems. *Percept Psychophysiol* 14:518–530, 1973.

Efron R, Yund EW: Dichotic competition of simultaneous tone bursts of different frequency. III. The effect of stimulus parameters on suppression and ear dominance functions. *Neuropsychology* 13:151–161, 1975.

Eisenson J: Developmental aphasia (dyslogia). A postulation of a unitary concept of the disorder. *Cortex* 4:184–200, 1968.

Evans EF: Neural processes for the detection of acoustic patterns and for sound localization. In Schmitt FO, Worden FG (eds): *The Neurosciences Third Study Program.* Cambridge, MA, M.I.T. Press, 1974, ch 13, pp 131–145.

Evans EF, Whitfield IC: Classification of unit responses in the auditory cortex of the unanaesthetized and unrestrained cat. *J Physiol* 171:476–493, 1964.

Exner S: Experimentelle untersuchung der einfachsten psychischen. *Processe Pflug Arch Physiol* 11:403–432, 1875.

Funkenstein HH, Winter P: Responses to acoustic stimuli of units in the auditory cortex of awake squirrel monkeys. *Exp Brain Res* 18:464–488, 1973.

Furth HG: Sequence learning in aphasic and deaf children. *J Speech Hear Disord* 29:171–177, 1964.

Furth HG, Youniss J: Sequence learning: perceptual implications in the acquisition of language. In Wathen-Dunn W (ed): *Models for the Perception of Speech and Visual Form.* Cambridge, MA, M.I.T. Press, 1967, pp 344–353.

Garner WR, Clement DE: Goodness of pattern and pattern uncertainty. *J Verb Learn Verb Behav* 2:446–452, 1963.

Garner WR, Gottwald RL: The perception and learning of temporal patterns. *Q J Exp Psychol* 20:97–109, 1968.

Goldberg JM, Diamond IT, Neff WD: Auditory discrimination after ablation of temporal and insular cortex in cat. *Fed Proc* 16:204, 1957.

Gordon HW: Hemispheric asymmetries in the perception of musical chords. *Cortex* 6:387–398, 1970.

Halperin Y, Nachshon I, Carmon A: Shift of ear superiority in dichotic listening to temporally patterned nonverbal stimuli. *J Acoust Soc Am* 53:46–50, 1973.

Handel S: Temporal segmentation of repeating auditory patterns. *J Exp Psychol* 101:46–54, 1973.

Handel S, Yoder D: The effects of intensity and interval rhythms on the perception of auditory and visual temporal patterns. *Q J Exp Psychol* 27:111–122, 1975.

Hirsh IJ: Auditory perception of temporal order. *J Acoust Soc Am* 31:759–767, 1959.

Hirsh IJ: Information processing in input channels for speech and language: the significance of serial order of stimuli. In Millikan CH, Darley FL (eds): *Brain Mechanisms Underlying Speech and Language.* New York, Grune & Stratton, 1967, pp 21–38.

Hirsh IJ, Fraisse P: Simultanéité et succession de stimuli hétérogénes. *Ann Psychol* 64:1–19, 1964.

Hirsh IJ, Sherrick CE: Perceived order in different sense modalities. *J Exp Psychol* 62:423–432, 1961.

Homick JL, Elfner LF, Bothe GG: Auditory temporal masking and the perception of order. *J Acoust Soc Am* 45:712–718, 1969.

Jerger J, Weikers NJ, Sharbrough FW III, Jerger S: Bilateral lesions of the temporal lobe. *Acta Otolaryngol* [Suppl] (Stockh) 258:1–51, 1969.

Karaseva TA: The role of the temporal lobe in human auditory perception. *Neuropsychology* 10:227–231, 1972.

Kimura D: Left-right differences in the perception of melodies. *Q J Exp Psychol* 16:355–358, 1964.

Konishi M: Comparative neurophysiological studies of hearing and vocalizations in songbirds. *Z Vergl Physiol* 66:257–272, 1970.

Krashen SD: An unbiased procedure for comparing degree of lateralization of dichotically presented stimuli. In Krashen S (ed): *Language and Left Hemisphere.* Working Papers in Phonetics, Los Angeles, U.C.L.A., 1972, vol 24.

Lackner J, Teuber H-L: Alterations in auditory fusion thresholds after cerebral injury in man. *Neuropsychology* 11:409–415, 1973.

Lashley KS: The problem of serial order in behavior. In Jeffress LA (ed): *Cerebral Mechanisms in Behavior.* New York, Wiley, 1951, pp 112–136.

Leeuwenberg EL: A perceptual coding language for visual and auditory patterns. *Am J Psychol* 84:307–349, 1971.

Leftoff S: Learning functions for unilaterally brain damaged patients for serially and randomly ordered stimulus material: Analysis of retrieval strategies and their relationship to rehabilitation. *J Clin Neuropsychol* 3:301–314, 1981.

Leshowitz B, Hanzi R: Auditory pattern discrimination in the absence of spectral cues. *J Acoust Soc Am* 52:166, 1972.

Levy-Agresti J, Sperry R: Differential perceptual capacities in major and minor hemispheres. *Proc Natl Acad Sci USA* 61:1151, 1968.

Lhermitte F, Chain F, Escourolle R, Ducarne B, Pillou B, Chedru G: Etude des troubles perceptifs auditifs dans les lesions temporales bilaterales. *Rev Neurol* 124:329–351, 1971.

Lomas J, Kimura D: Intrahemispheric interaction between speaking and sequential manual activity. *Neuropsychology* 14:23–33, 1976.

Massaro DW: Preperceptual images, processing time, and perceptual units in auditory perception. *Psychol Rev* 79:124–145, 1972.

Milner B: Laterality effects in audition. In Mountcastle VB (ed): *Interhemispheric Relations and Cerebral Dominance,* Baltimore, John Hopkins Press, 1962, chap 9, pp 177–195.

Milner B, Kimura D, Taylor LB: Nonverbal Auditory Learning after Frontal or Temporal Lobectomy in Man. Presented at a meeting of the Eastern Psychology Association, Boston, 1965.

Miscik JG, Smith JM, Hemm NH, Deffenbacher KA, Brown EL: Short term retention of auditory sequences as a function of stimulus duration, interstimulus interval, and encoding technique. *J Exp Psychol* 96:147–151, 1972.

Musiek FE, Geurkink NA: Auditory brain stem response and central auditory test findings for patients with brain stem lesions: a preliminary report. *Laryngoscope* 92:891–900, 1982.

Musiek FE, Kibbe K: Audiologic test results in patients with commissurotomy. *Epilepsy and the Corpus Callosum.* New York, Plenum Press, 1984.

Musiek FE, Pinheiro ML, Wilson DH: Auditory pattern perception in "split brain" patients. *Arch Otolaryngol* 106:610–612, 1980.

Musiek FE, Weider DJ, Mueller RJ: Audiologic findings in Charcot-Marie-Tooth disease. *Arch Otolaryngol* 108:595–599, 1982.

Musiek FE, Weider DJ, Mueller RJ: Reversible audiologic results in a patient with an extra-axial brain stem tumor. *Ear Hear* 4:169–172, 1983.

Neff WD: Discriminatory capacity of different divisions of the auditory system. *Brain* 1:205–224, 1961.

Neff WD: Temporal pattern discrimination in lower animals and its relation to language perception in man. In deRueck AVS, O'Connor M (eds): *Disorders of Language.* Boston, Little Brown, 1964, pp 183–199.

Neff WD, Diamond IT, Casseday JH: Behavioral studies of auditory discrimination: central nervous system. In Keidel WD, Neff WD (eds): *Handbook of Sensory Physiology.* New York, Springer-Verlag, 1975, vol 2, pp 307–400.

Neisser U: On the Perception of Auditory Sequences. Presented at a meeting of the American Psychological Association, Honolulu, 1972.

Nickerson RS, Freeman B: Discrimination of the order of the components of repeating tone sequences: effects of frequency separation and extensive practice. *Percept Psychophysiol* 16:471–477, 1974.

Papcun G, Krashen SD, Terbeck D, Remington R, Harshman R: The left hemisphere is specialized for speech, language and/or something else. *J Acoust Soc Am* 55:319–327, 1974.

Patterson JH, Green DM: Discrimination of transient signals having identical energy spectra. *J Acoust Soc Am* 48:894–905, 1970.

Peters RW, Wood TJ: Perceived order of tone pulses. *J Acoust Soc Am* 54:315, 1973.

Pinheiro ML: Auditory pattern perception in patients with left and right hemisphere lesions. *Ohio J Speech Hear* 12:9–20, 1976.

Pinheiro ML: Tests of central auditory function in children with learning disabilities. In Keith RW (ed): *Central Auditory Dysfunction.* New York, Grune & Stratton, 1977a, pp 223–254.

Pinheiro ML: Central auditory test profile in children with learning disabilities. In Burns MS, Andrews JR (eds): *Selected Papers in Language and Phonology.* Evanston, IL, Institute for Continuing Professional Education, 1977b, vol 1, pp 63–75.

Pinheiro ML: A central auditory test profile of learning disabled children with dyslexia. In Bradford LJ (ed): *Communication Disorders: An Audio Journal for Continuing Education.* New York, Grune & Stratton, 1978.

Pinheiro ML, Andrews LT: Perceptual Errors for Temporal Patterns Based on a Difference in Duration of Pattern Components. Presented at a meeting of the American Speech Hearing Association, Detroit, 1973.

Pinheiro ML, Jacobson GP, Boller F: Auditory dysfunction following a gunshot wound of the pons. *J Speech Hear Disord* 47:296–300, 1982.

Pinheiro ML, Ptacek PH: Reversals in the perception of noise and tone patterns. *J Acoust Soc Am* 49:1778–1782, 1971.

Pinheiro ML, Tinta T: Differences among response modes in pitch pattern perception. In Andrews JR, Burns MS, (eds): *Selected Papers in Language and Phonology.* Evasnton, IL, Institute for Continuing Professional Education, 1977, vol 2, pp 179–191.

Pinheiro ML, Weidner WE, Suren SM, Gaydos ML: Sequencing of Pitch Patterns with Competing Music and Competing Discourse by Patients with Right and Left Hemisphere Lesions. Presented at a meeting of the Academy of Aphasia, Montreal, 1977.

Pollack I: Discrimination of repeated auditory patterns of pulsed doppler sequences. *Am J Psychol* 81:480–487, 1968.

Preusser D: The effect of structure and rate on the recognition and description of auditory temporal patterns. *Percept Psychophysiol* 11:233–239, 1972.

Ptacek PH, Pinheiro ML: Pattern reversal in auditory perception. *J Acoust Soc Am* 49:493–498, 1971.

Royer FL, Garner WR: Response uncertainty and perceptual difficulty of auditory temporal patterns. *Percept Psychophysiol* 1:41–44, 1966.

Royer FL, Garner WR: Perceptual organization of nine-element auditory temporal patterns. *Percept Psychophysiol* 7:115–120, 1970.

Schuloff C, Goodglass H: Dichotic listening, side of brain injury and cerebral dominance. *Neuropsychology* 7:149–160, 1969.

Semmes J: Hemispheric specialization: a possible clue to mechanism. *Neuropsychology* 6:11–26, 1968.

Shankweiler D: Effects of temporal lobe damage on perception of dichotically presented melodies. *J Comp Physiol Psychol* 62:115–119, 1966.

Shulman HG, Greenberg SN: Perceptual deficit due to division of attention between memory and perception. *J Exp Psychol* 2:171–176, 1971.

Sternberg S, Knoll RL: The perception of temporal order: fundamental issues and a general model. In Kornblum S (ed): *Attention and Performance IV.* New York, Academic Press, 1973, pp 629–685.

Suga M: Functional properties of auditory neurones in the cortex of echolocating bats. *J Physiol* 181:671–700, 1965.

Suga N: Analysis of information bearing elements in complex sounds by auditory neurones of bats. *Audiology* 11:58–72, 1972.

Swisher L, Hirsh IJ: Brain damage and the ordering of two temporally successive stimuli. *Neuropsychology* 10:137–152, 1972.

Teuber H-L: Perception. In Field J, Magoun HW, Hall VE (eds): *Handbook of Physiology.* Washington, DC, American Physiology Society, 1960, vol 3, pp 1595–1678.

Thomas IB, Cetti RP, Chase PW: Effect of silent intervals on the perception of temporal order for vowels. *J Acoust Soc Am* 49:85, 1971.

Thomas IB, Fitzgibbons PJ: Temporal order and perceptual classes. *J Acoust Soc Am* 50:86–87, 1971.

Thomas IB, Hill PB, Carroll FS, Barcia B: Temporal order in the perception of vowels. *J Acoust Soc Am* 48:1010–1013, 1970.

Vitz PC, Todd TC: A coded element model of the perceptual processing of sequential stimuli. *Psychol Rev* 76:433–449, 1969.

Warren RM: Auditory temporal discrimination by trained listeners. *Cognit Psychol* 6:237–256, 1974.

Warren RM, Obusek CJ: Identification of temporal order within auditory sequences. *Percept Psychophysiol* 12:86–90, 1972.

Warren RM, Obusek CJ, Farmer RM, Warren RP: Auditory sequence: confusion of patterns other than speech or music. *Science* 164:586–587, 1969.

Watson CS, Kelly WJ: The role of stimulus uncertainty in the discrimination of auditory patterns. In Getty DJ, Howard JH Jr (eds): *Auditory and Visual Pattern Recognition.* Hillsdale, NJ, Lawrence Erlbaum, 1981, ch 3, pp 37–59.

Watson CS, Kelly WJ, Wroton HW: Factors in the discrimination of tonal patterns. II. Selective attention and learning under various levels of stimulus uncertainty. *J Acoust Soc Am* 57:1175–1181, 1975.

Wilcox G, Neisser U, Roberts J: Recognition of Auditory Temporal Order. Presented at a meeting of the East Psychological Association, Boston, 1972.

Wollberg Z, Newman JD: Auditory cortex of the squirrel monkey: response patterns of single cells to species-specific vocalizations. *Science* 175:212–214, 1972.

CHAPTER 14

Assessment of Central Auditory Disorders in Children

JACK A. WILLEFORD, Ph.D.

Dr. Willeford describes the behavioral, academic, and social characteristics of children who may present with central auditory problems. He addresses the clinical challenge in evaluating these children and discusses a test battery and results reported by researchers in this area.

INTRODUCTION

Manifestations

Large numbers of children are suspected of having subtle central auditory deficiencies even though their neurological test results are typically unremarkable. These children exhibit poor language and/or listening skills, and, although they are commonly found to have adequate to high intelligence, they present with academic performances below their estimated potential. Moreover, they routinely demonstrate normal peripheral hearing on traditional tests. Some do well in one-to-one conversations in quiet environments, but others show inordinate difficulty in comprehending speech. This is especially true in the presence of competing sounds. They may or may not exhibit a language disorder which is of sufficient severity or quality to qualify them for special education services in the public schools. An increasing number of audiologists and speech language pathologists throughout the United States are being asked to see such children because concerned parents and teachers have observed enough difficulty in communicating with them to cast suspicion on faulty auditory function of some nature. Children with central auditory processing disorders (CAPD)

are characterized as poor listeners, easily distractable, underachievers, with difficulty in following directions, short attention spans, poor memories for auditory information, and other behaviors that interfere with learning and communication processes. These behaviors are similar to those noted by other authors for the classification of children who are termed *learning-disabled*. This is not surprising since children with central auditory deficits commonly have learning difficulties, and many learning-disabled children have central auditory disorders as a contributing cause of their problems. However, these problems are not invariably concomitant (Willeford, 1980). Diagnosis in either case rests on confirmation of an auditory deficit through the use of appropriate measures of central auditory function. In the final analysis it is necessary to evaluate a given child's performance on *auditory tests* per se rather than on tests in which uncontrolled auditory stimuli theoretically play an integral part in the assessment of other skills such as oral, read, or written language. While there is little doubt that audition does play a role in these complex language processes, it is not presently possible to establish the precise nature of their contributions. That is particularly true for those tests that are administered when either the test environment or the test stimuli are not controlled. When professional workers are concerned about peripheral auditory skills (the measurement of pure tone sensitivity or simple speech discrimination ability), they generally expect the child to be evaluated in a sound-controlled test room with calibrated audiometric instruments.

The assessment of central auditory abilities demands similarly exacting conditions, since behavioral tests which are most commonly used for central auditory function are even more susceptible to the influences of ambient noise environments. Until all of the complex interrelationships of audition and language are resolved, one can merely hope to assess the functional integrity of a child's central auditory nervous system (CANS) by techniques that seek to isolate weaknesses somewhere in that system rather than simply implicate auditory deficiencies via measures of verbal linguistic processes. This is no simple task, since the elaborate network of the CANS affords the listener so many potential alternatives for processing complex auditory signals such as speech (Kiang, 1975; Panel on Communicative Disorders, U.S. Department of HEW, 1979; and Dr. Noback's chapter (2) in this book). Knowledge of that impressive system makes clear why traditional pure tone and speech discrimination tests performed in soundproof test rooms will generally fail to identify a central auditory dysfunction. Adequate auditory reception of verbal messages is possible for some children with CAPD during good ambient listening conditions in the audiology test room or in favorable social circumstances because of the redundant nature of speech and the syntactic and semantic cues from which one can synthesize the message.

The characteristics listed earlier cover a wide range of human behaviors observed in the daily lives of children with CAPD, but for practical purposes, they fall into three classifications which concern parents and teachers: auditory-communication behavior, academic performance, and social conduct.

Auditory-Communication Behavior

Children with CAPD exhibit a number of signs that can lead one to suspect a disorder in the auditory modality. They give the impression that they are not listening or that they fail to hear or understand what is said to them, even though they may be looking at the speaker. At other times they appear to hear, but apparently do not understand what they are told. However, under ideal circumstances, there are times when they do hear and understand quite well. For example, one mother told us that her first realization that her son might have some kind of special auditory problem (his hearing had been tested at school and found to be normal) came after she had to ask him four times to perform a simple household chore. When he did not obey, she asked him, "What's the matter; can't you understand me?" In spite of her exasperation, she reported that she suddenly realized what she was saying and wondered whether he really might have an auditory problem not revealed by the school's pure tone screening test. What confused her was the fact that the boy didn't seem to be willfully disobeying. The chain of events prior to clinical confirmation of the CAPD often has a profound psychological effect on the child. This leads him to a diminishing self-image, and he may become a management problem at school and in the home. As an unfortunate end result, in addition to academic deficiencies, the child may need psychological counseling, or he may even have a brush with delinquency. Referral of such children from mental health centers has become a common experience in some communities where central auditory diagnostic services are available. In summary, the child with normal hearing on traditional audiologic tests, but with a case history that leads one to suspect his auditory skills, is a prime candidate for central auditory evaluation.

Academic Performance

The major complaint of parents of a child with CAPD is that the youngster is performing below expected levels at school and doing so for reasons that are not clear, since his hearing is normal and his intelligence adequate. He may, or may not, meet the school diagnostic team's criteria for inclusion in special education services, since not all children with academic problems do so. The public schools simply cannot provide special services to every child with some deviation from expected norms of achievement. He may, nonetheless, still constitute a concern for his parents and/or classroom teachers. Major common concerns for these children are deficits in mathematical skills and/or in reading or other language proficiency, or simply an inability to function successfully in large, permissive, or "open" classrooms. Even when these children are enrolled in special education programs in the schools, the problems of some children may persist, and they may not respond to treatment strategies in the manner expected. Finally, there are children who progress adequately (if not well) except in discussion type classes where they cannot follow rapidly shifting conversation efficiently. That problem may be due to poor environmental listening conditions or to the classroom teacher's speaking skills, seating arrangements, or instructional protocols. When confirmation of a central auditory deficiency results in the proper awareness of the problem, and appropriate accommodations are made in the child's environments at home and at school, he may be able to cope adequately.

Social Conduct

The child with central auditory problems also has difficulty adjusting socially. It may be partially an outgrowth of his status in the classroom, but also can be the direct result of unfavorable interactions with family members and peers outside of school. Case histories reveal that the majority do not have friends or "buddies" of their own age. Rather, they seek out playmates who are usually two to three years younger than they are. Thus, they presumably avoid failures which may accompany competition with age-peers and cause them to become the butt of jokes or rejected in certain social activities. Some have confided that at times they haven't understood what friends said with the result that they responded in a way their friends thought was "dumb." A large number of children from our clinical experience are described by their parents as "loners" who prefer to play by themselves or to busy themselves with activities in the presence of parents or other tolerant adults.

Relation to Language Skills

A great deal has been written about the role which audition is thought to play in the development and use of language, and the degree to which it may be responsible for language disorders. Unfortunately, that relationship is still largely theoretical and often controversial. Although there seems to be no question that certain auditory and lan-

guage functions are uniquely interrelated in some highly complex manner, the essential parameters of that relationship elude us at present. Some of the reasons for our lack of solid information are: (1) confusions in terminology (for example, perceptual processing, conceptual processing, and auditory processing); (2) our inability to isolate and/or systematically control many of the theoretical subcomponents of audition (memory, sequencing, closure, association, etc.); (3) the enormous complexity of language phenomena (Witkin, 1971, Willeford and Billger, 1978); and (4) the variety of stimuli that have been employed to measure some aspect of audition (clicks, tones, consonant-vowels, nonsense syllables, words, and both meaningful and nonmeaningful sentences). The briefer and simpler the test stimulus, the easier it is to systematically control acoustic variables, such as frequency, intensity, and time. However, the more limited the verbal stimulus, the more segmented it becomes, and the further removed it is from functional language. Therefore, studies of isolated acoustic and phonetic features may have only limited value for understanding the necessary events that lead to semantic and syntactic processes. For a more detailed examination of the relationships between auditory processing and language skills, the reader is referred to an interesting literature review by Lubert (1981), and a subsequent exchange of views on these issues by Fuller (1982), O'Connell (1982), and Lubert (1982). In the final analysis there is wide agreement that there are children with CAPD, that there are also children with language disorders, and that some youngsters have both conditions. However, the fact that one condition can be present without evidence of the other (Willeford and Billger, 1978; Tallal et al, 1980; Ludlow, 1980) confirms the fact that the relationships between these phenomena are still poorly understood. Nonetheless, that void does not, and should not, keep us from our attempts to identify either CAPD or language disorders in children. However, it does mean that we should exercise caution in the way we view cause and effect relationships, and that treatment strategies selected for remediation of auditory/language disorders should be chosen and implemented with insight and care.

Etiological Implications

The suspected causes of most CAPDs in children are also poorly understood. The reason is that these disorders in the large number of children who fall under the rubric of the learning-disabled can seldom be traced to disease or injury. Similar disorders found in adults are usually specifically related to strokes, traumatic accidents, tumors, or other progressive disease processes. Although children are not immune to such causes, the discussion here is limited to the subtler type of disorder that involves poor listening skills, impedes learning, and interferes with social functioning. These children typically yield unremarkable neurological findings (Schain, 1977, p. 61) and show normal patterns of auditory brainstem response (Shimizu et al, 1981). Nonetheless, relationships have been proposed between neurological deficits, specific or behavioral, and low birth weight, birth damage, lead poisoning, food additives, excessive carbohydrate ingestion, otitis media, environmental deprivation, and delayed or arrested myelination (Schain, 1977; Barr, 1972; Academic Therapy, 1977). A traditional term for classifying such youngsters has been "Minimal Brain Dysfunction" (MBD). It includes a series of "soft" neurological signs that are thought to underlie many learning and behavioral disorders. They include such signs as awkward gait, problems with fine motor coordination, mixed laterality, and overflow movements. However, universal acceptance of soft neurological signs is lacking. Those who disagree with the concept point to the absence of acceptable norms and the fact that problems of attentiveness and distractability are present in enough children with learning disorders to confound interpretation according to Schain (1977, p. 53). He further notes (p. 61) that

... recourse to arguments that the traditional neurological evaluation fails to detect "subtle" disturbances of higher central nervous system functions is not an adequate substitute for providing solid evidence of neurological or neuropsychological abnormalities.

He takes the position that, if learning or disturbed behavior is the matter of prime concern, it should be categorized under a term descriptive of the observed disorder.

Apparently there has been strong sentiment for this position, since the *Diagnostic and Statistical Manual of Mental Disorders* (1980, p. 41) now recommends the term **"Attention Deficit Disorder" (ADD)** be used instead of MBD, and emphasizes inattention, impulsivity, and hyperactivity, although ADD may take another form that does not include hyperactivity. Unfortunately, many children with CAPD would not meet the specific criteria for the ADD classification in spite of their learning problems. Although many of them have problems of inattention, the fundamental feature which characterizes the heterogeneous CAPD population is an *auditory communication disorder*. To describe them as such is appropriate, because it is specific to their behavior as Schain (1977) recommends, is observable by many parents, teachers, and diagnosticians, and can be confirmed by central auditory tests.

The Clinical Challenge

Professional awareness of central auditory disorders is relatively new. It has been approximately 30 years since attention began to focus on the problem and on the uniqueness of the methods necessary for measuring the subtle and elusive characteristics of such disorders (Bocca et al, 1954, 1955; Bocca and Calearo, 1963). Diagnosis requires specialized test protocols with sufficient strength to identify deficiencies at various levels and in various functions of the CANS. Such tests remain experimental to some degree and need to be administered and interpreted with care. One reason is that central tests are largely behavioral measures, many of which tend to show wide ranges of performance among both normals and clinical patients, especially among younger children, and are not equally sensitive to all types of central auditory disorders.

Clinical attention was initially focused on neurologically impaired adults and was centered primarily on the use of specialized auditory tests for the purpose of confirming the presence and site of lesions in the CANS. Conversely, such tests are employed with children to assess the functional proficiency of their CANS with regard to their academic, social, and communication skills. The goal is to employ tests that will uniquely stress the auditory mechanisms at various levels of the CANS in order to identify weaknesses in the system. Stress is created by the special design of such tests, a design that requires more elaborate processing by the higher auditory centers than the simple traditional measures. Most central tests involve speech stimuli which have been modified in some fashion to make the stimuli more difficult to perceive. Thus, the listener must combine careful attention and listening skills with an efficient CANS in order to understand the test stimuli adequately. The object is to demonstrate an age-performance test deficiency that might account for the child's communication problems. Thus, in spite of the difference in purposes for administering central auditory tests to adults and children, both the principles and the nature of the tests are similar for both groups. Only the norms and certain aspects of test protocols differ. The following discussion describes some of the more widely used tests employed successfully with children. As mentioned, many of these measures should be considered experimental in nature, since one can point to limitations in each of them. Collectively, however, they represent a series of techniques by which certain central auditory strengths and weaknesses can be identified. As such, they have been found useful for both experimental and clinical purposes.

The Test Battery

The writer has long been persuaded by empirical evidence over many years of clinical practice that it is necessary to challenge the integrity of the central auditory system by an assortment of demanding tasks, i.e., with a well-chosen battery of tests. However, even the test battery approach is not without its critics (Duane, 1977), and clinical evidence to date suggests that there is no perfect single "preferred" measure. Although the developers of some tests might take issue with the fact that their particular test isn't an exemplary and all-encompassing instrument, it is quite easy to find fault with all present tests, the writer's included. Dempsey (1983) has recently critiqued a number of these measures. We still have a great deal to learn about the apparently vast variety of CAPDs. Both the science and the art in the clinical identification and management of

central auditory disorders in children is still evolving. For the present, it is recommended that those professionals responsible for the clinical evaluation of individual children with suspected CAPD select an age-appropriate series of tests, the success of which is supported by proper clinical and experimental evidence. It is then their responsibility to modify their approaches, or perhaps develop new tests, on the basis of their own experience and that of reports in the professional literature and other forums of professional knowledge exchanges.

CENTRAL TESTS APPLICABLE TO CHILDREN

The major central tests that have been used successfully with children fall into three general classifications: (1) behavioral tests that involve patterned or distorted monotic stimuli; (2) tests that present stimuli in a dichotic paradigm; and (3) binaural interaction tests. The descriptions of these tests illustrate the variety of strategies that seek to challenge the integrity of the CANS by subjecting it to stress. Modifications of speech stimuli are uniquely suited to this purpose.

Monotic Tests

Filtered Speech

Limiting the frequency content of speech stimuli degrades their natural intelligibility and makes them more difficult to perceive, especially by persons with lesions of the temporal lobe (see also Chapter 11). Frequency limiting of the test stimuli is accomplished by passing the material through electronic filters which attenuate some of the high frequency energy. Elimination of low frequency energy has not been found effective (Levy, 1981). Typically, the performance of the ear contralateral to the damaged hemisphere is poor in comparison to the ipsilateral ear, regardless of the side of cortical insult. It is this asymmetry which generally confirms an abnormality, since normal subjects show similar scores in both ears. However, some patients also show abnormally reduced scores in *both* ears. The technique has been validated on adults suffering from temporal lobe lesions (Bocca et al, 1954; Bocca and Calearo, 1963; Lynn

Table 14.1
Willeford Filtered Speech Norms

Age	N	Mean		Average ear difference[a]	SD		Range	
		LE	RE		LE	RE	LE	RE
5	Insufficient at present							
6	40	60.6	60.9	5.4	9.8	9.7	42/84	44/82
7	40	64.7	64.6	6.3	8.8	7.5	52/86	52/86
8	40	65.8	65.7	6.7	7.9	8.4	52/86	56/92
9	40	68.2	67.9	5.4	9.4	9.2	56/92	56/92
10	40	71.2	72.7	5.3	6.2	6.2	66/84	64/82
Adults[b]	20	87.6	87.4	0.2	6.3	5.7	74/98	74/98
Average:								
6–10	200	66.1	66.4	5.8	8.4	8.2	42/92	44/92

[a] Only 18 of the 200 subjects had ear differences which exceeded 10%. The greatest difference in any subject was 16%.
[b] College students; ages 18–29 yr (Ivey, 1969).

and Gilroy, 1972, 1975, 1977; Lynn et al, 1972). The same pattern of results obtained on adults may also be observed in children with CAPD (Willeford,1975, 1976, 1977a, 1977b, 1980; Willeford and Billger, 1978). Examples are shown in Tables 14.1, 14.2, and 14.3. Table 14.1 presents the norms for 40 children, ages 5 through 10 years of age, and for adults. Three features are notable in these data: (1) an age progression is observable, which suggests that task performance improves with maturation; (2) there is very little difference between left and right ears; and (3) there is a substantial range of skills at all age levels. In view of that wide range, quantitative scores are only considered abnormal when the score for one or both ears falls below the range boundary for the child's age group, or when there is a marked difference between the youngster's two ears. Table 14.2 presents the performances of six young people with long histories of auditory, academic, social, and emotional difficulties. Their ages (9 to 18 yr) are such that they should all have achieved scores of 56% or above (the lower boundary of the range for 9-yr-olds), with about equal skill in each ear. However, they all show either severely depressed scores bilaterally or marked asymmetries between ears.

In Table 14.3 the filtered speech scores for three children listed under A illustrate the great diversity of results that can be seen in such a population. These youngsters also had difficulty communicating both in and out of the classroom. All were referred by school systems. The last two subjects (B) in

Table 14.2
Clinical Results of Filtered Speech Tests on Youngsters with Learning, Auditory, and Social Difficulties

Subject	Age	Sex	Filtered speech score	
			LE (%)	RE (%)
CT	9	M	58	84
MB[a]	10.5	F	34	60
DL	13	M	54	74
GH	14	M	22	38
DS	16	M	18	20
DS	18	F	32	32

[a] Only subject with a diagnosed language disorder. All subjects except DL failed from one to four additional tests as well.

Table 14.3
Filtered Speech Results on a Younger Group of Patients with Learning, Auditory, and Social Difficulties

Subject	Age	Sex	Filtered speech score	
			LE (%)	RE (%)
A				
SP[a]	6.6	M	0	0
DM[a]	6.7	M	0	0
OW[a]	10	M	12	16
B				
DM[b]	6.5	M	70	72
RE[c]	9.10	M	92	84

[a] Also failed three other tests.
[b] Only test passed out of four tests administered.
[c] Passed three other tests as well, but failed a fourth.

this table were included to show that filtered speech is a task which some children with central auditory dysfunctions can perform quite well, while failing other stressful auditory tasks. This fact emphasizes the point that central auditory disorders may be expected to take a variety of forms, since all levels of the central auditory nervous system and corresponding mechanisms and/or functions are susceptible to disorder.

Compressed Speech

Another monotic measure applicable to central auditory assessment of children is compressed (accelerated) speech (see also Chapter 11). A disturbed temporal (time) factor has been widely acknowledged as a major characteristic observed in persons with central auditory disorders. This observation has served as a basis for the development of the concept of compressed speech as a test for central auditory dysfunction. It involves "speeded-up" versions of speech material in which the frequency factor is held constant in order to avoid peculiar vocal distortions that accompany standard speech recordings when they are played at rates faster than that at which they were recorded. Beasley and Freeman (1977) have provided a comprehensive review of the rationale for development and use of compressed speech as a diagnostic procedure. It has been employed in a wide range of studies which explored its relationship to such factors as hearing impairment (Kurdziel et al, 1976), articulation disorders (Orchik and Oelschlaeger, 1974), reading difficulties (Freeman and Beasley, 1976), auditory processing problems (Heard et al., reported by Beasley and Freeman, 1977), aging (Konkle et al, 1977), and cortical lesions (Kurdziel et al, 1976). We have used compressed speech tests developed by Beasley et al (1976) with many children as a supplement to the Willeford Test Battery (Willeford, 1975, 1980) that we employ for evaluating children with suspected central auditory dysfunction. It is a measure which uniquely evaluates a function that other tests do not. Table 14.4 includes results of clinical evaluations using the compressed WIPI test. Some children fail all measures in the test battery, whereas others fail only selected tests; and we have seen instances where the compressed speech test was the only test the child *could* perform

Table 14.4
Clinical Results in Which Children with Central Auditory Dysfunctions Showed Varied Responses on a Compressed WIPI (C-W) Test (Compression Rate Was 60%, SL = 32 dB)

Subject (Sex-Age)	Test				
	CS	FS	BF	AS	C-W
CT	L-80	58[a]	35[a]	100	68[b]
(M-90)	R-100	84	45[a]	100	76[b]
MP	L-80[a]	52[a]	30[a]	100	52[b]
(F-8.2)	R-80[a]	64	40[a]	100	60[b]
HS	L-90	68	85	100	54[b]
(M-9.4)	R-100	66	85	100	58[b]
BH	L-90	62	45[a]	80[a]	96
(F-10.2)	R-50[a]	48[a]	50[a]	70[a]	96

[a] Abnormal response (below normal range).
[b] Poor performance in relation to mean scores reported by Maki et al, 1973.

adequately, or the only one the child could *not* perform. Such results would seem to confirm that the population of children with central auditory dysfunctions is heterogenous and can be properly evaluated only by a test battery approach.

Pitch Pattern Sequences

This test was developed by Pinheiro (1977b) for the assessment of central auditory disorders (see Chapter 13). It has versions for both adults and children. This test is also unique in the sense that it is nonverbal and permits evaluation of both pattern perception skill and temporal sequencing ability. The children's version involves having the child report a pattern of three tone bursts (500 msec durations each, separated by 300 msec intervals between tones). The tone frequencies are 880 Hz (low) and 1430 Hz (high) which are played in six different combinations: HLH, LHL, HHL, LLH, HLL, and LHH. The test has provisions for training the subject with practice items, and then each ear may be tested under earphones, with 30 patterns presented to each ear. However, it may also be presented in sound field. Another novel feature of the test is that any of several response modes may be employed, depending on the ability of the child. Subjects may respond by whistling or humming the pattern perceived, by reporting the pattern verbally, or by pointing to or tapping high and low objects such as blocks.

There are no performance differences between response methods among normals. However, many subjects with brain lesions (Pinheiro, 1977a and Pinheiro et al, 1982) and learning disabilities (Pinheiro, 1978; Musiek and Geurkink, 1980; Musiek et al, 1982) are able to hum the patterns without difficulties but cannot perform efficiently when required to respond verbally or manually. The same is true for split-brain patients who were unimpaired on the task prior to surgery (Musiek et al, 1980, 1981). Figure 14.1 presents the pitch pattern results of normal and dyslexic children (Pinheiro, 1978). The group data shown in Figure 14.1 suggest that the pitch pattern test is an effective measure for assessing learning-disabled children with **dyslexia**. However, this test too has shown a wide range of performance by young children, and scores for some children under the age of 7 yr can be depressed by maturational factors, as well as by CANS deficiencies. Again, the use of a test battery is essential.

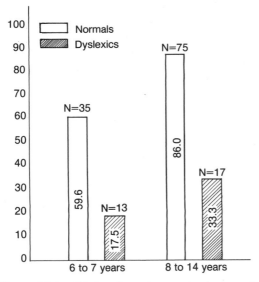

Figure 14.1. Pitch pattern sequencing in normal and dyslexic children. (From Pinheiro M: Central auditory test profile in children with learning disabilities. In Bradford L (ed): *Communication Disorders: An Audio Journal for Continuing Education.* New York, Grune & Stratton, 1978, vol 3.)

Synthetic Sentence Identification— Ipsilateral Competing Message

Another monotic test which is applicable to at least some children is the Synthetic Sentence Identification—Ipsilateral Competing Message (SSI-ICM) Test (Jerger and Jerger, 1974, 1975) which is discussed in Chapter 11. The competition derives from a monologue narrative competing with non-sense sentence stimuli at a series of message to competition ratios. Susan Jerger has reported successful use of the SSI-ICM on children (1980), and we have used this test successfully for some years in our clinic. However, it is limited in its use with many learning-disabled children who have difficulty reading even meaningful material. The subjects must be able to read (or recognize) the correct item from randomly ordered lists of 10 nonsense sentences. The procedure may be modified by having the child simply repeat what he hears, but the sentences are composed of noncoherent language which makes imprecise responses difficult to score.

Performance-Intensity Functions (PI-PB)

Susan Jerger (1983) also demonstrated the appropriateness of **performance-intensity functions** for phonetically balanced (PB) words for children with cerebral dysfunctions. One should be able to administer this test to any child who can perform a speech discrimination test, since it simply involves presenting the test material at increasing sensation levels in search of the "rollover" phenomenon.

Speech-in-Noise

Speech discrimination in the presence of competing noise is another monotic technique that can be used with children, but its value and the specific purpose for which it is administered is seldom detailed in the literature. The greatest use of this procedure is probably in educational evaluations or in estimations of how much difficulty a person may be anticipated to have when listening in noisy environments. Since children with central auditory deficiencies do indeed have difficulty communicating in noisy places and situations, the rationale seems quite sound. Unfortunately, **speech-in-noise** tests are often not administered in a standardized fashion for clinical use in terms of S to N ratios, type of speech stimuli and/or noise competition employed, or in protocol (some tests are presented monotically under phones, others binaurally under phones or in sound field). Moreover, fixed levels of white noise fail to simulate realistic auditory environments. Detailed reviews of speech-in-noise measures as tests for central auditory dysfunction have been presented by Willeford and Billger (1978) and McCroskey and Kasten (1980).

Dichotic Tests

Many of the **dichotic tests** discussed in Chapter 12 may also be used effectively with children. These include a variety of techniques and stimulus materials.

Digits

One such approach is with dichotic digits in which different pairs of numbers are presented simultaneously to the two ears. Although digits have been employed experimentally and clinically for many years, their effective clinical utilization with children has only recently been demonstrated by Musiek et al (1982).

Table 14.5 shows the results of a normal hearing 9-yr-old boy with a history of reading difficulty and a problem of hearing in noise. These results, adapted from Musiek and Geurkink (1980), show that the boy performed poorly in his left ear on compet-

ing sentences as well as on dichotic digits (Willeford, 1978) and on Katz' dichotic staggered spondee words (SSW) (Brunt, 1978). It is apparent that any of the three tests would have identified a central problem in this particular youngster. Unfortunately, such tests are not equally sensitive for all children with central disorders, as evidenced by the 9-yr-old learning-disabled girl shown in the same table. Such results are to be expected, since the tests are sufficiently different in a number of aspects to represent somewhat diverse auditory tasks, even though all employ a dichotic paradigm.

Staggered Spondaic Words (SSW)

Much has been written about the SSW Test in terms of its use with both adults and children. It was designed to present partially overlapping spondaic words so that the second syllable of the first spondee occurred simultaneously with the first syllable of the second word. A unique feature of this test is that the two uncontested syllables, at the beginning and end of the stimulus pairs, can be joined to constitute a new word.

	Noncompeting	Competing	Noncompeting
RE	up	stairs	
LE		down	town
New word:	up ....town

Most of the attention for this test has been directed toward its use with adults (Brunt, 1978). However, its adaptation for children is increasing. Detailed presentation of selected studies related to use of the SSW has been compiled in a recent book (Arnst and Katz, 1982). Studies reported in that source confirm the value of the SSW as a measure for assessing central disorders in children. The reader is also referred to other studies of the SSW (Pinheiro, 1977b; White, 1977; Sweitzer, 1977; Dempsey, 1977, 1983; Musiek and Geurkink, 1980; Musiek et al, 1982; Protti, 1983; Young, 1983).

Synthetic-Sentence Identification-Contralateral Competing Message (SSI-CCM

The clinical use of the SSI test in the ipsilateral mode (SSI-ICM) was presented earlier under discussion of monotic tests

Table 14.5
Results of Two Learning-Disabled Children on a Dichotic Digits Test, Willeford's Dichotic Sentences, and the SSW[a]

	Age	Sex	Dichotic test scores[b]					
			Digits		Sentences		SSW	
			L	R	L	R	L	R
1	9	M	35	80	40	80	50	78
2	9	F	92	96	55	95	78	96

[a] Data adapted from Musiek F, Geurkink N: Auditory perceptual problems in children: considerations for the otolaryngologist and audiologist. *Laryngoscope* 90:962–971, 1980.
[b] In percentage correct.

(Chapter 11). The SSI presented in a dichotic or contralateral mode (SSI-CCM) is also a test that can be administered to children (Chapter 12). This has been illustrated by Susan Jerger (1980). Apparently it is not widely used with children, however, because there are other measures which are more practical and easier for children to perform.

Competing Sentences

A dichotic test using natural sentences was developed by Willeford (1978) and validated initially on adults with cortical lesions as discussed in Chapter 12 on dichotic speech tests. This test subsequently has become rather widely used with children (Willeford, 1975, 1977a and b, 1978; 1980; Willeford and Billger, 1978; Dempsey, 1977, 1983; Protti, 1983; Pinheiro, 1977b; Musiek and Geurkink, 1980; Welsh et al, 1980; Protti and Young, 1980; McCroskey and Kasten, 1980; Musiek et al, 1982, Young, 1983). The test protocol is to present dichotic sentences which have similar length and semantic content such as, "Let's sit down on this bench," versus "Get me a chair so I can rest." One test option is to test one ear at a time, presenting the test ear sentence at 35 dB SL, while the other ear receives the competing sentence at 50 dB SL. Both ears can be tested in this manner. Another option is to present each of the sentences at 50 dB SL dichotically and have the subject attempt to repeat both of them, a task which often proves to be considerably more difficult. The norms for the single and double ear response protocols are presented in Tables 14.6 and 14.7, respectively. The single ear response mode shows a right ear advantage effect, and both test modes show improved performance as a function of age.

Ipsilateral-Contralateral Competing Sentence (IC-CS) Test

Another natural sentence test, developed recently by this writer and a colleague (Joan Burleigh), seeks to overcome some of the limitations of other tests and offers a comprehensive task paradigm. The IC-CS is patterned somewhat after the SSI, except that it doesn't require the subject to read and is not a closed set procedure. The task presents a female speaking sentences in competition

Table 14.7
Norms for Willeford Competing Sentences— Bilateral Response (N = 20 at each age level)[a]

Age	Score[b]	Range (%)	Mean ear response order[c]	
			L	R
6-yr-olds	46.0	20/70	3.5	6.5
7-yr-olds[d]	54.5	30/80	3.5	6.5
8-yr-olds	62.8	45/100	3.6	6.4
9-yr-olds	73.0	45/90	3.7	6.3
10-yr-olds	80.5	50/100	4.3	5.7
11-yr-olds	83.5	65/100	5.1	4.9
12-yr-olds	85.3	65/100	4.8	5.2

[a] From J. Willeford, Willeford Competing Sentence Test Norms-Bilateral Response, unpublished data, 1979.
[b] Single correct responses = 5%; double correct responses = 10%.
[c] Ear stimulus to which subject responded first.
[d] Seven-year-old data are interpolated.

Table 14.6
Norms for Willeford Competing Sentences—Unilateral Response

Age	N	Expected result		Mean		SD		Range	
		Weak ear	Strong[a] ear	Weak ear	Strong ear	Weak ear	Strong ear	Weak ear	Strong ear
5	25	20	90/100	24.8	94.0	35.9	4.4	0/80	90/100
6	40	60	90/100	59.5	96.5	33.2	4.0	0/100	90/100
7	40	70	100	67.8	97.5	31.2	3.6	0/100	90/100
8	40	80	100	83.0	98.0	22.2	3.2	10/100	90/100
9	40	90	100	93.0	98.8	9.8	2.6	70/100	90/100
10	40	100	100	98.4	99.2	3.6	2.6	90/100	90/100
5/10	225	70	100	71.6	95.9	22.7	3.5	0/100	90/100

[a] Strong ears were predominantly right ears. Left ears were the strong ears in only 13 of the 225 subjects.

with a male speaker. The test consists of five sets of ten sentence pairs each and is administered in the following manner:

Dichotic/Contralateral Competition:

List A: Male and female voices in opposite ears. *Response is required to the female voice* in test ear (right or left) at 35 dB SL (Re:SRT or PTA), while dichotic competition is supplied by the male voice at 50 dB SL.

List B: Test ear and competing ear are reversed so that the other ear is tested for reception of the female voice. The same signal to competition ratio (SCR) is used.

List C: Male and female voices are presented to opposite ears at 50 dB SL in each ear (SCR = 0 dB). The subject is asked to repeat *both* sentences (both female and male voices).

Nondichotic/Ipsilateral Competition:

List D: Both sentences are presented to the same ear. For children under the age of 12 response is required to the female voice only, as in lists A and B, and is presented at 50 dB SL, while the male-voice competition sentence is also presented at 50 dB SL (SCR = 0 dB). When the test is used with adults, the signal level is 45 dB SL for the female voice (SCR = −5 dB).

List E: The same procedure as in list D is utilized for testing subject's other ear.

As in the Willeford Competing Sentence Test, the sentences are similar in length, but each competing pair has a common word which is offset from its counterpart by one syllable, that is, they do not overlap. The purpose was to make them semantically more competitive by allowing both ears to hear the common word. The established norms for the female voice are shown in Table 14.8. Present plans include developing norms for the male voice and for a number of other variations in the test procedure, including norms for each test list for each of the five test protocols.

As with test materials of similar design described earlier, the contralateral (dichotic) test conditions primarily challenge the integrity of the auditory cortex according to studies on adults, whereas the ipsilateral conditions (specified in lists D and E) are believed to challenge the proficiency of the brainstem. While the precise nature and implications of subpar performance on these tests among children remain to be established in terms of linguistic processing events, such measures have been shown in previous discussion to be sensitive methods of identifying many children with learning disabilities. Scoring is based upon the degree to which the language in, and meaning of, each test item is preserved without being adversely

Table 14.8
Norms in Percent for the IC-CS Test[a]

Age		Test list				
		A	B	C	D	E
6 and 7	Mean	81.5	89.6	44.8	82.6	87.0
(N = 27)	SD	13.2	9.8	11.3	12.6	9.9
	Range	50/100	70/100	30/75	60/100	70/100
8 and 9	Mean	89.6	90.4	61.9	85.5	92.6
(N = 27)	SD	10.6	12.9	12.7	10.9	9.8
	Range	70/100	60/100	40/85	60/100	70/100
10 and 11	Mean	93.0	94.1	70.0	96.7	97.0
(N = 27)	SD	7.8	8.9	11.2	4.8	5.4
	Range	80/100	70/100	50/85	90/100	80/100
12 through adult	Mean	98.2	99.3	83.7	96.9	96.3
(N = 27)	SD	4.0	2.7	9.1	6.9	6.3
	Range	90/100	90/100	65/100	80/100	80/100

[a] From Willeford J, Burleigh J: *Handbook of Central Auditory Processing Disorders in Children.* New York, Grune & Stratton, in press, 1985.

influenced by the competing sentence. For example, *two* errors per sentence in any of the following combinations constitutes an incorrect response:

1. Borrowing from the competing sentence
2. Omitting a word
3. Adding a word
4. Substituting a word not found in either sentence
5. Any *single* word error that alters the meaning or intent of the sentence.

Some interesting aspects of the IC-CS are as follows: (1) it has not shown an ear dominance effect in the dichotic mode as observed with younger children on both the SSW and the Willeford Competing Sentences; (2) although scores increased with age while the range of scores decreased, both were less than the values observed in the Willeford Competing Sentences. The reason why an ear dominance effect was not observed on the IC-CS is unknown at this point, but it may be that the male voice is sufficiently different from the female voice that it doesn't offer the degree of competition presented by the same voice uttering different sentences to the two ears. Whether psychological factors may also play a role remains to be studied. Case examples of the IC-CS are shown in Table 14.9. One is a 9-yr-old boy who scored poorly on nearly every central test given him, but who has developed enough compensatory skills to manage acceptably well, except in classes where group discussion is required and in complex social environments. The two college students have difficulty in most lecture classes and require note takers. Continuing studies are underway on the IC-CS.

Consonant-Vowel Test

Dichotic consonant-vowel (CV) tests have been widely used for experimental purposes. Summaries of much of the experimental work may be found in the *Proceedings of the Symposium on Central Auditory Processing Disorders* at the University of Nebraska Medical Center (1975) and in Berlin and McNeil (1976). Norms have been established also for children (Berlin et al, 1973). However, on the basis of surveys by Katz (1978) and by the author (J. Willeford, Central Auditory Processing Questionnaire, An Unpublished Survey of Central Auditory Services in ASHA Accredited Programs, 1980), CV tests are apparently not used with any regularity for clinical purposes. Although they and others have found Berlin's CV test very sensitive and successful, Lynn and Gilroy (1977, p. 191) note that

. . . for most patients with brain tumors we have found that the dichotic CV test is often very difficult and we usually use it only in selected cases with excellent hearing levels and minimal neurological deficit.

Binaural Fusion

Binaural fusion (discussed by Tobin in Chapter 10) probably qualifies only as a special case of dichotic listening in the sense that, although the two ears are simultaneously stimulated, they are presented with complementary acoustic components of the same stimulus words as opposed to competing stimuli. For example, one ear receives selected high frequency energy of a given word, while the other ear receives selected low frequency components of that same word. The principle of the test is that high and low frequency messages, both poorly understood when presented individually, are fused into a relatively intelligible message when presented simultaneously, since their complementary components can be combined into meaningful words by an intact brainstem system. The principle for the test

Table 14.9
IC-CS Test Results in Percent for Three Patients with Learning Disabilities[a]

Subject/age	Ear	C-CS	Bilat C-CS	I-CS	Other tests failed
DS/9	L	20[b]		60[b]	
			45[b]		6
	R	100	45[b]	30[b]	6
TH/24	L			30[b]	
					5
	R			30[b]	
RF/27	L			30[b]/20[b,c]	
	R			30[b]/30[b,c]	

[a] One is an elementary school child, and the other two are college students who require note takers for class lectures.
[b] Abnormal response.
[c] Test repeated 6 months later.

was described by Matzker (1962), and it has since been constructed in modified versions and used clinically in different test protocols by Linden (1964), Smith and Resnick (1972), Ivey (1969), Willeford (1975, 1980), Pinheiro (1977b), and Musiek et al (1982). Some of the differences include type of stimulus words employed (spondees vs monosyllabic words), width of pass-bands, frequency region of pass-bands, sensation levels at which the bands are played, etc. While this type of test seems capable of identifying brainstem dysfunction, its sensitive stimuli are influenced by all of the foregoing factors, as well as by peripheral hearing loss, accuracy of pure tone threshold measurements on which the test SLs are set, calibration of the tape circuit in the audiometer, and by the care and use of the tapes themselves and their playback units. Of course, these factors are important considerations in administering any taped central auditory tests, but they are especially critical for tests of CVs, binaural fusion, filtered speech, compressed speech, or any other technique that involves a reduction in the natural redundancy of the test stimuli.

Competing Environmental Sounds

This is a nonlinguistic dichotic test developed by Katz (Katz et al 1975). Not a great deal of information is available on the test at present, but it involves the delivery of 14 pairs of dichotically competing environmental sounds on which performance can be compared with SSW results to provide a broader picture of auditory processing (linguistic and nonlinguistic) in the CANS. The available information may be found in Arnst and Katz (1982).

Binaural Interaction Tasks

Binaural interaction tasks provide still different kinds of challenges to the CANS. The two major tests in this classification follow.

Rapidly Alternating Speech

This test in which the stimulus material is switched alternately between the subject's two ears at rapid intervals is fully discussed in Chapter 10 by Tobin. One version of the test has been shown by Lynn and Gilroy (1977) to be particularly sensitive to certain lesions in the low pons and cerebellopontine angle. A similar version, which is a part of the Willeford battery, has been reported by Miltenberger et al (1979) to show remarkably low scores on deep sea divers with decompression sickness. However, Willeford and Billger (1978) have found positive results on this test in only a small percentage of learning-disabled children in comparison with other central tests. It is easily applicable to children and enjoyable for them to take, but it is not one of the more useful tests of central function for that population.

Masking Level Differences

The masking level difference (MLD) test is a binaural phenomenon which is described in Chapter 10 on binaural interaction tasks. It is a test which can be administered easily and quickly to children, but we have not found it to be one of the stronger tests for identifying central dysfunction in children. However, Sweetow and Reddel (1978) feel that it holds promise when used as part of a test battery. It is thought to measure low brainstem dysfunction when hearing is normal (Olsen et al, 1976).

Electrophysiologic Tests in Children

Aural Reflex Test

The measurement of the crossed and uncrossed stapedial muscle reflexes is another test for brainstem disorder (see also Chapter 7). It is simple, quick, and objective. The principle is that the uncrossed (ipsilateral) reflexes are present, but the crossed (contralateral) reflexes are absent whenever a brainstem pathology interferes with the reflex arc. Jerger et al (1975) have demonstrated this phenomenon clinically. It is occasionally observed in children with central auditory problems, but it is not common.

Auditory Brainstem Response (ABR)

The ABR is a method of objectively measuring processes in the central nervous system as discussed in Chapter 4 by Margaretta and Aage Møller. At present, it has been found to be of limited value in the case of children with auditory perceptual and learning problems. As mentioned in the section on "Etiological Implications," Shimizu et al (1981) were unable to demonstrate neurophysiological abnormality by ABR in the brainstem auditory systems in children with carefully defined MBD, a finding in contrast to that of Sohmer and Student (1978). However, Protti (1983) found positive ABR results in only 2 of 13 children who showed positive results on one or more behavioral tests. It appears that the ABR presently depends on test stimuli which do not offer sufficient stress to the elaborate CANS to detect subtle deficiencies.

Interpretation and Implications

When a central auditory disorder has been confirmed in a given child, it is crucial that the nature of that problem be defined as clearly as possible. However, that is a difficult task in view of limited present-day knowledge of such disorders. It is still not possible to translate test results directly into prescriptions for daily living and learning skills, because different children exhibit such diverse performances across central tests and display an equally broad range of communication, social, and academic behaviors. Nonetheless, it is out of these enigmatic relationships that eventual understanding of the problem may evolve. However, the child's diagnostic performance does isolate his auditory deficiencies and provides greater insight into his shortcomings and problems which might not have been previously appreciated. It seems reasonable to assume that the growing body of diagnostic data, when compared with psychosocial and academic information in carefully obtained case histories, will continue to provide us with fresh knowledge. We have a long-range study in progress at Colorado State University and, with the assistance of cooperating colleagues across the country, hope to clarify some of these relationships. This effort is being supported by the Royal Arch Masons, International, who have established auditory perceptual disorders in children as their primary philanthropic endeavor.

For the present, abnormal performances by children on central auditory tests can demonstrate successfully to parents and other professionals that a child does have limited auditory skills, in spite of a normal audiogram and good speech discrimination scores. Such results can serve as a basis for neurological referral and for modifications in management strategies for the child that have proven to be dramatically successful in many cases. For example, one parent reported

The staffing at the high school was the turning point for Bob. The staffing was very productive and informative in that there was a representative of all interested parties (your staff audiologist, the school district, the teachers, and the parents) present. Up to this point Bob hated school, was cutting classes, and just didn't give a damn! Now he likes school and is a little impatient for it to start again.

Such statements are commonplace from parents responding to a follow-up survey of children we have seen as clinical patients.

Present Limitations and Future Needs

Limitations

At the present time there are a number of limitations regarding assessment of central auditory problems in children. As noted earlier, there is a gaping void in our knowledge of the relationship between acoustic experience and the use of that experience by specialized areas of the brain for language functions. There is imprecise and incomplete data on the incidence of central auditory disorders among children, even though these problems are gaining increasing attention from professionals in a number of disciplines. Imprecise data may result from the variety of test instruments employed by audiologists, speech-language pathologists, neuropsychologists, and educational specialists. It may also be due partly to differences in the terminology used to describe both measured auditory behaviors and those theoretical aspects of audition which are presumed to subserve language functions. Still other difficulties include differences in the criteria by which judgments of abnormality are made, the wide ranges in test performances among normal subjects, variations in compensatory skills among individual subjects, and very likely a number of other factors. Fortunately, attention is being directed to many of these variables, and this relatively new clinical science will no doubt improve with time, experience, and research.

Needs

There are pressing needs in this area to understand the roles which heredity, disease, culture, diet, drugs, intelligence, maturation, stress, emotion, fatigue, and other factors play in auditory perceptual processes. We need to know why there appears to be an inordinately high incidence of poor central auditory skills in certain special populations of children, such as juvenile delinquents, those with emotional disorders, etc. There is an urgent need for greater public education about the existence and nature of central auditory disorders so that present misunderstanding is reduced. We need improved tests, more insightful test interpretation, and better treatment techniques. Yet, in spite of our present limitations and needs, we have made encouraging strides in diagnosing and managing central auditory disorders in children.

References

American Psychiatric Association: *Diagnostic and Statistical Manual of Mental Disorders*, ed 3. Washington, DC, APA, 1980.

Are the New Therapies Effective? Monograph. San Rafael, CA, Academic Therapy Publications, 1977.

Arnst D, Katz J: *Central Auditory Assessment: The SSW Test—Development and Clinical Use.* San Diego, College-Hill Press, 1982.

Barr D: *Auditory Perceptual Disorders.* Springfield, IL, Charles C Thomas, 1972.

Beasley D, Freeman B: Time altered speech as a measure of central auditory processing. In Keith R (ed): *Central Auditory Dysfunction.* New York, Grune & Stratton, 1977, pp 129–176.

Beasley D, Maki J, Orchik D: Children's perception of time-compressed speech using two measures of speech discrimination. *J Speech Hear Disord* 41:216–226, 1976.

Berlin C, Hughes L, Lowe-Bell S, Berlin H: Dichotic right ear advantage in children 5 to 13. *Cortex* 9:394–402, 1973.

Berlin C, McNeil M: Dichotic listening. In Lass N (ed): *Contemporary Issues in Experimental Phonetics.* New York, Academic Press, 1976, pp 327–388.

Bocca E, Calearo C: Central hearing processes. In Jerger J (ed): *Modern Developments in Audiology.* New York, Academic Press, 1963, pp 337–370.

Bocca E, Calearo C, Cassinari V: A new method for testing hearing in temporal lobe tumors. *Acta Otolaryngol (Stockh)* 44:219–221, 1954.

Bocca E, Calearo C, Cassinari V, Migliavacca F: Testing cortical hearing in temporal lobe tumors. *Acta Otolaryngol* 45:289–304, 1955.

Brunt M: The staggered spondaic word test. In Katz J (ed): *Handbook of Clinical Audiology.* Baltimore, Williams & Wilkins, 1978, pp 262–275.

Dempsey C: Some thoughts concerning alternate explanations of central auditory test results. In Keith R (ed): *Central Auditory Dysfunction.* New York, Grune & Stratton, 1977, pp 293–318.

Dempsey C: Selecting tests of auditory function in children. In Lasky E, Katz J (eds): *Central Auditory Processing Disorders.* Baltimore, University Park Press, 1983, pp 203–222.

Duane D: A neurologic perspective of central auditory dysfunction. In Keith R (ed): *Central Auditory Dysfunction.* New York, Grune & Stratton, 1977, pp 1–42.

Freeman B, Beasley D: Performance of Reading-Impaired and Normal Reading Children on Time-Compressed Monosyllabic and Sentential Stimuli. Paper presented at the American Speech and Hearing Association Convention, 1976.

Fuller C: Lubert and language disorders: a critique. Letters to the editor. *J Speech Hear Disord* 47:328–329, 1982.

Hurley R: The central auditory nervous system evaluation. In Rupp R, Stockdell K (eds): *Speech Protocols in Audiology.* New York, Grune & Stratton, 1980, pp 163–202.

Ivey R: Tests of CNS Function. Master's thesis, Colorado State University, 1969.

Jerger S: Evaluation of central auditory function in children. In Keith R (ed): *Central Auditory and Language Disorders in Children.* Houston, College-Hill Press, 1980, pp 30–60, 1980.

Jerger S: Speech audiology in young children. *Ear Hear* 4:56–66, 1983.

Jerger J, Jerger S: Auditory findings in brainstem disorders. *Arch Otolaryngol* 99:342–350, 1974.

Jerger J, Jerger S: Clinical validity of central auditory tests. *Scand Audiol* 4:147–163, 1975.

Jerger S, Neeley G, Jerger J: Recovery of crossed acoustic reflexes in brain stem auditory disorder. *Arch Otolaryngol* 101:329–332, 1975.

Johnson D, Enfield M, Sherman R: The use of the staggered spondaic word and the competing environmental sounds tests in the evaluation of central auditory function of learning disabled children. *Ear Hear* 2:70–77, 1981.

Katz J: Clinical use of central auditory tests. In Katz J (ed): *Handbook of Clinical Audiology.* Baltimore, Williams & Wilkins, 1978, pp 233–243.

Katz J, Kushner D, Pack G: The Use of Competing Speech (SSW) and Environmental Sound (CES) Test for Localizing Brain Lesions. Paper presented at the American Speech and Hearing Association Convention, 1975.

Kiang N: Stimulus representation in the discharge patterns of auditory neurons. In Tower D (ed): *The Nervous System, Volume 3: Human Communication and Its Disorders.* New York, Raven Press, 1975, pp 81–96.

Konkle D, Beasley D, Bess F: Intelligibility of time-altered speech in relation to chronological aging. *J Speech Hear Res* 20:108–115, 1977.

Kurdziel S, Noffsinger D, Olsen W: Performance by cortical-lesion patients on 40 and 60% time-compressed materials. *J Am Audiol Soc* 2:3–7, 1976.

Levy F: Central Auditory Testing in Learning-Disabled Children. Master's dissertation, University of Witwatersrand, 1981.

Linden A: Distorted speech and binaural speech resynthesis test. *Acta Otolaryngol (Stockh)* 58:32–48, 1964.

Lubert N: Auditory perceptual impairments in children

with specific language disorders. *J Speech Hear Disord* 46:3–9, 1981.

Lubert N: Reply to Fuller and O'Connell. Letters to the editor. *J Speech Hear Disord* 47:330, 1982.

Ludlow C: Impaired language development: hypothesis for research. *Bull Orton Soc* 130:153–169, 1980.

Lynn G, Benitez J, Eisenbrey A, Gilroy J, Wilner H: Correlates in cerebral hemisphere lesions: temporal and parietal lobe tumors. *Audiology* 11:115–134, 1972.

Lynn G, Gilroy J: Neuro-audiological abnormalities in patients with temporal lobe tumors. *J Neurol Sci* 17:167–184, 1972.

Lynn G, Gilroy J: Effects of brain lesions on the perception of monotic and dichotic speech stimuli. *Proceedings of a Symposium on Central Auditory Processing Disorders.* Omaha, University of Nebraska Medical Center, 1975.

Lynn G, Gilroy J: Evaluation of central auditory dysfunction in patients with neurological disorders. In Keith R (ed): *Central Auditory Dysfunction.* New York, Grune & Stratton, 1977, pp 177–222.

Maki J, Beasley D, Orchik D: Children's Perception of Time-Compressed Speech Using Two Measures of Speech Discrimination. Paper presented at the American Speech and Hearing Association Convention, 1973.

Matzker J: The binaural test, *J Int Audiol* 1:209–211, 1962.

McCroskey R, Kasten R: Assessment of central auditory processing. In Rupp R, Stockdell K (eds): *Speech Protocols in Audiology.* New York, Grune & Stratton, 1980, pp 339–390.

Miltenberger G, Caruso V, Correia M, Love T, Winkleman P: Utilization of a central auditory processing test battery in diagnosing decompression sickness. *J Speech Hear Disord* 90:110–120, 1979.

Musiek F, Geurkink N: Auditory perceptual problems in children: considerations for the otolaryngologist and audiologist. *Laryngoscope* 90:962–971, 1980.

Musiek F, Geurkink N, Keitel S: Test battery assessment of auditory perceptual dysfunction in children. *Laryngoscope* 92:251–257, 1982.

Musiek F, Pinheiro M, Wilson D: Auditory pattern perception in "split brain" patients. *Arch Otolaryngol* 106:610–612, 1980.

Musiek F, Wilson D, Reeves A: Staged commissurotomy and central auditory functions. *Arch Otolaryngol* 107:233–236, 1981.

O'Connell P: Response to Lubert. Letters to the editor. *J Speech Hear Disord* 47:329, 1982.

Olsen W, Noffsinger D, Carhart R: Masking level differences in clinical populations. *Audiology* 15:287–301, 1976.

Orchik D, Oelschlaeger M: Time-Compressed Speech Discrimination in Children and Its Relationship to Articulation. Paper presented at American Speech and Hearing Association Convention, 1974.

Panel on Communicative Disorders:Report of the Panel on Communicative Disorders to the National Advisory Neurological and Communicative Disorders and Stroke Council. Washington, DC, US Department of Health, Education and Welfare, 1979.

Pinheiro M: Auditory pattern perception in patients with left and right hemisphere lesions. *Ohio J Speech Hear* 12:9–20, 1977a.

Pinheiro M: Tests of central auditory function in children with learning disabilities. In Keith R (ed): *Central Auditory Dysfunction.* New York, Grune & Stratton, 1977, pp 223–256.

Pinheiro M: Central auditory test profile in children with learning disabilities. In Bradford L (ed): *Communication Disorders: An Audio Journal for Continuing Education.* New York, Grune & Stratton, 1978, vol 3.

Pinheiro M, Jacobsen G, Boller F: Auditory dysfunction following a gunshot wound of the pons. *J Speech Hear Disord* 47:296–300, 1982.

Protti E: Brainstem auditory pathways and auditory processing disorders: diagnostic implications of subjective and objective tests. In Lasky E, Katz J (eds): *Central Auditory Processing Disorders.* Baltimore, University Park Press, 1983, pp 117–140.

Protti E, Young M: The evaluation of a child with auditory perceptual deficiencies: an interdisciplinary approach. *Semin Speech Lang Hear* 1:167–180, 1980.

Schain R: *Neurology of Childhood Learning Disorders,* ed 2. Baltimore, Williams & Wilkins, 1977.

Shimizu H, Brown F, Capute A, Mahoney W: Auditory Brainstem Response in Children with Minimal Brain Dysfunction. Paper presented at the American Speech and Hearing Association Convention, 1981.

Smith B, Resnick D: An auditory test for assessing brainstem integrity; preliminary report. *Laryngoscope* 82:414–424, 1972.

Sohmer H, Student Q: Auditory nerve and brainstem evoked responses in normal, autistic, minimally brain damaged and psychomotor retarded children. *Electroencephalogr Clin Neurophysiol* 44:380–388, 1978.

Sweetow R, Reddell R: The use of masking level differences in the identification of children with perceptual problems. *J Am Audiol Soc* 4:52–56, 1978.

Sweitzer R: Team evaluation of auditory perceptually-handicapped children. In Keith R (ed): *Central Auditory Dysfunction.* New York, Grune & Stratton, 1977, pp 341–360.

Tallal P, Stark R, Kallman C, Mellits D: Perceptual constancy for phonemic categories: a developmental study with normal and language impaired children. *Appl Psycholinguistics* 1:49–64, 1980.

University of Nebraska Medical Center: *Proceedings of the Symposium on Central Auditory Processing Disorders.* Omaha, University of Nebraska Medical Center, 1975.

Welsh L, Welsh J, Healey M: Auditory testing and dyslexia. Laryngoscope 90:972–984, 1980.

White E: Children's performance on the SSW test and Willeford Battery: Interim clinical report. In Keith R (ed): *Central Auditory Dysfunction.* New York, Grune & Stratton, 1977, pp 319–340.

Willeford J: Central auditory function in children with learning disabilities. *Audiol Hear Educ.,* December-January:12–20, 1975–1976.

Willeford J: Differential diagnosis of central auditory dysfunction. In Bradford L (ed): *Audiology: An Audio Journal for Continuing Education.* New York, Grune & Stratton, 1976, vol 2.

Willeford J: Evaluation of central auditory disorders in learning disabled children. In Bradford L (ed): *Learning Disabilities: An Audio Journal for Continuing Education.* New York, Grune & Stratton, 1977a, vol 1.

Willeford J: Assessing central auditory behavior in children: a test battery approach. In Keith R (ed): *Central Auditory Dysfunction.* New York, Grune & Stratton, 1977b, pp 43–72.

Willeford J: Sentence tests of central auditory function. In Katz J (ed): *Handbook of Clinical Audiology.* Baltimore, Williams & Wilkins, 1978, pp 252–261.

Willeford J: Central auditory behaviors in learning disabled children. *Semin Speech Lang Hear.* 1:127–140, 1980.

Willeford J, Billger J: Auditory perception in children with learning disabilities. In Katz J (ed): *Handbook of Clinical Audiology.* Baltimore, Williams & Wilkins, 1978, pp 410–425.

Willeford J, Burleigh J: *Handbook of Central Auditory Processing Disorders in Children.* New York, Grune & Stratton, in press, 1985.

Witkin R: Auditory perception—implications for language development. In *Language, Speech and Hearing Services in the Schools*, Monograph 4. Washington, DC, American Speech and Hearing Association, 1971, pp 31–52.

Young M: Neuroscience, pragmatic competence, and auditory processing. In Lasky E, Katz J (eds): *Central Auditory Processing Disorders.* Baltimore, University Park Press, 1983, pp 141–162.

CHAPTER 15

Special Considerations in Central Auditory Evaluation

MARILYN L. PINHEIRO, Ph.D.
FRANK E. MUSIEK, Ph.D.

The most important goal of this final chapter is to point out the precautions and cautions necessary to successful central auditory evaluation. A number of these have been mentioned in previous chapters and will be reiterated here in somewhat greater depth and organized in one place to emphasize consequences to the student and clinician. A "gold standard" is badly needed for central auditory testing, and attention to the following should facilitate such an achievement in the future by making clinicians and researchers alike aware of present pitfalls and problems which may make central auditory results inadequate and noncontributory.

PROCEDURES

Instrumentation

The maintenance and calibration of the equipment as well as thorough knowledge of its proper use are tantamount to any reliable auditory evaluation procedure. Calibration should be careful and frequent with appropriate calibration equipment of good quality. This is one facet of central auditory evaluation which can be under complete control of the clinician and/or researcher.

Test Materials

Test materials should be carefully selected when either privately or commercially available tapes are used. Taped material often has a certain amount of noise in the background of the signals. The clinician/researcher should be aware of the signal to noise ratio. This may have to be taken into consideration when evaluating distractible children or adults who have even slight sensorineural decrements in hearing thresholds which may be at higher audiometric frequencies than the test material. (This topic will be discussed further when hearing losses and learning disabilities are considered in relation to central auditory evaluation later in this chapter.) A well-trained audiologist, psychoacoustician, psychophysicist, or neuropsychologist, i.e., anyone who presumes to do central auditory testing, should be familiar with and make use of a dual beam oscilloscope to examine the test material and/or signals employed. This is especially necessary when two channels of a tape are used as in some binaural and all dichotic stimuli (see Chapter 12). It has been noted that there often exist intensity differences between the two tape channels which may affect results. Audiometric adjustments may be necessary. Certainly the clinician/researcher must be well aware of all the parameters of any material he is using for central auditory tasks.

Taped material also becomes less clear and more noisy with age and usage. Therefore, it must be carefully monitored and newly recorded materials prepared or procured when necessary.

Need for Test Battery

The worker doing research may be limited to exploring the merits of only one central auditory procedure when it is being studied in great detail in one project with a large number of subjects involved. Such research can contribute greatly to present limited knowledge and help standardize tests and test methods and materials. This type of investigation is badly needed. However, even in this kind of project, complete audiological evaluation of each subject should precede use of the research tool. If the material to be evaluated is to be presented to the subject at suprathreshold hearing levels, hearing capability for this type of stimulus at these levels should be investigated in preliminary procedures (see Chapter 9).

On the contrary, when the clinician is attempting to measure central auditory competency in either a normal or a pathological subject, the use of a central auditory test battery is essential. No one test is adequate to determine a diagnosis of abnormal central auditory function other than for that particular test. It is enough to refer to the reviews of literature and clinical research covered in the various preceding chapters of this book to realize that the results of any one test might be normal in an individual who does have a brain lesion or might be abnormal in an individual who may not have any actual brain pathology. Further discussion later in this chapter on aging, maturation in children, et cetera, should make this need for a test battery even more emphatic.

After a complete audiological evaluation of peripheral hearing, which should include testing for eighth nerve and recruitment problems, a central auditory test battery should comprise the following: (1) several tasks known to involve different facets of brainstem auditory functions, including both objective (auditory brainstem response, ABR) and subjective procedures; and (2) several tests of various aspects of cortical functions, including both verbal and nonverbal materials and responses. (See discussion of relationship between language and central auditory evaluation later in this chapter.) Tasks used in the test battery should be based on firm normative data, as well as on as much previous knowledge from other workers as possible.

Normative Data

Normative data should be derived in general in the same audiological or acoustical environment with the same test equipment and materials used for central auditory evaluations in that setting. This normative data should represent results on a normal population as nearly matched as possible in as many ways as possible with the clinical population customarily evaluated. Several sets of normative data may be necessary, i.e., data on children, on adults with normal hearing and different types and degrees of hearing losses, and on various age groupings within these categories. There probably is no central auditory test on which *enough* normative data is available in these different categories so that more is not required. Occasionally an individual subject may serve as his own "control" when preoperative and postoperative results are to be compared or when progress or remission of disease is to be evaluated on a repetitive basis. This may also hold for certain individual tests such as Binaural Fusion (BF) and Rapidly Alternating Speech (RASP) discussed in Chapter 10. Even in these cases one must have normative data for comparison.

Standardization

At present standardization of central auditory tests and procedures is one of the greatest lacks in central auditory evaluation. A "gold standard" for this work cannot be established as long as different methods and different tests and/or test batteries are used in each and every clinical facility. It would be of great advantage to have various settings using the same procedures and central auditory tasks in order to accumulate larger bodies of both normative values and clinical data. Now it is difficult to compare results of one study to those of another because of significant dissimilarities in methods and test materials. Many bits and pieces of information on small numbers of subjects (who are also often dissimilar) appear in the literature, but it is difficult or impossible to organize these into a usable whole. Indeed, there is more confusion in the field, especially in relation to subjective central auditory tasks, than there is any real accumulation of reliable knowledge. This situation undoubtedly is to be expected in an area of clinical research as new as central auditory evaluation. However, this condition should not continue ad infinitum because real progress toward central auditory testing as a worthwhile contribution toward patient diagnosis can be made only when masses of similarly controlled data are available.

PROBLEMS AND PITFALLS

Age

As previously mentioned, normative data must be established for different age groups of normal hearing subjects before any central auditory tests can be applied reliably to individuals suspected of having central auditory pathology. Deriving normative data for both children and older adults is particularly difficult.

Children

In children we must consider the problems of brain maturation. This process is completed only over a number of years, and the age of maturation differs from individual to individual. Different areas of the brain mature at different rates, with the motor and sensory reception cortices developing earlier than the association cortices. Of special interest for central auditory evaluation is myelination of the corpus callosum. Myelin is the fatty insulating sheath that forms around the larger nerve fibers permitting rapid transfer of neural impulses (information). In the brain myelin forms the white matter while the actual cortex is made up of nerve cells or gray matter. The corpus callosum, the heavy band of nerve fibers which interconnects the two halves or hemispheres of the brain from anterior to posterior, is made up of myelin-covered nerve fibers. These fibers are responsible for interhemispheric transfer and comparison of information. According to Trevarthen (1974) the corpus callosum at birth is only one third of its adult size, and myelination may not be complete until adolescence in the human. Musiek et al (1984) have shown that any central auditory test that depends on interhemispheric interaction (such as dichotic and pitch pattern tasks) may show large standard deviations in normal hearing children, even in those within 1 or 2 yr of the same age. The younger the child, the greater the difficulty in establishing reliable norms. The larger right ear advantage found for dichotic tasks in younger children may be related to the delay in myelination of the corpus callosum.

It should be noted also that young children often are more sensitive to noise interference than are adults. Thus, one usually finds a wide variety of scores on normal children on speech-in-noise tasks. This can occur as well on low-pass filtered speech tests, especially if the taped stimuli have a background with some noise (which would not disturb a normal hearing adult).

Unfortunately one area in which central auditory evaluation is needed in young children is in the area of learning disabilities. Such children are particularly distractible by noise. Also, the earlier such children are identified, the better the prognosis for their remediation.

The clinician also must take into careful consideration the child's health history. Even if hearing is normal at the time of testing, any past middle ear infections could have caused a delay in language development which might, in turn, affect processing of central auditory tasks. (See material on the relationship between language and central auditory evaluation later in this chapter.)

Older Adults

Older adults also frequently have problems with signal to noise ratios, even when hearing is within normal limits. Speech-in-noise, low-pass filtered speech, and test tapes which have some background noise may result in false-positive scores on central auditory evaluation.

Hearing Loss

Conductive Hearing Loss

Possible effects of previous middle ear infections in children have just been mentioned. A conductive loss at the time of central auditory evaluation may not interfere with test results unless the loss is great enough so that the stimuli must be presented at intensity levels that might permit "crossover" by bone conduction from one ear to the other. Masking cannot be used in any binaural or dichotic central auditory task, and the effect, if any, of masking on monaural central auditory tests has not been adequately investigated. Therefore, a central auditory evaluation in any child or adult with a conductive hearing loss must be interpreted with more than the usual caution.

Sensorineural Hearing Loss and Presbycusis

The effects of sensorineural hearing loss in relation to monaural central auditory tests have been discussed in Chapter 11. The effects on binaural and/or dichotic tasks would be even more difficult to interpret; these have not been studied effectively. Even though the binaural hearing thresholds may appear to be similar, that is not enough to determine whether both ears have the same hearing capacity at suprathreshold levels. Recruitment or other problems relating to temporal factors may be present, even when the sensorineural hearing loss affects only the higher frequencies generally thought to be "above the speech frequency range." Of course, when the hearing loss is moderate to severe, the stimuli for central auditory tests cannot be presented at high enough intensity levels. This area needs much research as yet.

In presbycusis the audiologist may be dealing not only with a cochlear problem but also with a central auditory disability that is not related to a brain lesion. In the older adult central auditory evaluation scores may be depressed by a general loss of neurons throughout the central auditory system due to the aging process. Blood flow may be decreased because of fatty deposits in arteries supplying the brain. There are also changes in cerebral energy metabolism with age and/or in disease processes that do not necessarily affect peripheral hearing. Glucose metabolism and oxygen consumption in the brain decrease with aging (Smith, 1984), and enzymes are less active. Also, any sensory deprivation caused by hospitalization, social isolation, hearing loss, and other factors can bring about mental aberrations (usually reversible) in the older adult. All of these can affect central auditory evaluation results, even though there is no actual brain lesion. The age and a thorough health and social history of the patient should warn the clinician to be careful of his conclusions relative to central auditory tests.

Psychiatric Disorders

There is limited knowledge available on the effects of different psychiatric disorders on the results of central auditory evaluation. This problem will not be discussed at any length here, but the clinician/researcher should be alerted to the fact that certain of these disorders may affect central auditory tasks. Interhemispheric asymmetries have been reported for both schizophrenics (Gruzelier and Hammond, 1976) and for affective psychotics (Perris, 1974; Goldstein and Stoltzfus, 1973) on some auditory discrimination tasks and on objective measures. A 1978 study by Yozawitz and Bruder resulted in evidence of lateralized right temporal lobe dysfunction for dichotic tasks employing both speech (SSW) and nonspeech (binaural click summation) stimuli for affective psychotic patients. Their performances were similar to those of patients with right temporal lobe lesions or right temporal lobectomies. In this study schizophrenic patients had test results similar to those of normal subjects. When one peruses the neuropsychological literature for further information, it becomes evident that this is an area about which very little is known, and much research needs to be conducted.

Statistics in Central Auditory Evaluation

Some of the pitfalls of statistics have been pointed out in Chapter 9. Statistics may be applied easily to groups of normal subjects with the reservations suggested by Dr. Efron. However, the application of statistics to groups of abnormal individuals is a difficult matter. The authors have completed a number of studies on relatively large groups of patients on which the statistical results were nonsignificant because of large standard deviations representing wide ranges of scores due to individual patient differences. These studies often (and perhaps unfortunately) remain unpublished because of this lack of statistically significant results. Even though such investigations have included groups of patients in supposedly well defined categories (multiple sclerosis, right or left posterior hemispheric lesions, children with dyslexia), scores within groups have varied widely. Therefore, it has become obvious that the pathology needs to be even more carefully defined in research subjects. However, brain lesions are often difficult to describe with any exactness, even with modern diagnostic equipment. The effects of any lesion may exist far afield from the lesion itself. Even those patients who have had specific types of brain surgery may differ from one another because the preoperative pathology may have had different and enduring effects on the brain. Also, in one clinical/research location it is generally difficult to have available (even over a reasonable period of time) any very large group of patients with similar diagnoses that are specific enough to avoid wide deviations in test results. In individual clinical evaluations the central auditory scores for only one patient may be considered and may be of diagnostic value, but for research one needs a large group if one is to accumulate enough data to establish a central auditory profile for that type of lesion or central nervous system dysfunction. Again, cooperation among different facilities using the same central auditory test battery is essential in order to accrue greater quantities of data. In the literature we often find specific cases illustrated that may be more the extreme or "picture book perfect" case rather than the average example. Within any one group an individual patient may differ considerably from the "average" profile for that group. Thus, ranges of scores may be more valuable than averages or means.

In children with learning disabilities it is even more difficult to "match" individual subjects for group data. It is usually impossible to relate test results to any specific central nervous system pathology because the term "learning disability" itself covers a wide range of educational problems and, like the term "minimal brain dysfunction," has no known specific neuroanatomical or neurophysiological basis. This fact in itself may explain why different investigators obtain different results when the results of research are presented statistically. We still do not know the effects of possible lack of neuroanatomical and neurophysiological maturity in these children as previously discussed.

Site of Lesion

Most of the time it is not possible to determine an exact site of lesion from effects observed on a central auditory evaluation. A lesion may affect areas of the brain remote from its actual location by interference with neural transmission or the biochemistry of the brainstem or cerebrum. For example, when a nerve cell is damaged, its axon will not transmit an accurate "message" to a "receptor" neuron, nor will the message arrive if the interconnecting white fiber tracts (axons of nerve cells) are impaired. If the "receptor" neuron is damaged or destroyed, the same effect may occur. Also, the neurochemistry of the brain may become abnormal as the result of an insult, so that the neurotransmitters basic to synaptic conduction may no longer function adequately. Even when the location of a lesion is confirmed by objective neurological tests or by surgery, distant effects cannot be observed directly. These remote effects, as well as the lesion itself, may be responsible for impaired central auditory function. Therefore, the precise association between central auditory evaluation and site of lesion may be very difficult to determine. Of course, central auditory evaluation shares this problem with other neurodiagnostic procedures.

Some lesions may be so generalized (spread over various sites in the brain) that central auditory test results are mystifying, especially when there is no other observable neurological dysfunction. Multiple sclerosis, presenile dementias, and other systemic diseases or impairments which affect the brain fall into this category, contributing to difficulty in relating central auditory abnormalities to a specific site of lesion.

There are some disturbances of central auditory function observed on test procedures for which there is no known correlative lesion. This is especially true in the case of such disorders as learning disabilities which have not been associated with any specific anatomical site as yet. In fact, it is probable that there are many varied causes for the general category of learning disorders.

In many cases the central auditory clinician may be able to determine only that central auditory function is not normal and that the lesion or cause of dysfunction remains unknown.

Neuroanatomy and Neurophysiology

Much of our knowledge of the neuroanatomy and neurophysiology of the central auditory system comes from research on animals (see Chapters 2 and 3). Only a limited amount of this work has been accomplished on primates. Generally, investigations of the living human brain have been carried out only on those patients who have come to surgery for some brain abnormality. Other studies of the human brain have been done at postmortem examinations. We must realize that the brains of animals differ anatomically a great deal from those of humans. Man's brain is larger, and the cerebrum is more highly developed. Although the basic neurophysiology may be similar in animals and man, the latter's is much more complex and undoubtedly more greatly influenced by the cortex. Activities that are subserved by the brainstem in animals may involve processing at the cortical level in humans.

One must also be aware that central auditory processing apparently involves wide areas of the brain. Central auditory disorders have been related to lesions in frontal lobe, parietal lobe, both anterior and posterior temporal lobe, and corpus callosum. Brainstem dysfunction has also been found.

Therefore, the researcher/clinician must have as broad and detailed a knowledge as possible of human neuroanatomy and neurophysiology in order to understand what he is doing in a central auditory evaluation procedure. He must be able to comprehend fully the meaning of any medical and/or surgical findings, as well as results of neurodiagnostic examinations, and be able to relate these to the underlying structure and function of the brain. In other words, neither application nor interpretation of central auditory evaluation can proceed unless based upon thorough knowledge of the neuroanatomy and neurophysiology of the central auditory system and surrounding areas of the central nervous system.

CONTRIBUTION TO DIAGNOSIS

Since a central auditory test battery alone cannot pinpoint a specific site as the cause of an observed dysfunction, the clinician has been warned to use caution in diagnosis. However, we do believe that a central auditory evaluation can *contribute* to diagnosis of brain lesions. Also the clinician should be aware that he may be the first to observe that a patient has a brain dysfunction. The

authors have discovered central auditory impairment in patients who have not had any previous indications of neurologic disorder. The patient may come in for an audiological workup for an unrelated problem and be observed to have an as yet undiagnosed central nervous system pathology. These indications may be confirmed by referral to a neurologist and more objective neurological examinations, such as brain scan, ventriculography, arteriography, pneumoencephalography, etc. Generally, such tests are not undertaken unless there is some suspicion of central nervous system disease or damage, and the abnormal results of a central auditory evaluation may provide this indication. Occasionally a central auditory test battery shows that a patient has a brain dysfunction even when a number of neurological examinations have been negative. Although it may not be possible to localize the brain area responsible for the impairment, in such cases abnormal results on a central auditory evaluation may lead to further objective investigations to confirm that a problem exists. At times the discovery of a central auditory dysfunction may precede more objective neurological confirmation of a cerebral problem by months or years. For example, patients beginning to suffer from presenile dementia syndromes, such as Alzheimer's disease, may show central auditory abnormalities as long as 2 yr before other recognizable symptoms appear and there is confirmation of brain atrophy.

Another value of central auditory testing is in following the progress or remission of disease. Just as pre- and postsurgical central auditory scores can be compared, it is also possible to do repetitive test batteries on a patient who is recovering from disease or on one who needs to be monitored for spread of disease, such as a patient who might be prone to cerebral metasteses from primary tumor sites outside the brain.

It is obvious that central auditory evaluation offers a diagnostic technique that is noninvasive and comfortable for the patient.

RELATIONSHIP TO LANGUAGE

It is very important in the construction, application, and interpretation of any central auditory task to understand its relationship to language. It is common knowledge that speech or a speech-like signal is processed in the posterior left hemisphere of the brain in most right-handed individuals and in at least half of sinistrals. However, auditory stimuli other than speech also may be processed in the so-called language areas of the brain because "inner language" often is involved in the decision-making process or in the organization of a response. For example, most subjects performing a pitch pattern sequencing task reported that they labeled the sounds "in their heads" after they heard them and before initiating a verbal or manual response. Subjects used inner language labels of "high" and "low" or "up" and "down." Responses in this type of task (see Chapter 13) and in most other central auditory tasks are similarly thought out or prepared in language areas of the brain before any verbal or even a manual response is made. It has been observed that processing of most manual response tasks overlaps language function in the left hemisphere (Hicks, 1975; Lomas and Kimura, 1976). In fact, no differences were found on pitch pattern tasks between verbal and manual responses in several different studies of both normal subjects and patients with brain lesions. The right ear advantage observed on so many different auditory tasks probably is related to the involvement of language processing.

Even the so-called brainstem tasks require some language processing when speech stimuli or verbal responses are used. Also, in sound localization or lateralization, while the stimulus may be perceived and the fundamental physiologic localization process, according to phase and/or intensity differences at the two ears, may take place in one or more brainstem or other cortical areas, the thought/decision as to where to point (manual response) or what to answer verbally most probably is subserved by the left hemisphere language areas of the brain. All of the above emphasize the necessity of interpreting central auditory test results with care.

It is especially important to remember this relationship between central auditory tasks and language when evaluating children. Some normal children do not complete language development until about 8 yr of age. Children with developmental delays (the kind of child who may be a candidate for central auditory testing) may also be language-delayed. Since it is frequently of interest to assess the auditory abilities of young children of preschool age or during the first 2 yr of school, especially when measuring so-called learning disabilities, this problem must be considered. For example, the often used Willeford version of the BF test includes words that are difficult for normal children because they are not in everyday usage. It is difficult for children to recognize and repeat unfamiliar words. Normal children can hum pitch pattern sequences, but they do not perform at an adult level on verbal or manual responses until they are about 9 yr old. The hummed response is imitative and does not depend on language. (The hummed response does indicate that the pattern has been accurately perceived.) The verbal and manual response to pitch patterns require several central auditory functions including memory, sequencing, and language processing or organization of the response. The same problem has been noted with dichotic sentences, i.e., level of performance relates to age level in normal children. While the normal child can easily repeat a sentence presented monaurally and has little difficulty in repeating a sentence from one ear only when a simultaneous sentence is in competition, he cannot repeat both of the dichotically presented sentences easily until 9 yr of age. Again, memory is involved as well as language processing. These examples illustrate the fact that we do not know the precise relationship between some central auditory tasks and language ability in normal young children. This does not mean that we cannot evaluate them with central auditory tests. It does mean that we must proceed with great caution when we interpret test results.

One must also differentiate between auditory perception (occurring in the primary sensory regions of the brain) and auditory processing. Although the stimulus may be adequately perceived, the brain may not have the capability of processing the response. As an example, this becomes obvious in patients who can accurately hum pitch patterns but cannot respond either verbally or manually to the same stimuli. Thus, we must carefully distinguish, if possible, between perceptual dysfunction and a processing disorder, for these are subserved by different areas of the brain. In general, central auditory evaluations examine the processing of auditory stimuli. Diagnosis depends on the correct interpretation of *what* is occurring *where* in the brain.

FUTURE DIRECTIONS

Central auditory evaluation is still in its infancy. It has been slow to develop, and much progress needs to be made in improving central auditory tasks and procedures. The development of more objective tests would contribute importantly to this field, since most of the present tests are subjective and, therefore, prone to many influences outside the central auditory system. Also, there are many patients who do not have the ability to respond to such tests. These subjective tests require refinement and standardization.

With the rapid development of high technology industries and miniaturization, equipment should be better and less expensive. In the future we may see the computerized administration and/or interpretation of test results which would remove any effects of examiner error or bias.

The recent advent of positron emission tomography (PET) should contribute greatly to an understanding of the relationship between normal brain activities and tasks such as those used in central auditory evaluation. PET also should make the association between site of lesion and central auditory abnormalities easier to determine. The PET scan, developed over the past 8 yr, produces colored contour images of the living brain in a series of planes. It supposedly reveals areas of low and high neural activity by building up a profile of energy demand, demonstrated by different densities of glucose uptake. While there is still some controversy over the metabolism of glucose in the brain (Fox, 1984) and how quantitative PET really is, this technique is of increasing importance in diagnosis and may permit the observer to associate specific sites in the brain with specific cortical processing activities. Alternative techniques are also under development. These include single photon emission computed tomography and nuclear resonance spectrography.

In addition, the use of both psychophysical and electrophysiological assessment techniques may help in the detection and delineation of central auditory dysfunction. Some valuable relationships between ABR and various behavioral central auditory tests have already been shown in brainstem lesions (Hannley et al, 1983; Noffsinger et al, 1984; Musiek and Geurkink, 1982). Further development of correlations between psychophysical and electrophysiological tests in neuroaudiology will prove to be a very worthwhile direction for advancement.

Perhaps the greatest overall need is for knowledge. Most of the clinicians using central auditory tests have only limited understanding of the structure and function of the central nervous system and brain. University programs in the fields of communication and psychology frequently offer only a general course, often combining neuroanatomy and neurophysiology with emphasis on descriptions of peripheral structure and function. These courses are apt to be lacking in any concomitant laboratory work or experience with patients with brain disorders. Such programs may last only one academic semester or quarter and may meet for no longer than 3 hr each week. One textbook may be considered sufficient background material. Often the instructor has had very little acquaintance with the central nervous system himself. Medical students spend hours each day for months on combined lecture and laboratory work on these subjects, and that is considered to be only a basic foundation. Anyone sincerely interested in the brain must spend several more years of specialized study and practical training in this area. Lack of any but the most superficial background in the central nervous system makes suspect the clinician who proffers a diagnosis of brain abnormality based on a central auditory evaluation. He may be seen as an upstart by a neurological specialist. His inadequate knowledge may threaten the specialist's cooperation with and confidence in the clinician's ability. The greater the understanding one has of neuroanatomy and neurophysiology, the greater the respect the medical profession will develop for central auditory evaluation and its contribution to diagnosis. Just as there has come to be various subspecialties within the broad area of language and speech pathology, so hopefully there will develop more exacting subspecialties in audiology. It is suggested that the audiologist who wishes to involve himself in central auditory assessment make the study of neuroanatomy and neurophysiology an academic field of major concern in his pre- and postdoctoral training. Thus, there may be born the neuroaudiologist, just as there now exist the neurochemist, neurophysiologist, and neuropsychologist.

Greater cooperation among the professions whose interests overlap is necessary for progress in central auditory work. The audiologist cannot do it alone. Advancements will be forthcoming when the medical profession, the psychophysicist, the electrophysiologist, the psychoacoustician, and the neuroaudiologist cooperate for the advantage of all and the benefit of the patient.

An area that is especially in need of improvement is central auditory work with children. There are many difficulties in assessing auditory processing problems in children, some of which have been discussed earlier in this chapter. Unfortunately, there are very few centers concentrating on this problem and even fewer where more than one or two central auditory tasks are used with children. There is much criticism which can be directed at most studies of central auditory evaluation in children, especially in the area of the so-called learning disabilities, but research must be encouraged. Because of the many problems encountered in testing children and the great variability between different chronological ages and different levels of maturity in the same ages (and the difficulty in measuring this maturity), there is an even greater need for normative data and standardization.

In summary, it is obvious that much work needs to be accomplished in the area of central auditory evaluation. This includes the development and better control, refinement, and standardization of test materials and procedures, the use of an appropriate test battery, attention to the special problems in dealing with young children and older adults, and those with hearing losses or possible psychiatric disorders. We must have improved knowledge of neuroanatomy and neurophysiology and an understanding of the relationship between central auditory tasks and language in order to make central auditory evaluation a valuable contribution to neurodiagnosis.

References

Fox JL: PET scan controversy aired. *Science* 224:143–144, 1984.

Goldstein L, Stoltzfus NW: Psychoactive drug-induced changes of interhemispheric EEG amplitude relationships. *Agents Actions* 3:124–132, 1973.

Gruzelier JH, Hammond NV: Schizophrenia: a dominant hemisphere temporal-limbic disorder? *Res Commun Psychol Psychiatry Behav* 1:33–72, 1976.

Hannley M, Jerger J, Rivera V: Relationships among auditory brain stem responses, masking level differences and the acoustic reflex in multiple sclerosis. *Audiology* 22:20–33, 1983.

Hicks RE: Intrahemispheric response competition between vocal and unimanual performance in normal adult human males. *J Comp Physiol Psychol* 89:50–60, 1975.

Lomas J, Kimura D: Intrahemispheric interaction between speaking and sequential manual activity. *Neuropsychology* 14:23–33, 1976.

Musiek FE, Geurkink NA: Auditory brain stem response and central auditory test findings for patients with brain stem lesions: a preliminary report. *Laryngoscope* 92:891–900, 1982.

Musiek F, Gollegly K, Baran J: Myelination of the corpus callosum and auditory processing problems in children: theoretical and clinical correlates. *Semin Hear* 5:231–241, 1984.

Noffsinger D, Schaefer A, Martinez C: Behavioral and objective estimates of auditory brainstem integrity. *Semin Hear* 5:337–349, 1984.

Perris G: Averaged evoked response (AER) in patients with affective disorders. *Acta Psychiatr Scand* [Suppl] 255:89–98, 1974.

Smith CB: Aging and changes in cerebral energy metabolism. *Trends Neurosci* 7:203–208, 1984.

Trevarthen C: Cerebral embryology and the split brain. In Kinsbourne M, Smith W (eds): *Hemispheric Disconnection and Cerebral Function.* Springfield, IL, Charles C Thomas, 1974.

Yozawitz A, Bruder GE: Central Auditory Processing of Speech and Non-speech Stimuli in Affective Psychotics and Schizophrenics: A Neuropsychological Investigation. Paper presented at the 6th annual International Neuropsychology Society, Minneapolis, February, 1978.

Glossary

Acoustic reflex amplitude. The magnitude of the change in acoustic immittance, associated with reflexive contraction of the stapedius muscle, when compared to quiescent acoustic immittance.

Acoustic reflex decay. Decrease in acoustic reflex amplitude with continuous stimulation. Clinically significant decay is a decrement of over 50% of initial amplitude within 10 sec of stimulus onset.

Acoustic reflex latency. Time interval between the presentation of an acoustic stimulus and some index of acoustic reflex activity, usually detected as a change in acoustic immittance of the middle ear at the eardrum. Criteria for the index of acoustic reflex activity may vary.

Acoustic reflex pattern. The collection of acoustic reflex findings for crossed (contralateral) and uncrossed (ipsilateral) measurement conditions for the right and left ears. Analysis of patterns, in combination with other audiometric data, differentiates among abnormalities affecting the afferent (cochlea and eighth nerve), brainstem (caudal pons), and efferent (seventh cranial nerve and middle ear) portions of the acoustic reflex arc.

Acoustic reflex threshold. The lowest intensity level of a stimulus (in decibels) that produces reliable changes in acoustic immittance as measured close to the plane of the tympanic membrane.

Acoustic stapedial reflex. Bilateral contraction of stapedial muscle elicited by high intensity (greater than 75 to 85 dB) monaural or binaural acoustic stimulation.

Amplitude modulated tones and noise. Sounds of which the amplitude is varied around a certain value. The modulation is usually periodic and often sinusoidal, which means that the envelope has the shape of a sine wave. Other wave forms can be used to modulate a sound, such as triangular waves or square waves, or the modulation can be noise in which the envelope will have an irregular shape.

Anoxia. Absence or lack of oxygen; reduction of oxygen in body tissues below physiologic levels.

Apgar (score). A numerical expression of the condition of a newborn infant, usually determined at 60 sec after birth, being the sum of points gained on assessment of heart rate, respiratory effort, muscle tone, reflex irritability, and color.

Attention deficit disorder (ADD). Childhood disorders that include inattention, impulsivity, and hyperactivity. Such behaviors must be evident before the age of 7, have been present for 6 months, and not be the results of schizophrenia, affective, or severe or profound mental retardation.

Auditory brainstem responses (ABR). The farfield responses that can be recorded from scalp electrodes (usually placed on vertex or forehead and ipsilateral mastoid) within 10 msec after a click or short tone burst.

Auditory cortex. The auditory receiving area of the cerebral cortex located on the superior surface of the temporal lobe (transverse gyri of Heschl, cortical areas 41 and 42).

Axis of sensitivity. The directional axis of bending of hairs of hair cells; bending in one direction results in excitation, bending in opposite direction results in inhibition.

Bandpass-filtered clicks. Click sounds that have been passed through a bandpass filter. If the frequency range of the bandpass filter is within the flat part of the spectrum of the click, then the spectrum of the bandpass-filtered click is identical to the transfer function of the filter. The wave form of a band-pass-filtered click is a damped sinusoid, the frequency of which is equal to the center frequency of the filter.

Basal body. Organelle within the hair cells of the cochlea; location associated with axis of sensitivity of the cell.

Basilar membrane. The sensory epithelium on which the organ of Corti rests; it extends throughout the length of the cochlear spiral from the base near the oval window to the apex.

Brachium of inferior colliculus. Bundle of nerve fibers in midbrain extending from inferior colliculus to the medial geniculate body.

Bradykinesia. Slowness of movement implied, but in fact, slowness of initiation of movement is more correct.

Caudal regression syndrome. Also known as caudal dysplasia or sacral agenesis syndrome, this is a congenital malformation characterized by various degrees of developmental failure involving the legs, the lumbar, sacral, and coccygeal vertebrae, and the corresponding segments of the spinal cord.

Central auditory nervous system. Auditory nuclei and pathways from the synapse of eighth cranial nerve fibers with the cochlear nuclei rostral to the perisylvian region of the temporal lobe of cerebral cortex.

Central auditory processing disorder. Difficulty listening or comprehending auditory information.

Cephalopelvic disproportion. A condition in which the head of the fetus is too large for the pelvis of the mother.

Cerebral cortex. The mantle of gray matter on the outer surface of the cerebrum consisting of cell bodies, dendrites, axons, and glial cells.

Cesarean section. Incision through the abdominal and uterine walls for delivery of a fetus.

Characteristic frequency (CF). Frequency at which a nerve fiber or nerve cell has its lowest threshold when the ear is stimulated by pure tones.

Claustrum. A thin sheet of gray matter located between the cortex of central lobe (insula) and the lenticular nucleus of the basal ganglia.

Click sound. A brief sound produced by applying a short pulse (usually rectangular) to a sound transducer. The spectrum of the click is determined by the electrical signal that is aplied to the transducer and the characteristics of the sound transducer. In case the electrical signal is a rectangular wave, the spectrum is $P(\omega) = \dfrac{\sin(\omega T)}{\omega T}$ where $\omega = 2\pi f$ (f = frequency and T is the duration of the rectangular wave). This means that the spectrum is flat from low frequencies up to a certain frequency above which it falls gradually and it becomes zero at a frequency that is $\frac{1}{2} T$. the click becomes a rarefaction click if it is a short decrease in air pressure, and it is a condensation click if it is a short increase in pressure.

Cochlea. The spiral bony chamber curled $2\frac{1}{2}$ times which resembles a snail shell. It is partitioned into three spiral passageways called scala vestibuli, scala tympani, and cochlear duct. The latter contains the organ of Corti.

Cochlear microphonics (CM). Potentials that can be recorded in response to a sound from the cochlea (from inside or in its vicinity, e.g., at the round window). The wave form of the potential resembles the wave form of the sound, and hence its name. It is best seen in response to tones of low or moderate frequencies.

Cochlear nuclei. Nuclei containing neurons receiving direct input from peripheral neurons innervating the organ of Corti; located on outer surface of inferior cerebellar peduncle of medulla.

Commissural fibers. Axons of neurons passing from the one side of the brain usually to a similar structure on the other side of the brain.

Compound action potential (CAP). The potential that can be recorded from an electrode placed directly on a nerve. It is assumed to represent the summed action potentials from many nerve fibers. It is best seen in the auditory system when the stimulus is brief as represented by a click or a brief tone burst.

Condensation click. Click that causes a brief increase in air pressure.

Conjugate gaze. When both eyes move in unison as with vertical and horizontal gaze.

Contralateral (crossed) acoustic reflex. Measurement of reflex-related change in acoustic immittance in one ear, with acoustic stimulation of the opposite ear.

Corpus callosum. Commissure interconnecting the neocortices of the two cerebral hemispheres.

Cystic. Pertaining to a cyst (any closed cavity or sac, normal or abnormal, lined by epithelium, and especially one that contains a liquid to semisolid material).

Dichotic tests. Tests in which different verbal messages are presented to the two ears at the same time.

Differential recording. Recording of the difference in the potentials picked up by two electrodes.

Dipole. A model of a source of neurogenic potential which assumes that at any given instant the generator of such a potential can be likened to a source with its positive polarity located in one position and its negative polarity in a different position.

Dyslexia. Developmental reading disability.

Dysmetria. Overshoot- undershoot movements of limbs often associated with cerebellar disorders.

Electrocochleography (ECoG). Recording of the electrical response from the cochlea in human. Usually the recording electrode is placed on the promontorium near the round window. By the use of tone bursts, both the cochlear microphonic and the compound action potential can be recorded; and when clicks are used, the response is dominated by the neural response.

Encephalopathy. Any degenerative disease of the brain.

Extinction. Suppression of stimulus on one side on double simultaneous stimulation.

Extrinsic (extra-axial) brainstem pathology. Lesions arising outside of the brainstem and secondarily compressing or penetrating brainstem structures.

Farfield potential. Response recorded at large distances from the (neural) generator. The wave shape of the response is relatively independent of the exact location of the electrode, and only the amplitude varies with the movement of the electrode.

Frequency modulated tones. Tones, the frequency of which varies around a certain mean value. The modulation can be sinusoidal or any other wave form.

Frequency tuning curves (FTC). The sound pressure that gives a just noticeable increase in the firing rate of a single auditory nerve fiber or nerve cell in an auditory nucleus for pure tones plotted as a function of frequency of the tone.

Ganglion. Aggregation of nerve cells as in the spiral ganglion of the cochlear nerve.

Gyrus. Ridges on the surface of the cerebral cortex consisting of gray matter with an inner core of white matter.

Hair cells. Receptor cells of the auditory and vestibular systems, characterized by having numberous stereocilia and one kinocilium or basal body.

Homonymous. A bilaterally symmetrical defect, e.g., homonymous hemianopsia.

Hypoparathyroid(ism). The condition produced by greatly reduced function of the parathyroid glands. It leads to a fall in plasma calcium levels, resulting in increased neuromuscular excitability.

Hypoplastic. Marked by hypoplasia (incomplete development of an organ so that it fails to reach adult size; it is less severe in degree than aplasia).

Hypoxia. Low oxygen content or tension; deficiency of oxygen in the inspired air.

Hypsarrhythmic(mia) (EEG). An electroencephalographic abnormality sometimes observed in infants, with random high-voltage slow waves and spikes that arise from multiple foci and spread to all cortical areas. The disorder is usually characterized by spasms or quivering spells (myoclonus) and is commonly associated with mental retardation.

Inferior cerebellar peduncle. Bundle of fibers extending from the upper medulla to the cerebellum.

Inferior colliculus. Hillock on the roof of the lower midbrain, actually a major relay nucleus of the auditory pathway.

Intrinsic (intra-axial) brainstem pathol-

ogy. Lesions (e.g., neoplastic, vascular, demyelinating) arising from and remaining within the confines of the brainstem and midbrain.

Ipsilateral (uncrossed) acoustic reflex. Measurement of reflex-related change in acoustic immittance in the same ear that is acoustically stimulated.

Isofrequency strips. Areas of the auditory cortex in which cells respond preferentially to tones of nearly the same frequency.

Kinocilium. A true cilium of the hair cells of the vestibular system and developing auditory system; it remains as basal body of the auditory hair cells.

Koniocortex. Sensory neocortex with numerous small stellate (granular) neurons; when viewed through light microscope the small neurons appear as dust, hence konio (dust) cortex.

Latency. Time between the beginning of the stimulation and the earliest detectable response.

Lateral lemniscus. Bundle of fibers of the auditory pathway extending from lower pontine auditory nuclei to the medial geniculate body.

Lemniscus. Bundle of fibers within the central nervous system.

Medial geniculate body. Large nucleus of thalamus, which is the neural center of the auditory pathways projecting to the auditory cortex.

Morphology. The science of the forms and structures of organized beings.

Nearfield potential. Response recorded very close to the source. The wave shape is highly dependent on the location of the recording electrode.

Neocortex. Almost all of the cortex that can be seen on the outside surface of the cerebrum. "Neo" refers to the idea that it has appeared later in evolution. Of the total cortical area, neocortex accounts for 90%.

Nucleus. Functional group of neurons in the gray matter (not nucleus of cell); the dendrites and especially the axons of neurons may extend beyond the boundary of the nucleus.

Olivocochlear bundle. Fascicle of fibers originating in the superior olivary nuclear complex. Its fibers join the vestibulocochlear nerve and terminate in the organ of Corti.

Organ of Corti. Organ composed of epithelial cells (including inner and outer hair cells) arranged as a sheet following the cochlear spiral; it is the peripheral organ of hearing.

Performance-intensity functions (PI-PB). Verbal material is presented at a series of intensity levels.

Plasticky. Full range resistance of limb(s) to passive manipulation.

Porus acusticus. Intracranial orifice of the internal auditory meatus. It contains the eighth cranial nerve (vestiular and auditory parts), the seventh cranial nerve (facial nerve), and the cochlear artery.

Promontorium. The cochlear capsule as it protrudes between the round window and the oval window in the middle ear.

Pulvinar. Nucleus in the posterior part of thalamus.

Rarefaction click. Click that causes a brief decrease in air pressure.

Reticular formation. A diffuse, complex subcortical region of the CNS involved in activation of the cortex during sensory stimulation. Brainstem portions of the acoustic reflex arc may have reticular formation components.

Spastic. Hypertonic, so that the muscles are stiff and the movements awkward.

Speech-in-noise. Speech discrimination lists which are presented in the presence of masking noise—usually white noise.

Speech-on-fraction. The percentage of time speech is on vs off during each interruption cycle. For example, if interrupted speech has a speech-on-fraction of 25% at a rate of 10 interruptions per second (ips), the speech is on 25% of the time and off 75% of the time during 1 sec. Hence, speech-on-fraction corresponds to the duty cycle.

Sulcus. Infoldings on cerebral surface separating gyri.

Summating potentials (SP). Potentials that can be recorded from the cochlea in response to a sound (inside or in its vicinity, e.g., the round window). The potential follows the envelope of a sound and is best seen in response to bursts of high frequency tones.

Superior colliculus. Hillock on roof of upper midbrain, a nucleus involved with processing of visual stimuli and control of eye movements.

Supranuclear. Motor system above cranial nerve neurons (nuclei) and anterior horn cells of the spinal cord.

Synapse. Connection between a dendrite and a nerve cell, usually using a chemical transmitter substance in the transmission of information. There are also synapses that do not use chemical transmitters.

Synaptic transmission. Transmission of information between one part of the nervous system to another via a synapse.

Tegmentum. Continuous region of gray matter extending throughout brainstem located in front of cerebral aqueduct and fourth ventricle. It contains the reticular formation, nuclei of cranial nerves, brainstem nuclei, and many ascending and descending pathways.

Thalamus. Large egg-shaped diencephalic structure composed of many nuclei. One role is to act as processor of sensory information prior to its projection to the sensory cerebral cortex.

Toneburst. A tone that is switched on and off at certain intervals. Usually the switching is gradual whereby the tone burst builds up and diminishes over a certain time (rise and fall time).

Topography. The description of an anatomical region or of a special part.

Tract. Bundle of axons in the central nervous system which usually extends for relatively long distances. A lemniscus is a tract.

Trapezoid body. Transversely oriented fibers of the auditory pathways located in the tegmentum of the lower pons.

Vestibulocochlear nerve. The eighth cranial nerve consisting of the cochlear nerve (audition) and the vestibular nerve (balance).

Wernicke's area. Region of the cortex comprising supramarginal gyrus (area 40) and angular gyrus (area 39) of inferior parietal lobe and posterior portion of superior temporal gyrus. Damage to this area on left side results for most individuals in a disturbance in the comprehension of language, of objects seen, and of objects felt.

Index

Page numbers followed by "t" or "f" denote tables or figures, respectively.

273